SEXUALLY TRANSMITTED DISEASES

Topics In Clinical Dermatology

Series Editor: Larry E. Millikan, M.D.

SEXUALLY TRANSMITTED DISEASES
Tomasz F. Mroczkowski, M.D.

SEXUALLY TRANSMITTED DISEASES

Tomasz F. Mroczkowski, M.D.

Visiting Professor of Dermatology and Venereology
Department of Dermatology
Tulane University School of Medicine
And
Section of Infectious Diseases
Department of Medicine
Louisiana State University
New Orleans, Louisiana

Igaku-Shoin New York • Tokyo

Published and distributed by

IGAKU-SHOIN Medical Publishers, Inc.
1140 Avenue of the Americas, New York, N.Y. 10036

IGAKU-SHOIN Ltd.,
5-24-3 Hongo, Bunkyo-ku, Tokyo

Library of Congress Cataloging-in-Publication Data

Mroczkowski, Tomasz F.
  Sexually transmitted diseases / Tomasz F. Mroczkowski.
    p.   cm.—(Clinical guides in dermatology)
    1. Sexually transmitted diseases. I. Title. II. Series.
    [DNLM: 1. Sexually Transmitted Diseases. 2. Skin Diseases. WC
140 M939s]
RC200.M76   1990
616.95'1—dc20
DLC
for Library of Congress   89-26963
                                                                  CIP

ISBN: 0-89640-163-4 (New York)
ISBN: 4-260-14163-5 (Tokyo)

Printed and bound in the U.S.A.

10 9 8 7 6 5 4 3 2 1

PREFACE

This book, which is the first volume in the *Topics in Clinical Dermatology* series, is meant to be a relatively concise, well illustrated guide for physicians and students, dermatologists and non-dermatologists working with patients suffering from Sexually Transmitted Diseases (STDs).

The text is organized in a traditional manner, each chapter dealing with a single disease or a group of diseases, starting with overview, epidemiology and etiology sections, followed by clinical manifestations, diagnosis, differential diagnosis and treatment sections. Since the book was intended primarily for the clinicians, the emphasis is on clinical manifestations and differential diagnosis, whereas the etiology and epidemiology sections are rather short, consisting primarily of brief characteristics of the etiologic agents and current trends in morbidities. Realizing how often the selection of an appropriate sampling site or sampling technique(s), as well as storing of the specimens are crucial for accurate diagnosis, certain chapters are provided with illustrations or thorough descriptions of methods of sampling required to guarantee the highest isolated rates of causative microorganisms. In the laboratory diagnosis sections, a priority is given to well established, relatively easy to perform methods while the new, usually highly sophisticated methods, not yet used in routine practice, are only briefly discussed.

Contemporary venereology long ago crossed the boundaries of dermatology and entered the fields of many other specialties. Today's book on STDs, in addition to the chapters on traditional venereal diseases, must include information about pelvic inflammatory diseases and vaginitis-diseases which are strictly gynecologic, but whose etiologic agents are frequently sexually transmitted. The topic should also address certain pediatric problems which are the consequence of STD infection in the mother, not to mention the broad range of problems associated with homosexual behavior. Acquired immunodeficiency syndrome (AIDS) is a specific subject which goes far beyond the scope of this book. In the chapter on AIDS emphasis is made on cutaneous manifestations of the syndrome. They are often atypical or unique and frequently can be either the harbinger of the full blown disease or the first signs of HIV infection. Certain physicians especially non-dermatologists may have difficulties when faced with skin lesions of non-venereal origin located in the anogenital region. Chapter 15 "Skin Diseases Commonly Affecting the Anogenital Region", should aid them in differential diagnosis. For the same purpose, in each chapter there is a short section on differential diagnosis that should help to distinguish not only between the symptoms and signs of various sexually transmitted diseases but also between STDs and non-venereal skin conditions.

Treatment of STDs has been the subject of frequent revisions and updating. This should surprise no one since constant changes in microbial susceptibility require similar responses on the part of the therapist. Treatment recommendations presented in this book are based on, or in many instances are the exact copies of, the STD Treatment Guidelines issued by the Centers for Disease Control (CDC) in 1989. They should be, however, construed not as rules but as recommendations, which in time may require updating.

I wish to express my special thanks to Dr. Larry E. Millikan, the series editor, without whose inspiration and encouragement this volume would never have been possible. Moreover, I would like to express appreciation to my colleagues Drs. Wojciech A. Krotoski, David H. Martin, and George F. Risi for the time they devoted to reviewing certain chapters.

Many photographs included in this volume were taken at the Institute of Venereology, part of the Warsaw Medical Academy in Poland and I would like to express my gratitude to its director, Professor Andrzej Stapinski, for sharing them with me. Also, I would like to thank Professors Stefania Jablonska, Allan R. Ronald and Raju Thomas for letting me use some of the photographs from their collections.

Special thanks should also go to Dr. Willard Cates, Jr., from the Centers for Disease Control in Atlanta Georgia and to Professor Detlef Petzoldt from the University of Heidelberg in Germany for providing me with the new STD Treatment Guidelines developed recently by the CDC and the guidelines used in the Federal Republic of Germany.

I wish to thank Mrs. Ursula Hopkins for typing this manuscript and the entire Production and Editorial staff of Igaku-Shoin Medical Publishers for their efforts.

Tomasz F. Mroczkowski

CONTENTS

TOPICS IN CLINICAL DERMATOLOGY

SEXUALLY TRANSMITTED DISEASES

1

SEXUALLY TRANSMITTED DISEASES CAUSED BY *CHLAMYDIA TRACHOMATIS*

In recent years, an increasing number of sexually transmitted infections have been attributed to *Chlamydia* spp. Infections caused by *Chlamydia trachomatis* are more common than those caused by *Neisseria gonorrhoeae,* and it has been claimed that *C. trachomatis* is presently the most common sexually transmitted pathogen.[1,2]

Chlamydial infections are not reportable diseases in the United States. Nevertheless, it is estimated that there are over 3 million chlamydial infections annually in this country.[1-4] Numerous reports from Europe and Canada provide additional evidence for the dominant role of chlamydial infections among sexually transmitted diseases in developed countries.[4-8]

CHARACTERISTICS OF THE ORGANISM AND THE SPECTRUM OF INFECTIONS IT CAUSES

Based on their unique growth cycle, chlamydiae have been separated into their own order—Chlamydiales. There is only one family chlamydiaceae and one genus *Chlamydia,* which is made up of three species: *Chlamydia psittaci,* the causative agent of psittacosis, *Chlamydia trachomatis,* an etiologic agent of trachoma and a number of sexually transmitted diseases and recently identified TWAR-agent. *Chlamydia psittaci* can be differentiated from *C. trachomatis* on the basis of sulfonamide resistance and the type of intracellular inclusions. *Chlamydia trachomatis* produces glycogen-containing inclusions that stain with iodine and is sensitive to sulfonamides, whereas *C. psittaci* inclusions are glycogen negative, thus they do not stain with iodine, and this form is sulfonamide resistant.

The development of a microimmunofluorescence test (microIF) made it possible to differentiate *C. trachomatis* into 15 serotypes.[9] Types A, B, Ba, and C are associated with trachoma. Types D through K are associated with genital infections

TABLE 1.1. Some Characteristics of Chlamydiae That Distinguish Them from Viruses and Bacteria

Characteristic	Viruses	Chlamydiae	Bacteria
Size (nm)	15–350	350	300–3000
Obligately intracellular parasitism	+	+	−
Nucleic acids	RNA or DNA	RNA and DNA	RNA and DNA
Muramic acid in cell wall	−	Trace amounts	+
Reproduction	Eclipse, synthesis, and assembly	Complex cycle fission	Fission
Antibiotic sensitivity	−	+	+
Ribosomes	−	+	+
Metabolic enzymes	−	+	+
Energy production	−	−	+

Note: + = present, − = absent.
Source: Adapted from Thompson SE, Washington AE: Epidemiology of sexually transmitted *Chlamydia trachomatis* infections. *Epidemiol Rev* 5:96–123, 1983.

and, occasionally, eye infections. Types L_1, L_2, and L_3 cause lymphogranuloma venereum (LGV).

TWAR-strains are glycogen-negative and were previously considered strains of *C. psittaci*. However, based on different restriction endonuclease patterns and lack of substantial DNA homology with other chlamydia they were separated from *C. psittaci* and represent a third species. The new name proposed for TWAR-agent—*Chlamydia pneumoniae.*

Chlamydiae were formerly classified as viruses based on their size and obligatory intracellular parasitism. However, they possess characteristics which are not found among viruses, such as the presence of a cell wall and cell membrane similar to those of gram-negative bacteria, both RNA and DNA in the nucleus, and ribosomes and metabolic enzymes. Unlike viruses, they are sensitive to certain antibiotics (Table 1.1).

Chlamydiae are obligatory intracellular organisms which infect columnar and pseudostratified columnar epithelial surfaces. They depend on the host cell for nutrients and energy. Although they do not possess enzymes capable of generating ATP, they are capable of limited metabolic activity.

Chlamydiae have a unique growth cycle which distinguishes them from other microorganisms (Figure 1.1). Basically, the microorganism exists in two forms: (1) the elementary body, which is the infectious particle that attaches to the surface of the host cell, and (2) the initial (reticulate) body, representing the replicating phase of the organism, which multiplies by binary fission to form the inclusions

Figure 1.1. Chlamydial growth cycle. EB = elementary body, RB = reticulate body. From Thompson SE, Washington AE: Epidemiology of sexually transmitted *Chlamydia trachomatis* infections. *Epidemiol Rev* 5:96–123, 1983.

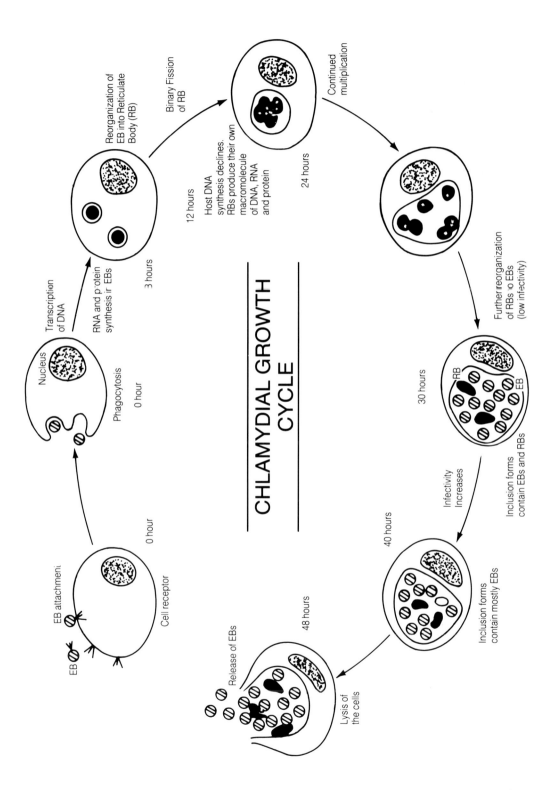

CHLAMYDIAL GROWTH CYCLE

EB
EB attachment
Cell receptor
0 hour

Nucleus
Phagocytosis
0 hour
Transcription of DNA
RNA and protein synthesis in EBs

Reorganization of EB into Reticulate Body (RB)
3 hours

Binary Fission of RB
12 hours
Host DNA synthesis declines. RBs produce their own macromolecule of DNA, RNA and protein

Continued multiplication
24 hours

Further reorganization of RBs to EBs (low infectivity)
30 hours
RB
EB
Inclusion forms contain EBs and RBs

Infectivity Increases
40 hours
Inclusion forms contain mostly EBs

Lysis of the cells
48 hours
Release of EBs

3

TABLE 1.2. Clinical Spectrum of *C. trachomatis* Infections

Men	Women	Infants
Serotype: D-K		
Infections		
Urethritis	Cervicitis	Conjunctivitis
Postgonococcal	Urethritis	Pneumonia
urethritis	Proctitis	Asymptomatic pharyngeal
Proctitis	Conjunctivitis	carriage
Conjunctivitis	Pharyngitis?	Asymptomatic gastrointestinal
Pharyngitis?		carriage
		Otitis media?
Complications		
Epididymitis	Salpingitis	
Prostatitis?	Endometritis	
Reiter's syndrome	Perihepatitis	
Perihepatitis	Ectopic pregnancy	
Sterility?	Infertility	
	Dysplasia?	
	Postpartum endometritis?	
	Prematurity?	
	Stillbirth?	
Serotype: L_1 L_2 L_3		
LGV	LGV	
Rectal stricture	Rectal stricture	
Rectal carcinoma?	Vulvar/Rectal carcinoma?	

Note: Question mark indicates that the relationship is not firmly established.

Source: Adapted from Centers for Disease Control. *Chlamydia trachomatis* infections policy guide-lines for prevention and control. *MMWR* 34 (suppl 35):53S–74S, 1985.

identifiable in properly stained cells. Intracellularly, chlamydiae exist within a cyto-plasmic vacuole and remain within this phagosome throughout their entire growth cycle, which lasts approximately 48 hours (Figure 1.1). After penetration into the cell cytoplasm the elementary body undergoes reorganization into the initial body, which possesses metabolic activity and represents the dividing form of the organ-ism. These forms are not infectious and cannot survive outside the host cell. Within the next 8–36 hours, the initial bodies undergo reorganization, during which they condense to form new infectious elementary bodies. Toward the end of the cycle the infectious particles are released when the infected cell bursts; the burst is probably what triggers the local inflammatory response.

    Chlamydia trachomatis has long been known as the etiologic agent of trachoma, a disease endemic in many developing countries as the cause of lymphogranuloma venereum and as the etiologic agent of inclusion conjunctivitis in newborns. In other parts of the world, predominantly in Europe and North America, *C. trachomatis* is the cause of numerous sexually transmitted diseases (Table 1.2).[10] In men *C. trachomatis* has been found to be the cause of urethritis, proctitis, epididy-mitis, prostatitis, and perihepatitis. In women chlamydiae can cause cervicitis, urethritis (acute urethral syndrome), and proctitis, and as a result of contiguous spread, they can infect the endometrium and the salpinges, being the frequent cause of pelvic inflammatory disease. *C. trachomatis* types D–K can cause conjunctivitis in adults (rarely) and have been frequently isolated in both male and female patients with Reiter's syndrome. The significance of the isolation of chlamydiae from the nasopharynx of adult patients is yet to be studied. As a result of vertical transmission, *C. trachomatis* may cause several diseases in neonates.[2,11-14] Among those most frequently encountered is conjunctivitis in newborns. *Chlamydia trachomatis* can also cause infantile pneumonia and, probably, otitis media. The causative role of *C. trachomatis* in other diseases is yet to be studied.

SEXUALLY TRANSMITTED DISEASES CAUSED BY *CHLAMYDIA TRACHOMATIS* IN MEN

Nongonococcal Urethritis

Nongonococcal urethritis (NGU) is a collective term for infections of the male urethra in which *Neisseria gonorrhoeae* cannot be recovered. The primary cause of NGU is *Chlamydia trachomatis* but other microorganisms can cause the disease as well.

Epidemiology

Nongonococcal urethritis in men is one of the most common sexually transmitted diseases (STDs). It is worldwide in distribution, but accurate data on its incidence are not available. NGU is not a reportable disease except in a few countries; one of them is the United Kingdom where it is two to three times as common as gonorrhea in men, and its incidence has nearly doubled in the last decade.[2,15] NGU is not a reportable disease in the United States; however, the Centers for Disease Control (CDC) estimate that over 2.5 million cases occur annually.[2] Since many men may be asymptomatic[16,17] or have symptoms which are mild enough to be ignored, the real prevalence of NGU actually may be much higher.

Comprehensive demographic data on NGU is not obtainable, and the information available comes from individual clinics or investigators. NGU seems to occur more often in heterosexual whites than in blacks or Hispanics.[18,19] The peak incidence is between the ages of 23 to 28, although the age range is from preteen to septuagenarian.[2] According to one large study, men with NGU, when compared with men with gonorrhea, have different socioeconomic profiles: they are better educated, are less likely to be unemployed, initiated sexual activity at an older age, and have fewer total lifetime sex partners.[20] Men with gonorrhea are more likely to have had gonorrhea in the past, whereas patients with NGU are more likely to give a history of prior episodes of NGU.[21]

Etiology

There is compelling evidence that *C. trachomatis* is the most important single cause of NGU and probably accounts for the majority of infections.[2,5,20,22-25] The second most common cause is *Ureaplasma urealyticum,* but the latter organism has also been found frequently in healthy individuals.[5,25-28] Other less frequent causes are *Trichomonas vaginalis* and *Herpesvirus simplex.* The etiologic aspect of NGU can-

TABLE 1.3. Microorganisms Isolated from Men with NGU

	Frequency of Occurrence
Chlamydia trachomatis	25–60%
Ureaplasma urealyticum	20–30%
Trichomonas vaginalis	1–7%
Neither	20–30%
Microorganisms rarely isolated from men with NGU	
Herpes virus hominis	
Gardnerella vaginalis	
Anaerobes	
Streptococcus group B	
Staphylococcus aureus	
Candida albicans	

not be identified in 20–30 percent of cases (Table 1.3).[20,25-27] *Chlamydia trachomatis* has been recovered from 25–60 percent of heterosexual men with untreated NGU.[28] The isolation rate among homosexuals with NGU is much lower. Men infected with *C. trachomatis* usually have clinical symptoms and signs of urethritis, but in some prevalence studies up to one third of these infections have been asymptomatic.[17,22,29] The average percentage of asymptomatic chlamydial infections among STD clinic patients is from 0 to 7 percent.[28] Female sex partners of men with chlamydial NGU have endocervical cultures positive for *C. trachomatis* in more than half of the cases.[20,30,31] Finally, the chlamydial etiology of urethritis has been confirmed by development of humoral antibodies in association with clinical disease, experimentally induced infection in primates, and selective antimicrobial treatment studies.[20,30-34]

The etiology of nonchlamydial NGU is uncertain, but there is evidence that *U. urealyticum* may be responsible for more than 30 percent of cases. However, its significance as a causative agent of NGU is not absolutely clear, since the microorganism is frequently present in apparently healthy men, and its presence in the male urethra is not, by itself, an indication for treatment. Data suggest that *U. urealyticum* is acquired by sexual contact and is a part of the vaginal flora of sexually active females. In one study, more than 40 percent of men who had vaginal sex with three to five sex partners harbored *U. urealyticum* in their urethras.[35] On the other hand, *U. urealyticum* has been isolated more often and in higher concentration from men with NGU than from healthy controls. The isolation rates of *U. urealyticum* usually have been greater in men without *C. trachomatis* than in men with concomitant chlamydial infection.[36] Since there are at least 14 serotypes of *U. urealyticum*, it is possible that only some of them might be pathogenic, whereas the others may colonize the genital tract without producing symptoms.[37] Treatment studies provide the evidence for the role of *U. urealyticum* in NGU. It has been demonstrated that persistent and recurrent nonchlamydial *U. urealyticum*–positive NGU resolved after successful treatment and elimination of this microorganism from the genital tracts of both sex partners.[38]

A small proportion of NGU may be caused by *T. vaginalis* and *H. simplex*.[20,25,27,39] The role of other microorganisms that have been isolated from NGU patients, i.e., *Gardnerella vaginalis, Staphylococcus aureus, S. epidermidis,* anaerobes, and yeasts, is uncertain,[40,41] and they probably play a marginal role, if any, in the etiology of NGU.

Although microbial infection is the most common cause of NGU, other conditions can produce urethral discharge and dysuria. Urethritis in men can be secondary to mechanical trauma, foreign bodies, or underlying congenital or acquired structural abnormalities such as urethral strictures, diverticuli, and valves. Urethral neoplasms, including benign polyps or malignant carcinomas, may also produce urethritis, but those causes are very rare.

Clinical Manifestations

After an incubation period ranging from 1 to 3 weeks (average 10–12 days), men with NGU complain of urethral discharge and/or dysuria. The discharge can be similar to that found in gonorrhea, but it differs in that it is usually watery, mucoid, or mucopurulent (Table 1.4), whereas in gonorrhea it is frequently thick and purulent. The simultaneous occurrence of discharge and dysuria in the same patient is more likely to occur in gonorrhea; either discharge or dysuria alone is more characteristic of NGU. In gonorrhea discharge is usually spontaneous or requires gentle penile compression for demonstration. In NGU the discharge is more likely to require penile stripping for its demonstration (Figure 1.2), or it is present only the first thing in the morning or when urine has not been passed for some hours. Dysuria in gonorrhea is usually more prominent and more persistent than in NGU. Many patients with NGU may have minimal or no discharge, and their only complaint may be a mild burning sensation which occurs only with urination. There is no distinguishing clinical feature that differentiates chlamydial from nonchlamydial infection.

TABLE 1.4. Clinical Characteristic of Gonococcal and Nongonococcal Urethritis in Men

	Gonorrhea	NGU
Incubation period	2–8 days (average 3–5 days)	1–3 weeks (average 10–12 days)
Onset	Rather abrupt	Rather gradual
Dysuria	+ + +	+ + or +
Discharge	Spontaneous, thick and purulent, present all time	Present after stripping; watery, mucoid, mucopurulent; frequently present only in the morning or after longer period without urination; often absent
Discharge or dysuria only	Infrequent	More likely

Note: + = mild, + + = moderate, + + + = severe.

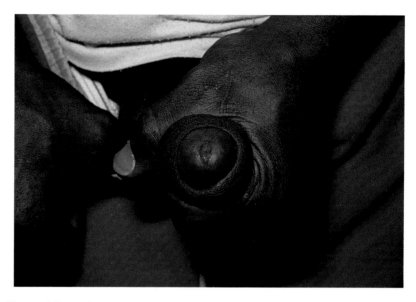

Figure 1.2. NGU in a male. Urethral discharge is visible after penile stripping.

Diagnosis

Although the clinical feature of the presentation may suggest either gonorrhea or NGU, they are not sufficiently specific. Therefore, laboratory testing is essential for accurate diagnosis.

Urethral Smear. A Gram-stained smear and culture of urethral exudate will permit accurate diagnosis in the majority of patients with NGU. If the smear contains polymorphonuclear leukocytes (PMN) and bacteria, but no intracellular or extracellular Gram-negative diplococci, then the diagnosis of NGU is very likely (Figure 1.3). However, current CDC recommendations are that all urethral specimens not showing Gram-negative diplococci should be cultured to definitely exclude gonorrhea. If the culture does not grow *N. gonorrhoeae,* then the diagnosis of NGU is established.

Gram-stained or other stained smears are also of value in the evaluation of patients with minimal signs or symptoms of urethritis and the detection of hypochondriacs or patients with venerophobia. The presence of four or more polymorphonuclear leukocytes (PMN) per oil high-powered field usually correlates with the diagnosis of NGU.

Urine Sediment. An alternative to Gram-stained smears is the examination of urine sediment.[42-45] The initial 10−15 ml of voided urine should be collected and centrifuged at 400 g for 5−10 minutes and all but 0.5 ml of the supernatant should be discarded. The sediment is then placed on the slide, and the number of PMN in each of five 400 × fields should be counted. The presence of more than 15 PMN in

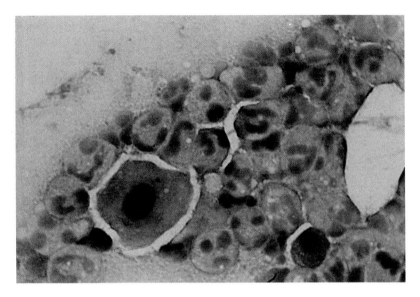

Figure 1.3. Gram-stained smear reveals polymorphonuclear leukocytes and no intracellular or extracellular diplococci. Diagnosis of NGU is very likely.

one or more of the five fields has been used by some investigators as confirmation of NGU.

For both tests, patients should be examined not earlier than 2 hours after the last voiding (the longer the interval, the better). In some instances symptomatic patients in whom the results of these tests are negative should be reexamined within 2 to 3 days, preferably before the day's first voiding.

If laboratory facilities are available, an attempt should be made to isolate *C. trachomatis, U. urealyticum,* and *T. vaginalis.* This is important in choosing appropriate therapy and especially for treatment failures or in cases of recurrent urethritis.

Detection of Chlamydia trachomatis

CELL CULTURE METHOD. The specimen should be obtained by insertion of a Dacron swab 3–4 cm into the urethra;* the swab is then placed into a specific transport medium. It should be transported to the laboratory as quickly as possible or kept in the refrigerator until delivered and then either immediately inoculated onto cell culture or frozen at −70°C. The culture is carried out in cycloheximide-treated McCoy cell monolayers using a modification of the procedure of Ripa and Mardh.[46] The preliminary results are available within 2 to 3 days after inoculation. Negative results may require passaging. Inclusions are identified either with iodine staining or with commercially available fluorescein-conjugated monoclonal antibodies (Figure 1.4).

---

*Obtaining specimens for *C. trachomatis* is exactly the same as for *N. gonorrhoeae.* For detailed description see Chapter 2 p. 42.

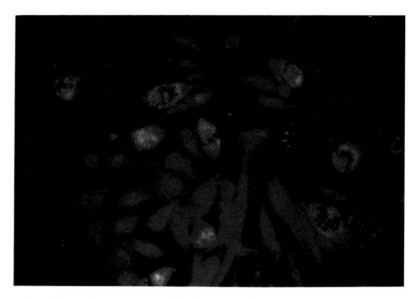

Figure 1.4. *Chlamydia trachomatis:* inclusions identified in tissue culture with fluorescein-conjugated monoclonal antibodies.

DIRECT IMMUNOFLUORESCENCE TEST. The direct fluorescent antibody assay (DFA) (MicroTrak; Syva CO., Palo Alto, CA) uses fluorescein-labeled *C. trachomatis*-specific monoclonal antibodies to detect elementary bodies in smears of genital secretions. The urethral specimen should be obtained in the same manner as described in the culture method section. However, instead of placing the swab into the transport medium, the specimen is rolled over a glass slide, air-dried, and fixed with acetone. Subsequently, the smears are stained with fluorescein-conjugated monoclonal antibodies for 15 minutes, rinsed with water, and air-dried. Specimens are screened using an epifluorescence microscope. Chlamydial elementary bodies are 350 nm in diameter and at $1000 \times$ magnification appear round or oval, with smooth edges and an apple-green even fluorescence (Figure 1.5).[47] This method is rapid and, in the hands of experienced technicians, sensitive and specific.

ENZYME IMMUNOASSAY. In enzyme immunoassay (Chlamydiazyme; Abbott Labs, Chicago, IL), the urethral specimen is obtained in the same manner as described above, placed into the collection tube, and extracted into the Chlamydiazyme specimen storage reagent. Positive results are determined with a spectrophotometer based on optical density.[48] The method is fairly rapid; however, it requires costly special equipment. Its sensitivity and specificity vary, depending on the population studied.[49]

Just recently we had an opportunity to test a new enzyme-linked immunoassay (EIA) (Syva CO., Palo Alto, CA) which is based on the detection of chlamydia genus cross-reactive lipopolysaccharide antigens in clinical specimens with rabbit polyclonal antibody. This test, according to our results, seems to be highly sensitive and specific.

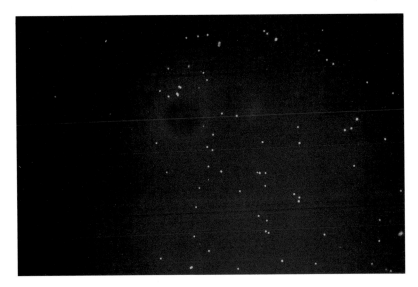

Figure 1.5. Elementary bodies of *Chlamydia trachomatis* identified in direct specimen stained with fluorescein-labeled monoclonal antibodies.

Given the relative ease of EIA testing of large numbers of specimens, it is likely that for screening purposes this approach and/or DNA probe techniques will be widely used in the future.

Detection of Chlamydial DNA. Several methods of detection of chlamydial DNA including DNA-hybridization analysis and polymerase chain reaction technique are under investigation (Unpublished data). These methods, currently being investigated by us, appear to be very sensitive and as soon as their specificity improves they should be useful methods of detection of *chlamydiae* in clinical specimens.

Detection of Ureaplasma urealyticum. Since *U. urealyticum* is frequently detected in apparently healthy men, the usefulness of the identification of this microorganism in men with NGU is questionable. It should be considered primarily in treatment failures or in males with persistent urethritis. A specimen obtained with a urethral swab, or the first voided urine, is cultured in broth and on agar medium. On agar plates *U. urealyticum* produces typical colonies, which can be confirmed by a positive urease test. In broth *U. urealyticum* is identified by a change in color due to decreased pH.

Detection of Trichomonas vaginalis

CULTURE. A direct urethral specimen or urine sediment is inoculated onto Diamond's or other media for *T. vaginalis*. Positive results are available within 2–3 days; negative results require 6–7 days of incubation.

WET MOUNT. A drop of urethral secretion or urine sediment mixed with warmed saline can be examined under low power for motile trichomonads. (The sensitivity of this method in men is questionable.)

TRICHOMONAS DIRECT SPECIMEN TEST. The urethral specimen is incubated with fluorescein-labeled monoclonal antibodies specific to *trichomonas.* The trichomonads appear as apple-green, pear-shaped organisms against a red background of counterstained cells.

STAINED SMEARS. A variety of staining techniques have been described, including Giemsa, Wright's, Papanicolaou, and acridine orange; the last requires a fluorescence microscope. All of these methods, when applied in men, have disadvantages and lack sensitivity.

Complications

Epididymitis. In heterosexual men under 35 years of age, *C. trachomatis* is the leading known cause of infectious epididymitis.[50,51] The condition is frequently preceded or accompanied by urethritis. Chlamydial etiology of epididymitis has been confirmed by direct isolation of this microorganism from epididymal aspirates[50] and from urine.[52] It has been estimated that epididymitis occurs in 1–3 percent of patients with NGU and that more than half of the cases in young heterosexual men are due to *C. trachomatis.*[53]

Chlamydial epididymitis clinically presents as scrotal pain, swelling, and tenderness over the affected part of the scrotum. The condition is usually unilateral; however, the other epididymis may be affected later. The patient may have fever. Generally, symptoms and signs of chlamydial epididymitis tend to be less severe than with gonococcal infection, (see chapter 2 p. 54) and patients improve rapidly after administration of tetracycline.[53]

Prostatitis. Since the prostate gland is in continuity with the urethra, it is not surprising that the sexually transmitted microorganisms that infect the urethra may also infect the prostate. Besides *N. gonorrhoeae,* microorganisms that can be the cause of NGU are suspected of causing prostatitis as well. These include *C. trachomatis,*[52,54,55] *U. urealyticum,*[56] and *T. vaginalis.*[57,58] This theory, however, has its critics, who conclude that *C. trachomatis* is a rather rare cause of prostatitis,[59] whereas the role of *U. urealyticum* and *T. vaginalis* is still uncertain. Further studies are clearly needed to elucidate the role of these microorganisms in prostatitis.

Acute prostatitis is very rare, and in most cases, the process seems to be chronic from the beginning. Patients usually complain of discomfort on passing urine and vague, dull aches in the perineum, groin, penis, suprapubic region, and lower part of the back. Some patients complain of painful ejaculation, rectal fullness, dysuria, and urinary urgency and frequency. Hematospermia and a history of penile discharge with bowel movements also have been reported. Since all of these symptoms may be attributable to entities other than prostatitis, an accurate diagnosis is very difficult and should be based on more objective findings.

On examination, the prostate may feel firm, slightly tender, and nodular.

Prostatic secretions, obtained by expression during transrectal massage, should be examined for pus cells and pathogenic microorganisms. Unfortunately, culture of the prostatic fluid is usually either sterile or may frequently show commensal microorganisms.

Urethral stricture.   Urethal stricture, frequently described in the preantibiotic era, is now a rare complication. It is more likely to occur in long-standing or recurrent NGU and can be identified by urethroscopy or urethrogram. The presence of an asymptomatic stricture, due either to previous gonorrhea or NGU, may be the cause of treatment difficulties or relapse of the disease.

Differential Diagnosis

- *Gonorrhea:* Although the symptoms and signs of gonorrhea are quantitatively different (see Table 1-4), the diagnosis ultimately requires laboratory confirmation, including positive Gram-stained smear and positive culture.
- *Genital herpes:* Genital herpes is characterized by the frequent presence of external lesions, marked dysuria, inguinal lymphadenopathy, and systemic symptoms accompanying the primary episode. In the absence of external lesions, a definitive diagnosis may be almost impossible without laboratory tests.
- *Balanitis/balanoposthitis:* Physicians suspecting NGU in uncircumcised men have to make sure that the discharge and dysuria reported by the patient originate from the urethra, not the preputial sac. The glans of the penis and the interior side of the prepuce must be examined for possible lesions. Partners of women with vaginal candidiasis or nonspecific vaginitis frequently complain of irritation or erythema and develop discharge from the preputial sac. Microscopic examination of discharge plus culture may help to establish the diagnosis.
- *Cystitis:* Cystitis usually involves a history of frequency, urgency, nocturia, suprapubic and/or low back pain, hematuria with or without fever, and chills. Urine examination should be done and a urine culture taken.
- *Prostatitis:* Symptoms of prostatitis include a history of penile discharge with bowel movements, complaints of scrotal or inguinal discomfort, and altered frequency or force of voiding. Rectal examination may reveal a painful and often an enlarged gland. Culture of the prostatic fluid may be helpful.
- *Urethral trauma:* The patient may have a history of recent catheterization, self-instrumentation, or instillation of foreign bodies or chemicals. The physician should be alerted to this possibility when dealing with mentally unstable, debilitated, or psychiatric patients unresponsive to antimicrobial treatment.

Treatment

Infections caused by *C. trachomatis* or *U. urealyticum* should be treated with *doxycycline,* 100 mg by mouth, twice daily for 7 days or *tetracycline hydrochloride,* 500 mg by mouth, 4 times a day for 7 days. Patients for whom tetracyclines are contraindicated should be given *erythromycin base* or *stearate,* 500 mg by mouth, 4 times a day for 7 days. For *T. vaginalis* urethritis, *metronidazole,* 2.0 g by mouth, in a single dose, *or metronidazole,* 250 mg by mouth, 3 times daily for 7 days, is recommended.

Management of Sex Partners

All persons who are sex partners of men with NGU should be examined and treated promptly, depending on the cause of the disease found in index cases. Since the majority of NGU is caused by *C. trachomatis* and *U. urealyticum,* tetracyclines or erythromycin is recommended for symptomatic as well as asymptomatic sex partners. Epidemiologic treatment of contacts of men with NGU not caused by these organisms is of questionable value.[60]

Postgonococcal Urethritis

Postgonococcal urethritis (PGU) is a form of NGU which is believed to result from concomitant infection with *N. gonorrhoeae* and microorganisms causing NGU. Diagnosis of PGU is made in the presence of persistent or remitting symptoms and signs of urethritis in men treated for proved gonorrhea and whose posttreatment cultures for *N. gonorrhoeae* are negative.

Most studies indicate that more than two thirds of the cases of PGU are caused by *C. trachomatis.*[20,61,62] Other microorganisms, such as *U. urealyticum* and *T. vaginalis,* have also been found to be the cause of PGU but in a small proportion of patients.[62] Additional support for multiple infection is provided by therapy trials in which patients treated for gonorrhea with penicillin or spectinomycin (which have no activity against chlamydiae and other pathogens causing NGU) develop PGU much more often than those treated with tetracyclines and their derivatives.[63,64]

Treatment of PGU is the same as for NGU. The sex partners of men who developed PGU should be examined and treated with regimens effective for *N. gonorrhoeae* and *C. trachomatis.* Tetracyclines or erythromycin are the antibiotics of choice.

Reiter's Syndrome

A small proportion of men with NGU have symptoms of Reiter's syndrome at the time of presentation or will develop them later. The condition may be preceded not only by nongonococcal urethritis but also by enteric infections caused by *Shigella dysenteriae, S. flexneri,*[65] *Salmonella typhimurium,*[66] and *Yersinia enterocolitica.*[67] The specific cause of the syndrome is not known, and the etiology seems to be multifactorial, with infective, immunologic, and genetic factors taking part. *Chlamydia trachomatis* has been recovered from up to 60 percent of cases of the syndrome with urethritis and may act as a trigger of an autoimmune reaction.[68,69]

Serologic evidence for *C. trachomatis* infection has been found in about one half of cases,[70,71] and there is a higher antibody response to *C. trachomatis* in men with chlamydiae-associated acute Reiter's syndrome than in men with acute *C. trachomatis*-associated NGU.[72] The lymphocyte transformation response to *C. trachomatis* was also higher in patients with acute chlamydiae-positive Reiter's syndrome than among patients with acute chlamydiae-associated NGU without joint or skin involvement.[71] Additional support for the role of *C. trachomatis* in Reiter's syndrome comes from a recently published report in which chlamydiae were identified by electron microscopy in the synovial tissue of a patient with arthritis associated with Reiter's syndrome.[73] The genetic susceptibility is based on the fact that more than three fourths of patients with Reiter's syndrome possess the histocompatibility determinant HLA-B27.[74] Of particular interest to dermatologists is the extremely strong association of Reiter's syndrome and psoriasiform lesions. There is also a strong association between psoriatic arthritis and pustular psoriasis with HLA-B27.[75,76]

Reiter's syndrome is predominantly a male disease. A recent report indicates that the ratio of men to women with Reiter's syndrome is 3:2.[77] The syndrome affects mainly young, sexually active persons with multiple sex partners.

Clinical Features

In the venereal form of Reiter's syndrome, *urethritis* is the first manifestation, followed within a few days by conjunctivitis and, usually after 3–4 weeks, by arthritis. The urethritis may be symptomatic with a characteristic mucoid discharge and/or dysuria, or asymptomatic, detected only in early morning smears after urine has been held overnight or by pyuria in first-voided urine. Urethritis may also be a feature among patients with dysenteric onset.

Conjunctivitis occurs in less than one half of cases and is often mild and self-limited, with the lower eyelids being mainly involved. The discharge varies from mucoid to merely purulent. *Iritis* is uncommon and is more likely to occur in subsequent rather than initial episodes of the syndrome. *Polyarthritis* is common, involving large joints of the lower extremities and/or sacroiliac joints. At times, small joints of the hands or wrists and the temporomandibular joint may be affected. The arthritis is usually subacute, characterized by moderate erythema, edema, and painful and tender joints with or without effusion. Involvement of sacroiliac joints may be asymptomatic or may be manifested by a backache. Some patients develop fasciitis, tenosynovitis, and myositis. Pain, tenderness, and, occasionally, erythema close to the heel are characteristic manifestations of plantar fasciitis. *Skin and mucous membrane* involvement occurs in a small proportion of cases. Lesions of the penis are found in about 25 percent of the cases and usually appear on the glans and inner aspect of the prepuce. Clinically and histologically these lesions may resemble psoriasis. In uncircumcised men they are rounded, shallow erosions with slightly raised edges, becoming circinate in outline as adjacent lesions coalesce (*Balanitis circinata*) (Figure 1.6). In the circumcised, the glans of the penis is dry and the lesions begin as vesicles. Later becoming pustules, and subsequently forming keratodermic crusts. Circinate lesions may also appear on the vulva in women. *Stomatitis* presents as painless, superficial erosions of the tongue and buccal mucosa have been observed in patients with Reiter's syndrome. Occasionally, they are seen on the soft palate and uvula; however, this manifestation is rare and occurs in less than 10 percent of cases. The lesions of *keratoderma blennorrhagica* start as dull-red macules and develop into dry, scaly pustules or nodular keratotic patches, which may form limpet-like, soft masses of scales. They are usually confined to the soles of the feet (Figure 1.7), but in severe cases they may spread to the limbs, trunk, and scalp resembling psoriasis. The lesions usually heal within a couple of months. Besides the manifestations of urethritis, conjunctivitis, arthritis, and dermatitis, involvement of the nervous[78] and cardiovascular[79,80] systems has been reported. Fortunately, these complications are infrequent.

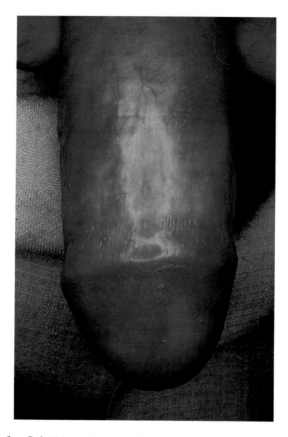

Figure 1.6.   *Balanitis circinata:* circinate lesion on the glans of the penis.

The natural history of Reiter's syndrome is variable. It is characterized by exacerbations and remissions of some or all of the clinical features.[81,82] The recurrences are usually more severe than the first episode. The frequency of recurrences is as unpredictable as the interval between them.

Treatment

Treatment of Reiter's syndrome is empirical and directed at the reduction of pain and other symptoms. If possible, severely ill patients should be hospitalized until the active phase of the disease has passed. The assistance of an experienced rheumatologist or ophthalmologist is frequently desirable.

Urethritis should be treated with *doxycycline* in the usual way (100 mg by mouth, 2 times a day), but administration of the antibiotic should be extended to 14 days. Conjunctivitis is usually self-limited and clears up without any local treatment. In more severe cases, administration of corticosteroid eye drops, with or without an anti-infective agent, is helpful. Sulfacetamide or tetracycline ophthalmic ointment may be used to control secondary infection.

Management of the arthritis consists of rest, physical therapy, analgesics, and treatment with systemically administered anti-inflammatory drugs. Nonsteroidal

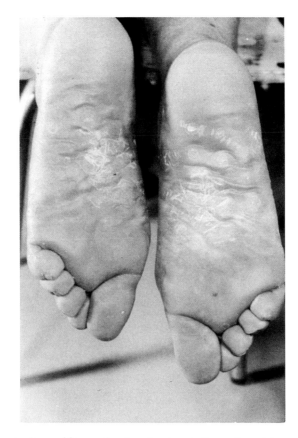

Figure 1.7.   *Keratoderma blennorrhagica:* dry, keratotic, scaly patches on the soles.

anti-inflammatory agents are usually effective for this purpose; however, in more severe or nonresponding cases, prednisone or methotrexate is recommended.[83] Skin lesions (balanitis circinata, keratoderma blennorrhagica) generally do not require topical treatment, although some authors recommend topical low or medium-potency corticosteroid creams.

Proctitis

Proctitis due to *C. trachomatis* infection has been reported in both homosexual men and heterosexual women.[84-89] In homosexuals, transmission presumably occurs via receptive anal intercourse with a partner who has chlamydial urethral infection. In women, infection can be acquired through anal intercourse or as a result of contamination with discharge caused by chlamydial cervicitis.

The clinical spectrum of the disease ranges from asymptomatic infection to severe proctocolitis,[84-90] and clinical manifestations seem to depend on the immunotype of *C. trachomatis* causing the disease. Both lymphogranuloma venereum (LGV) and nonlymphogranuloma venereum (non-LGV) strains can cause the disease.[85,90,91]

Patients infected with LGV strains (L_1, L_2, or L_3) usually develop severe proctocolitis clinically resembling Crohn's disease of the rectum,[90,92,93] whereas infection with non-LGV strains is associated with mild symptoms or is asymptomatic.[85]

Severe proctocolitis (due to LGV strains) usually presents with mucopurulent or bloody discharge, lower abdominal and rectal pain, tenesmus, hematochezia, and diarrhea and/or loose stools.[85,91,94] Fever and adenopathy may be present in some cases. Sigmoidoscopy may reveal mucopus and diffuse rectal friability and superficial ulceration in the rectum and, occasionally, in the sigmoid colon.[91,94] Histopathology shows diffuse inflammation with crypt abscesses, granulomas, and giant cells.[85,91,94] If not treated, this form of proctitis may cause serious sequelae.[95]

Non-LGV strains which account for 75 percent of chlamydial rectal infections in the United States produce either asymptomatic infection or mild proctitis characterized by moderate rectal pain, discharge, rectal irritation, and bleeding.[96] Anoscopy and sigmoidoscopy show minimal abnormalities such as erythema and/or focal friability or a mucopurulent discharge. Rarely, there are small ulcerations. Biopsy specimens usually reveal mild inflammation of rectal mucosa.[85,94] Gram-stained fecal smears may reveal leukocytes even in asymptomatic cases.[85]

The diagnosis of chlamydial proctitis is based on the identification of *C. trachomatis* in rectal specimens either by culture or direct immunofluorescent testing. Positive anoscopy and the finding of leukocytes on a rectal Gram's stain may support diagnosis. Serodiagnosis may be helpful in some cases, but its results should be interpreted with caution. The differential diagnosis includes proctitis due to *N. gonorrhoeae* and herpes simplex virus (HSV). Gonococcal proctitis can be confirmed by isolation of *N. gonorrhoeae*. Proctitis caused by HSV may produce severe constipation, sacral radiculopathy, and radiating pain in the legs. Positive culture for HSV or other tests confirms the diagnosis.

Treatment of proctitis consists of doxycycline, 100 mg orally 2 times a day or tetracycline hydrochloride, 500 mg tablets 4 times a day, both for 14–21 days. For mild or asymptomatic chlamydial infection of the rectum, a 7-day course of doxycycline or tetracycline may be sufficient.

When cultures cannot be performed, empirical therapy with ceftriaxone 250 mg IM in a single dose followed by 100 mg of oral doxycycline twice daily for 7 days, may be considered. This regimen should be effective especially in homosexual men in whom *C. trachomatis* and *N. gonorrhoeae* are frequent causes of proctitis.[96] However, it will be of no value in cases in which herpes simplex virus is the cause of infection.[97]

Pharyngeal Infection

Although pharyngeal colonization with *C. trachomatis* has been reported by numerous authors, "chlamydial pharyngitis" as a clinical entity is still a controversial issue.[84,87,88,98] The organism has been isolated from a female sexual partner of a man with recurrent NGU,[98] and women practicing fellatio should be at increased risk for pharyngeal infection. However, Bowie and coworkers were unable to isolate *C. trachomatis* from women who practiced fellatio and whose partners were known to have NGU due to *C. trachomatis*.[99]

Homosexual men, who frequently practice orogenital sex, should be another high-risk group for pharyngeal infection, but *C. trachomatis* has been isolated from them in only 1–4 percent of cases.[87,88] In view of the high isolation rates of *C. trachomatis* in urethritis and cervicitis, the low isolation rate of this organism from the pharynx is somewhat surprising. It may be possible that the oropharyngeal mucosa is less well suited to colonization by chlamydiae than urethral or cervical epithelium. Animal studies have revealed that the pharynx is much more difficult to infect than the urethra and that much larger inocula of *C. trachomatis* are necessary to establish infection in the pharynx.[32] An alternative possibility is that investigators have sampled the wrong site by performing oropharyngeal cultures. In infants with chlamydial conjunctivitis or pneumonia, nasopharyngeal cultures frequently reveal the organism.[12]

The question of whether *C. trachomatis* is capable of causing acute symptomatic pharyngitis or if the infection is mainly asymptomatic still needs to be answered. Based on serologic data, Komaroff and coworkers suggested that *C. trachomatis* is an important pharyngeal pathogen and may be responsible for a large proportion of symptomatic pharyngitis.[100] Unfortunately, the organism has not been isolated in these patients, and the serologic evidence of infection could be due to cross-reactivity to antigens from another microorganism or chlamydial infection elsewhere in the body.

Chlamydia trachomatis in the pharynx is best isolated by means of culture; however, direct immunofluorescence is also useful. Interestingly, the number of inclusions as well as the number of elementary bodies is low.[88]

There are insufficient data on treatment of chlamydial pharyngitis. Based on the high efficacy of tetracyclines in the treatment of chlamydial infection of other sites, doxycycline, 100 mg tablets twice daily or tetracycline HCl, 500 mg 4 times a day both for 7 days is recommended.

SEXUALLY TRANSMITTED DISEASES CAUSED BY *CHLAMYDIA TRACHOMATIS* IN WOMEN AND NEONATES

Mucopurulent Cervicitis

Endocervicitis is the most common form of chlamydial infection of the urogenital tract in women. From the epidemiologic point of view, it is regarded as an equivalent of nongonococcal urethritis in men.

Epidemiology

Chlamydial infection appears to be common in every sexually active group of women and the prevalence of chlamydial endocervicitis varies from one geographic area and clinical population to another. In clinics treating sexually transmitted diseases, the prevalence of endocervical chlamydial infection has ranged from 19 to 33 percent.[2] *Chlamydia trachomatis* infections have been shown to be more prevalent in young unmarried women under 20 years of age,[101,102] women using oral contraceptives,[103] and partners of men with NGU.[101,104] However, not all investigators confirm these observations.[105] *Chlamydia trachomatis* was isolated more often from women who had intercourse with a new partner within the preceding 2 months[106] and those with multiple sex partners.[102] Also, women from lower socio-economic groups[107] and those who are at highest risk for other STDs had higher isolation rates.[108,109]

It has been demonstrated that chlamydial infection of the cervix, despite causing inflammatory changes, was also associated with cervical intraepithelial neoplasia (CIN).[110] Another study showed that patients with cervical neoplasia had a significant excess of antichlamydial antibodies as compared with a control group of patients.[111] The prevalence of chlamydial infections of the cervix in pregnant women has been reported to be between 8 and 37 percent.[112-116] These observations should be of special concern in view of possible vertical transmission with adverse pregnancy outcomes.

The effect of maternal chlamydial infection on pregnancy and perinatal complications is still controversial, although several studies have suggested a link between chlamydial infection of the cervix and perinatal mortality, preterm premature rupture of the membranes, preterm labor, and low birth weight.[112,117,118]

Clinical Features

The clinical features of chlamydial cervical infection range from a clinically normal appearance (asymptomatic infection) to severely hypertropic erosions of the cervix with mucopurulent discharge.[105,119]

Folliclelike lesions, similar to those seen in the conjunctiva, have been described,[120] and severe inflammatory atypia, with or without dyskeratotic changes, have been observed in Papanicolaou's smears.[121]

However, the frequent feature of chlamydial cervicitis is the presence of yellow, mucopurulent endocervical discharge (Figure 1.8), or the finding of a yellow

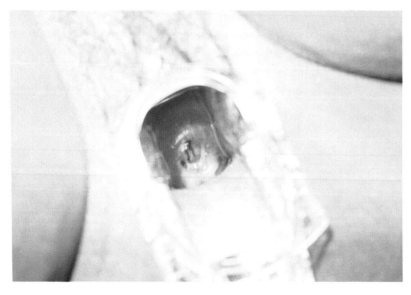

Figure 1.8. Mucopurulent cervicitis. Notice mucopurulent discharge and friability characteristic of chlamydial infection of the cervix.

or green exudate of endocervical secretions on a white cotton-tipped swab.[122,123] In women without visible mucopus, the presence of more than 10 polymorphonuclear leukocytes per oil high-power field on a Gram-stained specimen of endocervical mucus (without contamination by vaginal cells) also allows a presumptive diagnosis. Other clinical criteria include erythema or edema within a zone of cervical ectopy and/or cervical friability (bleeding when the first swab culture is taken).

Diagnosis and Differential Diagnosis

Since, basically, only two microorganisms, *N. gonorrhoeae* and *C. trachomatis*, are found associated with mucopurulent cervicitis, one may approach the differential diagnosis of cervicitis in a manner analogous to that for NGU in men. Nongonococcal cervicitis may be suspected on the basis of the aforementioned symptoms and the presence of more than 10 PMNs per high-power field of stained cervical mucus and confirmed by a negative Gram's stain and culture for *N. gonorrhoeae*.

Definitive diagnosis (as to the causative agent) is made by successful isolation of *C. trachomatis* in cervical specimens.

Complications

Complications of chlamydial cervical infection include pelvic inflammatory disease, Fitz-Hugh-Curtis syndrome (see Chapter 3), and others (see below).

Treatment

Patients should be given *Doxycycline*, 100 mg by mouth, twice daily or *tetracycline HCl*, 500 mg by mouth, 4 times daily for 7 days. For patients in whom tetracyclines are contraindicated, administer *erythromycin base* or *erythromycin stearate*, 500 mg by mouth, 4 times daily for 7 days. If *N. gonorrhoeae* is found along with *C. trachomatis*, a treatment regimen effective against both gonococcal and chlamydial infection should be used.

Management of Sex Partners

Men exposed to women with cervicitis attributed to *C. trachomatis* should be evaluated for STD and treated (even if asymptomatic) with one of the above regimens. If concomitant gonorrhea is found, treatment should be with a regimen effective against gonococcal and chlamydial infection.

Endometritis

Nonpuerperal Endometritis

Another manifestation of chlamydial infection in nonpuerperal women is endometritis.[124-127] It has been suggested that chlamydiae ascend from the cervix and affect the uterine mucosa. Spread from the endocervix to the endometrium presumably precedes, or occurs simultaneously with, spread to the fallopian tubes. Interestingly, *C. trachomatis* was also recovered in endometrial cultures despite negative cervical cultures.[124,125] It has been shown that one third of women with mucopurulent cervicitis caused by *C. trachomatis* have histologic evidence of endometritis.[128] *Chlamydia trachomatis* has also been recovered from the endometrial cavity of women with salpingitis.[125,129,130]

Most women with endometritis do not have clinical symptoms or signs of genital tract infection, and the clinical diagnosis of nonpuerperal endometritis is based on the finding of intermenstrual bleeding, lower abdominal pain, cervical motion tenderness, and uterine tenderness—but not adnexal tenderness. Histopathologic examination of endometrial biopsy specimens reveals plasma cells. The sedimentation rate and WBC count may be elevated. Some patients may complain of fever, chills, and malaise.

Postpartum Endometritis

Late postpartum endometritis is a clinically mild disease caused by the ascent of bacteria from the lower genital tract (vulva, vagina, and cervix) into the endometrium after delivery. A variety of microorganisms are found in association with the disease, including *C. trachomatis, Ureaplasma urealyticum,* and *Mycoplasma hominis* as well as aerobic and anaerobic bacteria.[131,132]

Pregnant women with chlamydial infection detected during their prenatal visit are at risk for developing late onset endometritis following vaginal delivery.[119,133,134] More than half of the women whose infants had chlamydial conjunctivitis developed intrapartum pelvic infection within the first 2–5 weeks postpartum.[119] *Chlamydia trachomatis* infection was also correlated with intrapartum fever in women who delivered vaginally[133] and with severe pelvic disease following cesarean section.[135] In contrast, the performance of a cesarean section is associated with early postpartum infection, usually occurring within 48 hours of delivery.[133] Nevertheless several studies have failed to demonstrate an association between postpartum endometritis and *C. trachomatis.*[136-138] They found a strong correlation between *M. hominis* or *M. hominis* infection combined with *C. trachomatis* infection and intrapartum and postpartum fever but not with *C. trachomatis* alone.[136,137] Further research must define the role of *C. trachomatis* and other microorganisms in postpartum endometritis.

The onset of late postpartum endometritis occurs between 1 and 6 weeks postpartum (mean time of 3 weeks). The course of the disease is mild. Women with late postpartum endometritis usually have a mild to moderate degree of pain and tenderness, a mildly elevated temperature, and no other systemic signs.

Patient Management

Women with suspected endometritis should have cervical *C. trachomatis* and *N. gonorrhoeae* cultures obtained. The treatment regimen should include antibiotics effective against *N. gonorrhoeae* and *C. trachomatis* (see treatment of PID in Chapter 3).

Proctitis in Women

Chlamydial proctitis in women is rare but should be anticipated in patients who have practiced anal sex. Symptoms and signs occur usually a few weeks after exposure and may present as severe inflammation with painful defecation, constipation with bloody and purulent discharge, or as a mild process with minimum symptoms and mild mucoid discharge. In one case, chlamydial proctitis in a woman presented as a symptomatic vaginal mass.[139] Both LGV serotypes as well as genital strains of *C. trachomatis* may cause the disease. (For detailed description of chlamydial proctitis see p. 17)

Urethritis/Acute Urethral Syndrome

There is no doubt that cervicitis is the most common form of chlamydial infection in women, although *C. trachomatis* was also found in the female urethra with or without concomitant cervical infection. Many women with chlamydial infection of the urethra have no apparent symptoms. However, some of them may complain of dysuria and frequency. Dysuria occurs more frequently in females who have simultaneous cervical and urethral infection than in females with cervical infection only. In contrast to clinical findings of women with mucopurulent cervicitis, women with chlamydial urethritis have no signs of urethral inflammation (urethral discharge, edema,and erythema of the urethral orifice) or these signs are infrequent. Often chlamydial urethritis can be suspected on epidemiological grounds (e.g. in young, sexually active women complaining of dysuria and frequency), especially if the person had been named as a sex partner of men with NGU or had sex with a new partner recently. Despite frequent asymptomatic infection of the female urethra, *Chlamydia trachomatis* has been implicated as a possible cause of the so-called acute urethral syndrome (AUS). The syndrome is one of the newly recognized clinical entities in which the role of *C. trachomatis* is seriously discussed. Even though the etiology of the syndrome is unclear and more than one pathogen or factor may be involved, it is appropriate to consider AUS here since it can be the form of chlamydial infection of the female urethra.

The acute urethral syndrome in women presents as urgency, frequency, and dysuria. Urine examination reveals pyuria, but the bladder urine is usually sterile or contains less than 10^5 microorganisms per milliliter.

The cause of the syndrome in women without appreciable bacteriuria is uncertain, and the frequent presence of multiple pathogens or potential pathogens in sexually active women makes the cause of the syndrome even more difficult to ascertain.

Although structural and functional abnormalities of the bladder neck, urethral injury during intercourse, and other noninfectious causes have been implicated, it is generally believed that, in most instances, AUS is due to infections, especially with sexually transmitted microorganisms.

Many suggestions for an infective basis for AUS have been proposed. There is some data to suggest that *Mycoplasma hominis* and *Ureaplasma urealyticum* may cause the disease.[140,141] Dysuria without frequency or urgency may result from vulvovaginitis caused by *Candida albicans* or *Trichomonas vaginalis*.[142] *Neisseria gonorrhoeae* and *Chlamydia trachomatis* can infect the female urethra with or without concomitant infection of the cervix, and some women with these infections may complain of dysuria and frequency as well.[143-145] Other uropathogens such as *Escherichia coli*, and sometimes *Staphylococcus epidermidis* and *Klebsiella*, have been found in women with AUS and pyuria.[146]

Several investigators have placed *C. trachomatis* infections among the most likely causes of AUS. This microorganism can infect the female uretha with or without concomitant infection of the cervix,[145,147] causing urethral discharge with dysuria or dysuria alone. *Chlamydia trachomatis* has been found in symptomatic women who had pyuria and sterile urine.[146,148] Several findings of the medical history, such as recent change in sexual partners, the use of oral contraceptives, and prolonged duration of symptoms, are suggestive of *C. trachomatis* being the causative agent of the syndrome.[148] Finally, antimicrobial therapy which utilized an agent effective against *C. trachomatis* was significantly more effective than placebo in eradicating the urethral syndrome with pyuria.[149] However, a recently published study, in which the authors investigated the correlation between urinary symptoms (dysuria, frequency) and pyuria and infection of the lower urogenital tract among sexually active women, found no association between urinary symptoms and sexually transmitted infections.[150]

All these findings highlight the complexity of the etiology of AUS and raise questions as to whether other urethral pathogens,[151] noninfectious causes (including autonomically mediated smooth muscle spasm of the sphincter),[152] or even psychological factors alone[153] should be considered.

Diagnosis

To establish the diagnosis, an attempt should be made to differentiate patients with AUS from patients with vulvovaginitis and cystitis. Cultures for *C. trachomatis* and *N. gonorrhoeae* and microscopic examinations and/or cultures for *Candida albicans* and *T. vaginalis* should be performed in any sexually active women complaining of dysuria. Cultures for genital mycoplasmas do not seem to be useful, but careful examination for the presence of genital warts and herpetic lesions, including the Tzanck test or culture if necessary, may be required since sexually transmitted viral infections may be the cause of dysuria.

Culture of midstream urine should be performed to differentiate AUS and cystitis. A bacterial count of 10^5 or fewer microorganisms per milliliter is being used currently as a cutoff for diagnosis of AUS. Other findings that may help to distinguish AUS and cystitis are suprapubic tenderness, hematuria, history of previous episodes, and the presence of prominent urgency and frequency characteristic of cystitis.[148]

Treatment

Patients should be given *doxycycline,* 100 mg twice daily or *tetracycline HCl,* 500 mg 4 times daily, both for 7 days. These regimens are effective not only against *C. trachomatis* and *N. gonorrhoeae* but also against other common urethral pathogens which may be the cause of the syndrome.[150] Alternatively, patients may be treated with *erythromycin,* 500 mg 4 times daily for 7 days.

Management of Sex Partners

The sex partners of women with AUS should be examined for sexually transmitted infections and treated concomitantly.

Chlamydial Infections in Neonates

It is well documented that infants born through an infected birth canal are at risk of developing chlamydial conjunctivitis and pneumonia.[13,109,154-156] Until recently, it has been thought that intrauterine transmission of *C. trachomatis* did not occur. A report of four newborns with chlamydial conjunctivitis delivered by cesarean section in the presence of intact membranes may change this view. If it is confirmed, it would indicate that infants might acquire *C. trachomatis* by routes other than passage through an infected birth canal, possibly by ascending cervical infection. Some of the infants who developed chlamydial conjunctivitis after cesarean section might, however, be infected after birth, since both parents of two of them had *C. trachomatis* genital infection.[156]

Conjunctivitis

Chlamydia trachomatis is the most common cause of conjunctivitis in the first month of life. The disease usually develops 5–14 days after birth and begins with a watery eye discharge, which rapidly progresses to become mucopurulent or purulent (Figure 1.9). The eyelids are swollen and conjunctiva become reddened and somewhat thickened throughout. *Chlamydia trachomatis* may be demonstrated in conjunctival scrapings. If the disease is treated early, no sequelae will develop. In untreated cases, spontaneous resolution usually occurs during the first few months of life. Sequelae are rare and include scarring and micropannus. Occasionally, infants have persistent conjunctivitis.

Treatment. Oral erythromycin syrup, 50 mg/kg body weight per day in 4 divided doses for 14 days, can be administered. There is no indication that topical therapy provides additional benefit.

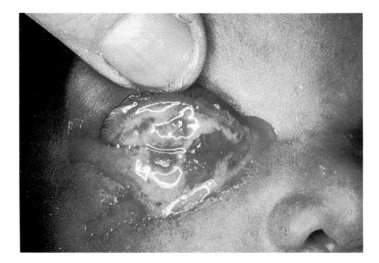

Figure 1.9. Severe chlamydial conjunctivitis in a neonate.

Pneumonia

Chlamydial pneumonia is probably one of the three most common pneumonias seen in infancy. The infection is presumably acquired during birth. However, the infected conjunctiva or nasopharynx may be the initial site of infection in some cases.

The disease usually occurs between 4 and 11 weeks of life and presents initially with upper respiratory symptoms, which include congestion and obstruction of nasal passages. An abnormal bulging eardrum can be found in about half of the cases. Some patients may have concomitant conjunctivitis. Lower respiratory tract symptoms consist of tachypnea and repetitive staccato cough. Crepitant inspiratory rales may be heard. Roentgenologic examination may reveal hyperinflated lungs with bilateral interstitial infiltrates. Patients usually have normal body temperature or minimal fever with no other signs of systemic illness. Laboratory tests demonstrate eosinophilia with a normal white blood cell count. IgG and IgM are generally elevated.[13,14]

The diagnosis is made on clinical features of an afebrile pneumonitis confirmed by the presence of antichlamydial IgM antibodies and/or demonstration of *C. trachomatis* in clinical specimens.

Treatment.   Oral erythromycin syrup, 50 mg/kg per day in 4 divided doses for 14 days should be given.

Other Infections

Chlamydia trachomatis has been proposed as a cause of otitis media in infancy.[157] Nasopharyngeal infections and bronchiolitis have also been associated with chlamydial infections. Subclinical chlamydial infections of the rectum and vagina were detected in infants born to mothers with positive cervical cultures for *C. trachomatis.*[155] Nevertheless, chlamydial conjunctivitis and pneumonia are the only two firmly established clinical entities, and in the aforementioned conditions a definite role of *C. trachomatis* has not been established.

REFERENCES

1. Washington AE, Johnson RE, Sanders LL, et al: Incidence of *Chlamydia trachomatis* infections in the U.S.: Using reported *Neisseria gonorrhoeae* as a surrogate, in Oriel JD, Ridgway G, Schachter J, Taylor-Robinson D, Ward M (eds): *Chlamydial Infections. Proceedings of the 6th International Symposium on Human Chlamydial Infections.* Cambridge, Cambridge University Press, 198:487–490, 1986.

2. Thompson SE, Washington AE: Epidemiology of sexually transmitted *Chlamydia trachomatis* infections. *Epidemiol Rev* 5:96–123, 1983.

3. Schachter J, Grossman M: Chlamydial infections. *Annu Rev Med* 32:45–61, 1981.

4. Judson FN: Assessing the number of genital chlamydial infections in the United States. *J Reprod Med* 3(Suppl):269–272, 1985.

5. Bowie WR, Wang S-P, Alexander ER, et al: Etiology of nongonococcal urethritis: Evidence for *Chlamydia trachomatis* and *Ureaplasma urealyticum. J Clin Invest* 59:735–742, 1977.

6. Forsey T, Kazar J, Dines RJ, et al: A seroepidemiological survey of chlamydial infections in Czechoslovakia, in Oriel JD, Ridgway G, Schachter J, Taylor-Robinson D, Ward M (eds): *Chlamydial Infections. Proceedings of the 6th International Symposium on Human Chlamydial Infections.* Cambridge, Cambridge University Press, 198:507–510, 1986.

7. Mardh P-A, Moller BR, Paavonen J: Chlamydia infection of the female genital tract with emphasis on pelvic inflammatory disease: A review of Scandinavian studies. *Sex Transm Dis* 8:140–155, 1981.

8. Stapinski A, Mroczkowski TF, Gede K, et al: Epidemiology of nongonococcal urethritis. *Przegl Derm* 72:43–50, 1985.

9. Grayston JT, Wang SP: New knowledge of chlamydiae and the diseases they cause. *J Infect Dis* 132:87–105, 1975.

10. *Chlamydia trachomatis* infections: Policy guidelines for prevention and control. *MMWR Suppl* 34(3S):53s–74s, 1985.

11. Schachter J, Lum L, Gooding CA, et al: Pneumonitis following inclusion blennorrhea. *J Pediatr* 87:779–780, 1975.

12. Beem MO, Saxon EM: Respiratory tract colonization and distinctive pneumonia syndrome in infants infected with antepartum *Chlamydia trachomatis* infection. *N Engl J Med* 296:306–310, 1977.

13. Harrison HR, English MG, Lee CK, et al: *Chlamydia trachomatis* infant pneumonitis: Comparison with matched controls and other infant pneumonitis. *N Engl J Med* 298: 702–708, 1978.

14. Tipple MA, Beem MO, Saxon EM: Clinical characteristics of the afebrile pneumoniae associated with *Chlamydia trachomatis* infection in infants less than 6 months of age. *Pediatrics* 63:192–197, 1979.

15. Sexually transmitted diseases. Extract from the Annual Report of the Chief Medical Officer of the Department of Health and Social Security for the year 1978. *Br J Vener Dis* 56:178–181, 1980.

16. Stamm WE, Cole B: Asymptomatic *Chlamydia trachomatis* urethritis in men. *Sex Transm Dis* 13:163–165, 1986.

17. Karam GH, Martin DH, Flotte TR, et al: Asymptomatic *Chlamydia trachomatis* infections among sexually active men. *J Infect Dis* 154:900–903, 1986.

18. Wiesner PJ: Selected aspects of the epidemiology of nongonococcol urethritis, in Hobson D, Holmes KK (eds): *Nongonococcal Urethritis and Related Infections.* Washington DC, American Society for Microbiology, 1977, pp. 9–14.

19. Judson FN: Epidemiology and control of nongonococcal urethritis and genital chlamydial infections: A review. *Sex Transm Dis* 8:117–126, 1981.

20. Holmes KK, Handsfield HH, Wang S-P, et al: Etiology of nongonococcal urethritis in men. *N Engl J Med* 292:1199–1206, 1975.

21. Jacobs NF, Kraus SJ: Gonococcal and nongonococcal urethritis in men: Clinical and laboratory differentiation. *Ann Intern Med* 82:7–12, 1975.

22. Stamm WE, Koutsky LA, Benedetti JK, et al: *Chlamydia trachomatis* urethral infections in men—Prevalence, risk factors, and clinical manifestations. *Ann Intern Med* 100:47–51, 1984.

23. Oriel JD, Reeve P, Thomas BJ, et al: Infection with *Chlamydia* group A in men with urethritis due to *Neisseria gonorrhoeae*. *J Infect Dis* 131:376–382, 1975.

24. Schachter J: Chlamydial infections. *N Engl J Med* 298:423–490, 1978.

25. Mroczkowski TF, Dajek Z, Stapinski A, et al: The role of Chlamydias, Mycoplasmas

and *Trichomonas vaginalis* in nongonococcal urethritis in men. *Przegl Derm* 71:47–50, 1984.

26. McCormack WM, Lee T-H, Sinner SH: Sexual experience and urethral colonization with genital mycoplasmas: A study in normal men. *Ann Intern Med* 78:696–698, 1973.

27. Bowie WR: Nongonococcal urethritis, in Felman YM (ed): *Symposium on Sexually Transmitted Diseases. Dermatol Clin* 1:53–64, 1983.

28. Bowie WR: Nongonococcal urethritis and lymphogranuloma venereum. *Cutis* 33:97–110, 1984.

29. Podgore JK, Holmes KK, Alexander ER: Asymptomatic urethral infections due to *Chlamydia trachomatis* in male U.S. military personnel. *J Infect Dis* 146:828, 1982.

30. Paavonen J, Kousa M, Saikku P, et al: Examination of men with nongonococcal urethritis and their sexual partners for *Chlamydia trachomatis* and *Ureaplasma urealyticum. Sex Transm Dis* 5:93–96, 1978.

31. Worm A-M, Petersen CS: Transmission of chlamydial infections to sexual partners. *Genitourin Med* 63:19–21, 1987.

32. Jackobs NJ, Arum ES, Kraus SJ: Experimental infection of the chimpanzee urethra and pharynx with *C. trachomatis. Sex Transm Dis.* 5:132–136, 1978.

33. Richmond SJ, Oriel JD: Recognition and management of genital chlamydial infection. *Br Med J* 2:480–482, 1978.

34. Mroczkowski TF, Dajek Z: Nongonococcal urethritis in men: Modern diagnostic and treatment. *Przegl Derm* 68:577–583, 1979.

35. Taylor-Robinson D, McCormack WM: The genital mycoplasmas. *N Engl J Med* 302:1003–1010, 1980.

36. Bowie WR: Nongonococcal urethritis, in Felman YM (ed): *Sexually Transmitted Diseases.* New York, Churchill Livingstone, 1986, p. 65.

37. Shepard MC, Lunceford DC: Serological typing of *Ureaplasma urealyticum* isolates from urethritis patients by an agar growth inhibition method. *J Clin Microbiol* 8:566–574, 1978.

38. Arya OP, Pratt BC: Persistent urethritis due to *Ureaplasma urealyticum* in conjugal or stable partnership. *Genitourin Med* 62:329–332, 1986.

39. Corey L, Adams HG, Brown ZA, et al: Genital herpes simplex virus infections. Clinical manifestations, course and complications. *Ann Intern Med* 98:958–972, 1983.

40. Fontaine EA, Taylor-Robinson D, Hanna NF, et al: Anaerobes in men with urethritis. *Br J Vener Dis* 58:321–326, 1982.

41. Lawrynowicz R, Dajek Z, Mroczkowski TF: Anaerobic flora of male's urethra and its significance in urethritis. *Przegl Derm* 71:47–51, 1984.

42. Desai K, Robson HG: Comparison of gram-stained urethral smears and first-voided urine sediment in the diagnosis of nongonococcal urethritis. *Sex Transm Dis* 9:21–25, 1982.

43. Stamm WE: Diagnosis of *Chlamydia trachomatis* genitourinary infections. *Ann Intern Med* 108:710–717, 1988.

44. Bowie WR: Comparison of Gram stain and first voided urine sediment in the diagnosis of urethritis. *Sex Transm Dis* 5:39–42, 1978.

45. Schwartz SL, Kraus SJ, Herrmann KL, et al: Diagnosis and etiology of nongonococcal urethritis. *J Infect Dis* 138:445–454, 1978.

46. Ripa KT, Mardh P-A: Cultivation of *Chlamydia trachomatis* in cycloheximide-treated McCoy cells. *J Clin Microbiol* 6:328–331, 1977.

47. Tam MR, Stamm WE, Handsfield HH, et al: Culture-independent diagnosis of *Chlamydia trachomatis* using monoclonal antibodies. *N Engl J Med* 310:1146–1150, 1986.

48. Jones MF, Smith TF, Houglum AJ, et al: Detection of *Chlamydia trachomatis* in genital specimens by the chlamydiazyme test. *J Clin Microbiol* 20:465–467, 1984.

49. Chernesky MA, Mahony JB, Castriciano S, et al: Detection of *Chlamydia trachomatis* antigen by enzyme immunoassay and immunofluorescence in genital specimens from symptomatic and asymptomatic men and women. *J Infect Dis* 154:141–148, 1986.

50. Berger RE, Alexander ER, Monda GD, et al: *Chlamydia trachomatis* as a cause of acute "idiopathic" epididymitis. *N Engl J Med* 298:301–304, 1978.

51. Hawkins DA, Taylor-Robinson D, Thomas BJ, et al: Microbiological survey of acute epididymitis. *Genitourin Med* 62:342–344, 1986.

52. Bruce AW, Chadwick P, Willett WS, et al: The role of chlamydiae in genitourinary disease. *J Urol* 126:625–629, 1981.

53. Berger RE, Alexander ER, Harnish JP, et al: Etiology, manifestations and therapy of acute epididymitis: Prospective study of 50 cases. *J Urol* 121:750–754, 1979.

54. Ballard RC: Delayed hypersensitivity to *Chlamydia trachomatis:* Cause of chronic prostatitis. *Lancet* 2:1305–1306, 1979.

55. Colleen S, Mardh P-A: Complicated infections of the male genital tract with emphasis on *Chlamydia trachomatis* as an etiologic agent. *Scand J Infect Dis* (Suppl) 32:93–99, 1982.

56. Weidner W, Brunner H, Krauze W: Quantitative cultures of *Ureaplasma urealyticum* in patients with chronic prostatitis or prostatosis. *J Urol* 124:622–625, 1980.

57. Kuberski T: *Trichomonas vaginalis* associated with nongonococcal urethritis and prostatitis. *Sex Transm Dis* 7:135–136, 1980.

58. Krieger JN: Urologic aspects of trichomoniasis. *Invest Urol* 18:411–417, 1981.

59. Mardh P-A, Ripa KT, Colleen S, et al: Role of *Chlamydia trachomatis* in nonacute prostatitis. *Br J Vener Dis* 54:330–334, 1978.

60. Fitzgerald MR: Effect of epidemiological treatment of contacts in preventing recurrences of non-gonococcal urethritis. *Br J Vener Dis* 60:312–315, 1984.

61. Richmond SJ, Hilton AL, Clarke SKR: Chlamydial infection: Role of chlamydia subgroup A in nongonococcal and postgonococcal urethritis. *Br J Vener Dis* 48:437–444, 1972.

62. Stapinski A, Dajek Z, Mroczkowski TF, et al: Gonorrhea, accompanied by chlamydial and mycoplasmatical infection. Their effect on the development of post-gonococcal urethritis. *Przegl Derm* 71:449–461, 1984.

63. Mroczkowski TF: Postgonococcol urethritis in men, Part I. *Przegl Derm* 63:53–57, 1976.

64. Karney WW, Pedersen AHB, Nelson M, et al: Spectinomycin versus tetracycline for the treatment of gonorrhea. *N Engl J Med* 296:889–894, 1977.

65. Davies NE, Haverty JR, Boatwright M: Reiter's disease associated with shigellosis. *South Med J* 62:1011–1014, 1969.

66. Warren CPW: Arthritis associated with *Salmonella* infections. *Ann Rheum Dis* 29:483–487, 1970.

67. Winblad S: Arthritis associated with *Yersinia enterocolitica* infections. *Scand J Infect Dis* 7:191–195, 1975.

68. Kousa M, Saikku P, Richmond SJ, et al: Frequent association of chlamydial infection with Reiter's syndrome. *Sex Transm Dis* 5:57–61, 1978.

69. Amor B, Kahan A, Orfila J, et al: Immunological evidence of chlamydial infection in Reiter's syndrome. *Ann Rheum Dis* 38 (Suppl):116–118, 1979.

70. Keat AC, Maini RN, Nkwazi GC, et al: Role of *Chlamydia trachomatis* and HLA-B27 in sexually acquired reactive arthritis. *Br Med J* 1:605–607, 1978.

71. Martin DH, Pollock S, Kuo C-C, et al: *Chlamydia trachomatis* in men with Reiter's syndrome. *Ann Intern Med* 100:207–213, 1984.

72. Keat AC, Thomas BJ, Taylor-Robinson D, et al: Evidence of *Chlamydia trachomatis* infection in sexually acquired reactive arthritis. *Ann Rheum Dis* 39:431–437, 1980.

73. Ishikawa H, Ohno O, Yamasaki K, et al: Arthritis presumably caused by *Chlamydia* in Reiter syndrome. Case report with electron microscopic studies. *J Bone Joint Surg* 68:777–779, 1986.

74. Brewerton DA, Caffrey M, Nicholls A, et al: Reiter's disease and HL-A27. *Lancet* 2:996–998, 1973.

75. Zachariae H, Peterson HO, Nielsen FK, et al: HL-A antigens in pustular psoriasis. *Dermatologica* 154:73–77, 1977.

76. Marcusson J: Psoriasis and arthritis lesions in relation to the inheritance of HLA genotypes. *Acta Derm Venerol* (Stockh) 59 (Suppl 82):1–48, 1979.

77. Neuwelt CM, Borenstein DG, Jacobs RP: Reiter's syndrome: A male and female disease. *J Rheumatol* 9:268–272, 1982.

78. Oates JK, Hancock JAH: Neurological symptoms and lesions occurring in the course of Reiter's disease. *Am J Med Sci* 238:79–84, 1959.

79. Rodnan GP, Benedek TG, Shaver JA, et al: Reiter's syndrome and aortic insufficiency. *JAMA* 89:889–894, 1964.

80. Paulus HE, Pearson CM, Pitts W: Aortic insufficiency in five patients with Reiter's syndrome: A detailed clinical and pathological study. *Am J Med* 53:464–472, 1972.

81. Butler MJ, Russell AS, Percy JS, et al: A follow-up study of 48 patients with Reiter's syndrome. *Am J Med* 67:808–810, 1979.

82. Sharp JT: Reiter's syndrome (reactive arthritis), in McCarty DJ (ed): *Arthritis and Allied Conditions.* Philadelphia, Lea & Febiger, 1985, p. 841.

83. Lally EV, Ho G: A review of methotrexate therapy in Reiter's syndrome. *Semin Arthritis Rheum* 15:139–142, 1985.

84. Goldmeier D, Darougar S: Isolation of *Chlamydia trachomatis* from throat and rectum of homosexual men. *Br J Vener Dis* 53:184–185, 1977.

85. Quinn T, Goodell S, Mkrtichian E, et al: *Chlamydia trachomatis* proctitis. *N Engl J Med.* 305:1984–2000, 1981.

86. Schachter J: Confirmatory serodiagnosis of lymphogranuloma venereum proctitis may yield false-positive results due to other chlamydial infections of the rectum. *Sex Transm Dis* 8:26–28, 1981.

87. McMillan A, Sommerville RD, McKie PMK: Chlamydial infection in homosexual men: Frequency of isolation of *Chlamydia trachomatis* from the urethra, ano-rectum and pharynx. *Br J Vener Dis* 57:47–49, 1981.

88. Sulaiman MZC, Foster J, Pugh SF: Prevalence of *Chlamydia trachomatis* infection in homosexual men. *Genitourin Med* 63:179–181, 1987.

89. Munday PE, Cardfer JM, Taylor-Robinson D: Chlamydial proctitis? *Genitourin Med* 61:376–378, 1985.

90. Levine JS, Smith PD, Brugge WR: Chronic proctitis in male homosexuals due to lymphogranuloma venereum. *Gastroenterology* 79:563–565, 1980.

91. Bolan RK, Sands M, Schachter J, et al: Lymphogranuloma venereum and acute ulcerative proctitis. *Am J Med* 72:703–706, 1982.

92. Annamuthodo H: Rectal lymphogranuloma venereum in Jamaica. *Dis Colon Rectum* 4:17–26, 1981.

93. Abrams AJ: Lymphogranuloma venereum. *JAMA* 205:199–202, 1968.

94. Stamm WE: Proctitis due to *Chlamydia trachomatis,* in Ma P, Armstrong D (eds): *The Acquired Immunodeficiency Syndrome and Infections of Homosexual Men.* New York, Yorke Medical Books, 1984, pp. 40–47.

95. Levin I, Romano S, Steinberg M, et al: Lymphogranuloma venereum: Rectal stricture and carcinoma. *Dis Colon Rectum* 7:129–134, 1964.

96. Rompalo AM, Price CB, Roberts PL, et al: Potential value of rectal screening culture for *Chlamydia trachomatis* in homosexual men. *J Infect Dis* 153:888–892, 1986.

97. Rompalo AM, Roberts P, Johnson K, et al: Empirical therapy for the management of acute proctitis in homosexual men. *JAMA* 260:348–353, 1988.

98. Schachter J, Atwood G: Chlamydial pharyngitis? *J Am Vener Dis Assoc* 2:12, 1975.

99. Bowie WR, Alexander ER, Holmes KK: Chlamydial pharyngitis? *Sex Transm Dis* 4:140–141, 1977.

100. Komaroff AL, Aronson MD, Pass TM, et al: Serologic evidence of chlamydial and mycoplasmal pharyngitis in adults. *Science* 222:927–929, 1983.

101. Sweet RL, Gibbs RS: *Infectious Diseases of the Female Genital Tract.* Baltimore, Williams & Williams, 1985, p. 109.

102. Chacks MR, Lovchik JC: *Chlamydia trachomatis* infections in sexually active adolescents: Prevalence and risk factors. *Pediatrics* 73:838–840, 1984.

103. Kinghorn GR, Waugh MA: Oral contraceptives use and prevalence of infection with *Chlamydia trachomatis* in women. *Br J Vener Dis* 57:187–190, 1981.

104. Oriel JD, Powis PA, Reeve P, et al: Chlamydial infections of the cervix. *Br J Vener Dis* 50:11–16, 1974.

105. Oriel JD, Johnson AL, Barlow D, et al: Infection of the uterine cervix with *Chlamydia trachomatis. J Infect Dis* 137:443–451, 1978.

106. Handsfield HH, Jasman LL, Roberts PL, et al: Criteria for selective screening for *Chlamydia trachomatis* infection in women attending family planning clinics. *JAMA* 255:1730–1734, 1986.

107. Alexander ER, Chandler J, Pheifer TA, et al: Prospective study of perinatal *Chlamydia trachomatis* infection, in Hobson D, Holmes KK (eds): *Nongonococcal Urethritis and Related Disorders.* Washington DC, America Society for Microbiology, 1977, p. 148.

108. Wiesner PJ, Thompson SE, Dratman DP: Confusing correlates of chlamydial infection. *JAMA* 247:1606–1607, 1982.

109. Thompson SE, Dretler RH: Epidemiology and treatment of chlamydial infections in pregnant women and infants. *Rev Infect Dis* 4 (Suppl):5747–5757, 1982.

110. Paavonen J, Meyer B, Vesterinen E, et al: Colposcopic and histologic findings in cervical chlamydial infection. *Lancet* 2:320, 1980.

111. Schachter J, Hill EC, King E, et al: *Chlamydia trachomatis* and cervical neoplasia. *JAMA* 248:2134–2138, 1982.

112. Harrison RH, Alexander ER, Weinstein L, et al: Cervical *Chlamydia trachomatis* and mycoplasmal infections in pregnancy: Epidemiology and outcomes. *JAMA* 250:1721–1727, 1983.

113. Hardy PH, Hardy JB, Nell EE, et al: Prevalence of six sexually transmitted disease agents among pregnant inner-city adolescents and pregnancy outcome. *Lancet* 2:333–337, 1984.

114. Martin DH, Pastorck JG, Faro S: Risk factors for *Chlamydia trachomatis* infection in a high risk population of pregnant women in chlamydial infections, in Oriel D, Ridgway G, Schachter J, Taylor-Robinson D, Ward M (eds): *Proceedings of the 6th International*

Symposium on Human Chlamydial Infections. Cambridge, Cambridge University Press, 189–192, 1986.

115. Schachter J, Grossman M, Sweet RL, et al: Prospective study of perinatal transmission of *Chlamydia trachomatis. JAMA* 255:3374–3377, 1986.

116. Pastorek JG, Mroczkowski TF, Martin DH: Fine-tuning the fluorescent antibody test for chlamydial infections in pregnancy. *Obstet Gynecol* 72:957–960, 1988.

117. Martin DH, Koutsky L, Eschenbach DA, et al: Prematurity and perinatal mortality in pregnancies complicated by antepartum maternal *Chlamydia trachomatis* infections. *JAMA* 247:1585–1588, 1982.

118. Gravett MG, Nelson HP, DeRouen T, et al: Independent association of bacterial vaginosis and *Chlamydia trachomatis* infection with adverse pregnancy outcome. *JAMA* 256:1899–1903, 1986.

119. Rees E, Tart IA, Hobson D, et al: Chlamydia in relation to cervical infection and pelvic inflammatory disease, in Holmes KK, Hobson D (eds): *Nongonococcal Urethritis and Related Infections.* Washington DC, American Society for Microbiology, 1977, pp. 67–76.

120. Dunlop EMC, Harper IA, Al-Hussaini MK, et al: Relation of TRIC agent to "nonspecific" genital infection. *Br J Vener Dis* 42:77–87, 1966.

121. Paavonen J: Chlamydial infections: Microbiological, clinical and diagnostic aspects. *Med Biol* 57:135–151, 1979.

122. Brunham RC, Paavonen J, Stevens CE, et al: Mucopurulent cervicitis—The ignored counterpart in women of urethritis in men. *N Engl J Med* 311:1–6, 1984.

123. Mucopurulent cervicitis STD treatment guidelines. *MMWR* 34(4S):1035–1045, 1985.

124. Mardh P-A, Moller BR, Ingerselv HJ, et al: Endometritis caused by *Chlamydia trachomatis. Br J Vener Dis* 57:191–195, 1981.

125. Tomioka ES, Anzai RY, Kwang WN, et al: Endometrial damage in acute salpingitis. *Sex Transm Dis* 14:63–68, 1987.

126. Gump DW, Dickstein S, Gibson M: Endometritis related to *Chlamydia trachomatis* infection. *Ann Intern Med* 95:61–63, 1981.

127. Jones RB, Mammel JB, Shepard MK, et al: Recovery of *Chlamydia trachomatis* from the endometrium of women at a risk for chlamydial infection. *Am J Obstet Gynecol* 155:35–39, 1986.

128. Paavonen J, Kiviat N, Brunham RC, et al: Prevalence and manifestations of endometritis among women with cervicitis. *Am J Obstet Gynecol* 152:280–286, 1985.

129. Sweet RL, Schachter J, Robbie MO: Acute salpingitis: Role of *Chlamydia trachomatis* in the U.S., in Mardh P-A, Holmes KK, Oriel JD, et al. (eds): *Chlamydial Infections.* Amsterdam, Elsevier Biomedical Press, 1982, p. 175.

130. Sweet RL, Schachter J, Robbie MO: Failure of β-lactam antibiotics to eradicate *Chlamydia trachomatis* in the endometrium despite apparent clinical cure of acute salpingitis. *JAMA* 250:2641–2645, 1983.

131. Lamey JR, Eschenbach DA, Mitchell SH, et al: Isolation of mycoplasmas and bacteria from blood of postpartum women. *Am J Obstet Gynecol* 143:104–112, 1982.

132. Hoyme UB, Kiviat N, Eschenbach DA: Microbiology and treatment of late postpartum endometritis. *Obstet Gynecol* 68:226–232, 1986.

133. Wagner GP, Martin DH, Koutsky L, et al: Puerperal infections morbidity. Relationship to route of delivery and to antepartum *Chlamydia trachomatis* infection. *Am J Obstet Gynecol* 138:1028–1033, 1980.

134. Eschenbach DA, Wagner GP: Puerperal infections. *Clin Obstet Gynecol* 23:1003–1037, 1980.

135. Cytryn A, Sen P, Chung HR, et al: Severe pelvic infection from *Chlamydia trachomatis* after cesarean section. *JAMA* 247:1732–1734, 1982.

136. Thompson SE, Lopez B, Wang KH: A prospective study of chlamydia and mycoplasmal infections during pregnancy, in Mardh P-A, Holmes KK, Oriel JD, Piot P, Schachter J (eds): *Chlamydial Infections.* Amsterdam, Elsevier, vol. 2, 1982, pp. 155–158.

137. Harrison HR, Alexander ER, Weinstein L, et al: Cervical *Chlamydia trachomatis* and mycoplasmal infections in pregnancy: Epidemiology and outcomes. *JAMA* 250:1721–1727, 1983.

138. Sweet RL, Landers DV, Walker CH, et al: *Chlamydia trachomatis* infection and pregnancy outcome. *Am J Obstet Gynecol* 156:824–833, 1987.

139. Schuch RJ, Musich JR, Nelson RL: Chlamydial proctitis—Unusual presentation as a symptomatic vaginal mass. *Obstet Gynecol* 63:132–134, 1984.

140. Greenberg RN, Rein MF, Sander CV, et al: Urethral syndrome in women. *JAMA* 245:1106–1109, 1981.

141. Stamm WE, Running K, Hale J, et al: Etiologic role of *Mycoplasma hominis* and *Ureaplasma urealyticum* in women with the acute urethral syndrome. *Sex Transm Dis* 10:318–322, 1983.

142. Komaroff DL, Pass TM, McCue JD, et al: Management strategies for urinary and vaginal infections. *Arch Intern Med* 138:1069–1073, 1978.

143. Wiesner PJ: Gonorrhoea. *Cutis* 27:249–254, 1981.

144. Curran JW: Gonorrhoea and the urethral syndrome. *Sex Transm Dis* 4:119–121, 1977.

145. Paavonen J: *C. trachomatis* induced urethritis in female partners of men with nongonococcal urethritis. *Sex Transm Dis* 6:69–71, 1979.

146. Stamm WE: Etiology and management of the acute urethral syndrome. *Sex Transm Dis* 8:235–238, 1981.

147. Woolfitt JMG, Watt L: Chlamydial infection of the urogenital tract in promiscuous and non-promiscuous women. *Br J Vener Dis* 53:93–95, 1977.

148. Stamm WE, Wagner KF, Amsel R, et al: Causes of the acute urethral syndrome in women. *N Engl J Med* 303:409–415, 1980.

149. Stamm WE, Running K, McKevitt M, et al: Treatment of the acute urethral syndrome. *N Engl J Med* 304:956–958, 1981.

150. Feldman RG, Johnson AL, Schober PC, et al: An etiology of urinary symptoms in sexually active women. *Genitourin Med* 62:333–341, 1986.

151. Maskell R, Pead L, Pead PJ, et al: Chlamydial infection and urinary symptoms. *Br J Vener Dis* 60:65, 1984.

152. Barbalias GA, Meares EM: Female urethral syndrome: Clinical and urodynamic perspectives. *Urology* 23:208–212, 1984.

153. O'Dowd TC, Smail JE, West RR: Clinical judgment in the diagnosis and management of frequency and dysuria in general practice. *Br Med J* 288:1347–1349, 1984.

154. Schachter J, Holt J, Goodner E, et al: Prospective study of chlamydial infection in neonates. *Lancet* 2:377–380, 1979.

155. Schachter J, Grossman M, Sweet RL, et al: Prospective study of perinatal transmission of *Chlamydia trachomatis*. *JAMA* 255:3374–3377, 1986.

156. Barry WC, Teare EL, Uttley AHC, et al: Lim KS, Gamsu H, Price JF: *Chlamydia trachomatis* as a cause of neonatal conjunctivitis. *Arch Dis Child* 61:797–799, 1986.

157. Schaefer C, Harrison HR, Boyce WT, et al: Illnesses in infants born to women with *Chlamydia trachomatis* infections. *Am J Dis Child* 139:127–133, 1985.

2

GONORRHEA

Gonorrhea is a common sexually transmitted disease caused by gram-negative diplococci, *Neisseria gonorrhoeae*. The primary sites of infection are the genitals, rectum, and oropharynx directly involved in sexual activity. Nongenital tract disease results from direct, contiguous, or hematogenic spread. Newborns may acquire infection from their mothers during passage through the infected birth canal.

EPIDEMIOLOGY

In the United States and Europe, gonorrhea is the most frequently reported communicable disease. Nearly 1 million cases are reported in the United States, whereas the number of unreported cases of gonorrhea probably equals or exceeds the number reported.[1,2] The current epidemic began in 1957, and the number of reported cases increased steadily for both men and women from 1965 to 1975. Beginning in 1976, the number of cases and rates began to decline, with the tendency persisting into the 1980s[3] (Figure 2.1).

In the United Kingdom, after a steady rise for nearly 20 years, the number of cases of gonorrhea leveled in 1973 at 66,000 cases, and beginning from 1977, there was a steady decline.[4]

The incidence of gonorrhea in developing countries is not known because of incomplete reporting; however, according to some authors, the prevalence of gonococcal infection in some areas of Africa was estimated to be much higher than that of developed countries.[5,6] In Africa the disease is considered to be the major cause of infertility.

In the United States, 80 percent of reported cases occur in individuals between 15 and 29 years of age, with the heaviest concentration in the 20- to 24-year-old group. The male to female ratio is 1.5:1, but among young teenagers this trend is reversed in favor of female predominance.

The risk factors for the acquisition of gonorrhea include multiple sex partners, young age, race (gonorrhea is most prevalent among blacks), and socioeconomic

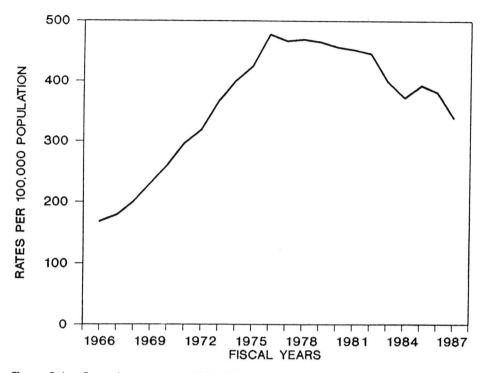

Figure 2.1. Gonorrhea rates per 100,000 population United States fiscal years 1966–1987. From STD Statistics 1987. No. 136. US DHHS, PHS. Centers for Disease Control.

status. However, the last two factors may reflect a skewing of the data because gonorrhea is most likely to be reported by STD clinics predominantly attended by nonwhites and poor people.[7]

Transmission of gonorrhea is almost entirely by sexual contact. The chance of an uninfected man acquiring an infection from an infected woman is 19 percent during a single episode. The risk increases significantly with the number of episodes to 57 percent after four or more exposures.[8] The risk of transmission from men to women is much higher and is estimated at 80 to 90 percent.[9,10]

Infection acquired from anorectal coitus, whether homosexual or heterosexual, as well as from oral intercourse is not uncommon. Anorectal gonorrhea in a male is almost always a result of passive anal intercourse. Gonococcal pharyngitis results from either fellatio or cunnilingus; however, the latter form of transmission of gonorrhea is less common.[11]

ETIOLOGY

Gonorrhea is caused by *Neisseria gonorrhoeae*, a gram-negative diplococcus naturally pathogenic only in men. *Neisseria gonorrhoeae* is a fastidious organism with specific nutrient and environmental needs. Its growth is optimal at pH 7.4 in a

2–10 percent carbon dioxide atmosphere at a temperature of 35°C. On solid media, *N. gonorrhoeae* grows as four morphologically distinct types of colonies, which correlates with infectivity.[12,13] Of the four types of colonies, types 1 and 2, which contain pili, are more virulent to man. Pili appear to be involved in the adhesion of gonococci to epithelial cells[14,15] and play a role in the ingestion process of gonococci by polymorphonuclear leukocytes.[16,17] Pili are involved in genetic aspects of the organism, and it was found that piliated gonococci have much higher levels of competence for transformation than nonpiliated variants.[18] They are also immunogenic, capable of inducing production of specific antibodies.[19,20]

Neisseria gonorrhoeae may be subdivided by means of auxotyping based on the pattern of growth requirement for various amino acids and nucleic acid bases.[21] It is important for a clinician to note that, among the many types that have been identified, one auxotype that requires arginine, hypoxanthine, and uracil (AHU) and is also highly susceptible to penicillin has been associated with 89 percent of the cases with disseminated gonococcal infection presenting in Seattle.[22] Auxotyping also contributed to epidemiologic studies, since the prevalence of certain auxotypes varies among geographic regions.[23] Serologic methods based on the antigenic determinants of protein 1A or 1B have been used to differentiate further between gonococcal strains.[24,25] This classification is carried out using coagglutination techniques and permits the classification of strains of *N. gonorrhoeae* into three serogroups called WI, WII, and WIII. As a further step, monoclonal antibodies against *N. gonorrhoeae* have been developed to facilitate subdivision within the three serogroups into serovars.[26] Serotyping is also possible using enzyme-linked immunosorbent assay (ELISA).[27] This short description elucidates tremendous heterogenicity among gonococci.

Since the introduction of penicillin for the treatment of infections caused by gonococci, their susceptibility to penicillin and other antibiotics has changed a great deal. There are at least two mechanisms of resistance to penicillin that gonococci have developed. The first mechanism is chromosomally mediated, and the second results from β-lactamase production by *N. gonorrhoeae*. Constantly increasing numbers of chromosomally mediated, resistant strains of *N. gonorrhoeae* (CMRNG) in the late 1960s and early 1970s prompted medical authorities in many countries to raise the single dose of procaine penicillin G from 2.4 million units to the currently recommended dose of 4.8 million units, with a concomitant 1.0 g of probenecid. Even though this regimen has been successfully used for many years, reports of CMRNG resistant to this dose[28,29] as well as an increasing number of β-lactamase-producing gonococci, in addition to other factors (e.g., procaine reaction), have caused penicillin to gradually lose its privileged role in the treatment of gonorrhoea.

In 1976, the first penicillinase-producing strains of *N. gonorrhoeae* (PPNG) were reported in the United States and England. They were isolated from patients who had become infected in Southeast Asia and Africa respectively.[30,31] Since then, the number of cases of gonorrhea caused by PPNG has significantly increased throughout the world. The prevalence of PPNG depends on the geographic region and the population studied. The prevalence of PPNG among prostitutes in the Philippines and Singapore was 30–40 percent and 19 percent, respectively, and the prevalence was 29 and 20 percent among men with gonococcal urethritis in Thailand, and Nigeria.[32-34] In the United Kingdom, Canada, and the United States, the overall prevalence of PPNG is less than 1 percent, although in some areas of the United Kingdom, the prevalence in early 1981 reached 5 percent.[34,35] In the United States, PPNG strains have been reported from at least 43 states, with the majority of cases reported from Florida, California, and New York.[36] PPNG strains produce TEM-1 type β-lactamase, which is coded on plasmids of 3.2 or 4.4 megadaltons (MDa).[37] These strains are believed to have originated in Southeast Asia and Africa as two separate but related clones. Asian strains carried a 4.4 MDa penicillinase-encoding plasmid with or without a 24.5 MDa plasmid coded for conjugation. Those strains required proline or were prototropic and were resistant to antibiotics such as tetracycline. African-type strains that carried a 3.2 MDa penicillinase-coding plasmid (some may contain a 24.5 MDa plasmid as well) required arginine for growth and were more sensitive to antibiotics. A majority of PPNG isolates from the United States and also from the Netherlands contain the Asian type of plasmid, while the majority of isolates from the United Kingdom have the African type.[38] Since detection of PPNG strains and the identification of β-lactamase-encoding plasmids, new plasmids different in size from the Asian and African types recently have been identified.[39,40]

Constantly improving techniques, especially those based on molecular genetics and modern serology, have gradually opened new horizons in the bacteriology and epidemiology of gonococcal infection. They have made possible not only the identification of new combinations of auxotypes, plasmids and serovars, but also have permitted the study and analysis of temporal changes in the gonococcal population. As a result of these advances it has also been possible to follow the migrations of gonococci between different geographical areas.[41-45] The gonococcus is no longer the same organism as originally described, and despite the tremendous amount of knowledge accumulated about it there still remains much more to learn.

PATHOLOGY

Gonococci have a predilection for columnar epithelium which is readily available after bacteria have gained entrance at any of the body's orifices, such as the urethra, endocervix, rectum, pharynx, or conjuctiva. Both transitional and stratified squamous epithelia are more resistant to gonococcal invasion. The gonococci, presumably with the help of pili and perhaps some proteins, attach themselves to the epithelial cells and to the secretory surface of the mucous cells.[44,46,47] This attachment prevents them from being dislodged by urine flow or mucous secretions. Some of them become embedded within the epithelial cells. The infection produces a marked polymorphonuclear response, which along with partial destruction of the epithelium, results in purulent discharge.

From the port of entry, the infection can spread to the other structures lined with columnar epithelia, such as Littré's and Cowper's glands, the prostate, the seminal vesicles and epididymis in men and Skene's and Bartholin's glands and the fallopian tubes in women. Infections of the bladder, preputial sac, vulva, and vagina (except in prepubertal girls) are extremely rare.

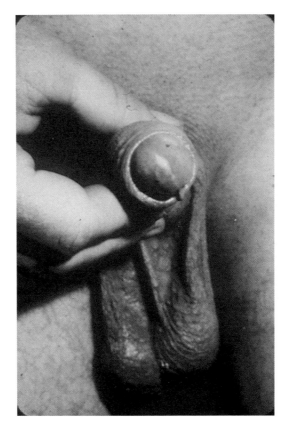

Figure 2.2. Spontaneous urethral discharge (purulent) in men with gonorrhea.

CLINICAL MANIFESTATION IN ADULTS

Uncomplicated Infection in Men

Gonococcal Urethritis

In most cases of gonococcal urethritis, the incubation period is 2 to 5 days, with a range of 36 hours to 14 days. The earliest symptom is usually irritation at the urinary meatus, followed by burning or stinging when passing urine and urethral discharge, which in typical cases is purulent, yellow to green in color, and profuse (Figure 2.2). In some cases, the discharge may be mucoid or mucopurulent, but this kind of exudate is more characteristic of nongonococcal urethritis. The amount of discharge may depend on the time interval since the patient last passed urine and is usually more profuse the longer the interval since the last voiding. (Examination of an uncircumcised patient requires retraction of the foreskin to distinguish sub-preputial discharge from that coming from the urethra.) The lips of urinary meatus may be reddened and swollen (meatitis). The patient may also notice stains on his underwear. Occasionally, inguinal lymph nodes may be slightly enlarged and tender.

If the infection has reached the posterior urethra, the patient may complain of increasing dysuria, frequent micturition, and strangury. Rarely there may be a few drops of blood at the end of micturition, but considerable hematuria is even less common.

Gonococcal urethritis in males may be asymptomatic. The accurate incidence of asymptomatic gonococcal infection among sexually active men is difficult to establish and is probably somewhere between 1.5 and 5 percent.[48,49] However, in selected groups (such as among sex partners of women with symptomatic gonorrhea), the prevalence of asymptomatic infection may be as high as 40 percent.[48] Asymptomatic men are more important in epidemiologic terms because those with symptoms usually seek treatment while those who are asymptomatic usually do not and may proceed to infect others.

Uncomplicated Infection in Women

The incubation period of gonorrhea infection in women is not well defined, and it is believed that the average range is between 7 and 14 days. Uncomplicated gonorrhea in women involves primarily the endocervix, but the anus, urethra, and, to a lesser extent, Skene's and Bartholin's glands may be involved as well. Asymptomatic endocervical infection is common; however, symptomatic infection occurs more frequently than is commonly appreciated.[50,51] Probably 40 to 60 percent of women who have gonorrhea develop some symptoms.[50] As a result of cervicitis, there may be an increase in vaginal discharge, and infection of the urethra is followed by dysuria, and frequent micturition. Some women may complain of abnormal uterine bleeding, lower abdominal or pelvic pain, and occasionally, of low backache.

On examination, the cervix is congested and enlarged in about half of the cases. Purulent or mucopurulent discharge may be seen exuding from the endocervix. Other abnormalities include cervical edema, erythema, and friability. In case of urethral infection, the meatus may be reddened, and pouting and pus may be expressed on massaging the urethra. Pus exudate may be seen at the orifices of the paraurethral ducts if Skene's glands are infected. Bartholin's duct involvement is common but often asymptomatic. Occasionally, the duct orifice may be inflamed, and a bead of pus may be visible. Physical examination of an adult female for genital gonorrhea should include a bimanual pelvic examination. If adnexal and lower abdominal tenderness is found, the clinician must consider the possibility of pelvic inflammatory disease (PID).

Extragenital Gonorrhea

Anorectal Gonococcal Infection

Anorectal gonorrhea is common in women and homosexual men. About 30–60 percent of women with endocervical gonorrhea may have positive rectal cultures[52-54] usually, but not always, as a result of secondary contamination with cervicovaginal discharge. Involvement of only the anorectum occurs in about 2–9 percent of infected women.[55,56] Gonococcal proctitis in males nearly always results from passive homosexual anal intercourse.[56,57] The disease rarely, if ever, occurs in men who are strictly heterosexual. Secondary infection of the rectum is very rare and may result from rupture of the prostatic abscess or Cowper's gland. In both sexes, accidental infection by contaminated fingers, rubber gloves, thermometers, or other instruments is possible, but extremely rare.

There are minimal differences in the symptoms between men and women, except in the percentage of asymptomatic cases, which account for 18–34 percent of rectal infections among men.[58,59] Although anorectal gonorrhea can produce a severe proctitis, many patients have either no symptoms or minimal symptoms, and the evidence of infection is found on routine examination or culture. In a few cases, the onset of proctitis may be acute, with a rapid change in bowel habits; there may be complaints of burning pain in the anorectum, tenesmus, and mucoid, purulent, or blood-stained discharge. Rectal itching and a feeling of pressure and fullness are also common sensations. There may be blood or mucus, or both, in the stool. In other cases, the onset may be less acute, with symptoms and signs that are less specific. Patients may complain of anal irritation, moisture around the anus, and the presence of mucus in the stool. In acute cases, anoscopic examination reveals an inflamed and edematous rectal wall which bleeds easily. Pus or mucopus may be seen on the surface of the rectum. Ulcerations are rare. In less acute cases, rectal mucosa may look normal, or there may be a minor degree of congestion with or without streaks of mucopus on the rectal wall and in the columns of Morgani. The differential diagnosis of rectal infection is more important for homosexual men than for women. Proctitis among homosexuals is quite common, and a number of sexually transmitted pathogens have been implicated as the cause, including *Chlamydia trachomatis, Herpes virus simplex, Shigella, Giardia lamblia,* and *Entamoeba histolytica.*[60,61] The same agents may, of course, produce proctitis in women, but this is very rare.

Pharyngeal Gonococcal Infection

Pharyngeal infection with *N. gonorrhoeae* occurs predominantly in homosexual men and women practicing fellatio.[62,63] The mode of infection is orogenital contact, with fellatio being the common mean of transmission.[63,64] The infection can be acquired by cunnilingus,[65] albeit rarely. Mouth-to-mouth transmission seems to be unlikely; however, *N. gonorrhoeae* was isolated from the saliva of 67 percent of patients with oropharyngeal gonorrhea.[66] The problem as to whether gonorrhea can be acquired by ordinary kissing has not been solved as yet.[67]

Among patients presenting with gonorrhea in STD clinics in the United States, the frequency of pharyngeal infection was 3.2 percent among heterosexual men, 10.3 percent among women, and 20.9 percent among homosexual men.[62] Other investigators have reported higher and lower rates depending on the populations studied.[68-70]

Gonococcal infection of the pharynx is often asymptomatic, although an acute exudative pharyngitis or tonsillitis with sore throat, pyrexia, and cervical lymphadenopathy may occur. In the majority of cases, however, the symptoms have been slight or almost absent. There seems to be no characteristic features of pharyngeal gonorrhea, and the symptoms of pharyngitis correlate better with fellatio than with gonococcal infection of the pharynx.[62] The real significance of pharyngeal gonococcal infection is unclear; however, several serious conditions have been ascribed prior to pharyngeal colonization with *N. gonorrhoeae*. These include disseminated gonococcal infection (DGI) and gonococcal meningitis.[62,71,72] Diagnosis of pharyngeal gonorrhea may create certain problems, since the Gram's-stained smear is useless and cultures on selective media are insufficient. The microorganism has to be differentiated from other *Neisseria* commonly present in the oropharynx: *N. meningitidis* and *N. lactamica*. The sugar fermentation test or immunofluorescence or coagglutination methods are necessary to confirm the presence of gonococci in the pharynx.

Adult Gonococcal Conjunctivitis

Gonococcal conjunctivitis, or ophthalmia, is primarily an infection of newborns but may rarely occur in adults or children.[73] The infection mainly results from a lack of hygiene and frequently is caused by direct contamination of the eye with gonococci by fingers or towels. The source of infection may be the patient's own genital secretion, or it may be transferred from a sexual partner or, rarely, from another member of the household with the symptomatic disease.

The symptoms and signs may be mild to severe and include purulent discharge, redness of the conjunctiva, and edema of the eyelids, accompanied by photophobia (Figure 2.3). The infection is unilateral in two thirds of cases.

If the disease is recognized and treated promptly, patients recover within a couple of days without any sequelae. In untreated cases, a gonococcal conjunctivitis may proceed to involve the cornea, with subsequent damage to sight.

Adults with gonococcal ophthalmia should be hospitalized for parenteral therapy because of the potential complication of blindness (see Treatment of Uncomplicated Gonorrhea).

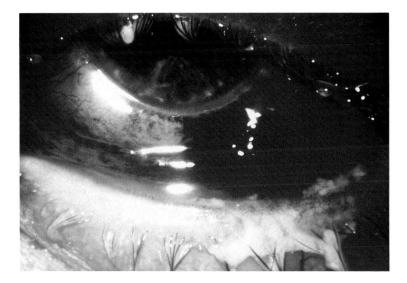

Figure 2.3. Gonococcal ophthalmia with hyperemic conjunctiva and purulent discharge.

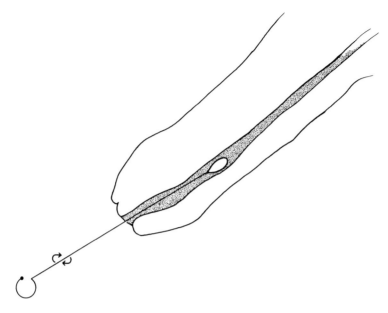

Figure 2.4.   Insert a sterile urethral swab or wire loop about 3 cm into the anterior urethra. Gently rotate the swab or scrape the mucosa with the wire loop to obtain an adequate specimen.

DIAGNOSIS

In all forms of gonococcal infection, diagnosis depends on identification or isolation of *N. gonorrhoeae*. However, the accuracy of diagnosis depends a great deal on the quality of the specimen.

Sampling Techniques

Urethral Specimen

A urethral specimen either in men or women can be obtained by means of urethral swabs or a sterile wire loop (Figure 2.4). In men the swab or loop should be inserted about 3 cm into the anterior urethra. The specimen should be collected by gently rotating the swab or scraping the mucosa with the wire loop. The male patient may be asked to press the urethra or to "milk" it forward prior to specimen collection. In asymptomatic cases or where exudate is minimal, it is necessary to strip the urethra toward the orifice in order to obtain a maximum amount of the exudate. In order to obtain a urethral specimen in female patients, the examiner should insert the index finger into the vagina and massage the urethra from below anteriorly toward the urinary meatus (Figure 2.5). Next, a urethral swab is inserted 2 to 3 cm and gently rotated to obtain an adequate specimen (Figure 2.6). The specimen should be immediately rolled on the glass slide (for Gram's staining) or streaked on selective medium (Thayer-Martin medium).

Urine specimens from males yield positive results comparable to urethral cultures,[74] but this method has been used mainly for research purposes.

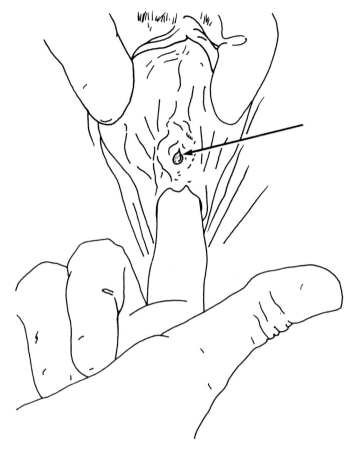

Figure 2.5. A small bead of pus can be expressed after gentle massage of the urethra through the vaginal wall.

Endocervical Specimen

An endocervical specimen may be obtained at any point in the menstrual cycle and should not be delayed because the patient is menstruating. The speculum used to expose the cervix should be moistened with water only. Lubricants are to be avoided, since they may contain antibacterial substances. Some investigators recommend removing the mucous covering the cervical orifice or cleaning vaginal contamination from the cervix prior to insertion of the swab. The sterile cotton-tipped swab should be inserted into the endocervical canal and gently rotated for about 10 seconds to allow absorption of the endocervical exudate into the cotton (Figure 2.7). In pregnant women, the cervical os rather than the endocervix should be sampled. The specimen should be inoculated immediately on selective medium or applied on a glass slide for Gram's staining. The sensitivity of Gram-stained endocervical specimens has been questioned because of many false negative and false positive results. However, in my opinion, when the examination is performed by experienced personnel, the method is quite reliable.

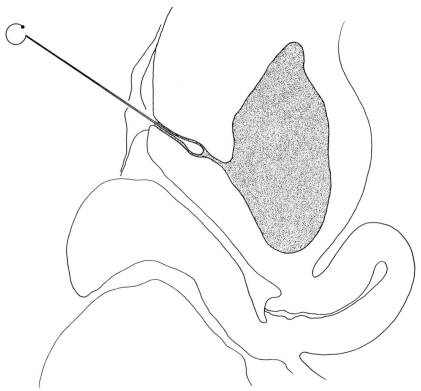

Figure 2.6. Insert a sterile urethral swab or wire loop about 2–3 cm into the urethra and gently rotate the swab or scrape with the wire loop to obtain an adequate specimen.

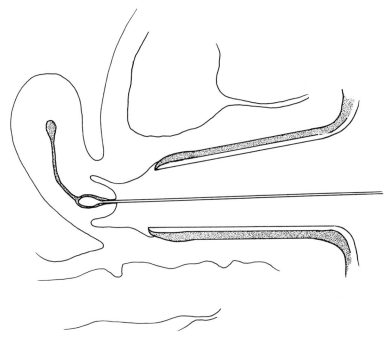

Figure 2.7. Insert a sterile cotton-tipped swab into the endocervical canal and rotate it slowly for about 10 seconds to allow absorption of the organism onto the swab.

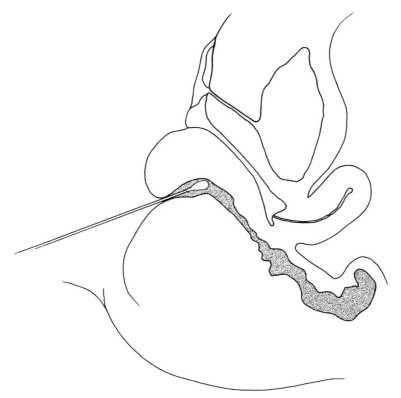

Figure 2.8.   Insert a sterile, cotton-tipped swab approximately 2–3 cm into the anal canal and keep it there for about 20 seconds to absorb the organisms. Slowly move the swab from side to side to contact the crypts, avoiding heavy fecal contamination.

Anorectal Specimen

An anorectal specimen should be obtained by inserting a sterile cotton swab approximately 2 to 3 cm into the anus (Figure 2.8). The swab should be slowly rotated to contact the cryps, kept in the anal canal for about 20 seconds to absorb enough material, and inoculated on selective media. The Gram-stained specimens are not recommended, and although many may reveal gonococci, their sensitivity and specificity are low.

Pharyngeal Specimen

Pharyngeal specimens are obtained with sterile cotton-tipped swabs applied vigorously on the posterior pharyngeal wall and the tonsillar crypts (Figure 2.9). The specimens should be inoculated on the selective media, but later the microorganism must be differentiated from other *Neisseria* that might be present in the oropharynx. Gram-stained smears are useless.

Conjunctival Specimens

Conjunctival specimens should be obtained before the application of any topical anesthetics or chemotherapeutic drops that may diminish the bacterial in-

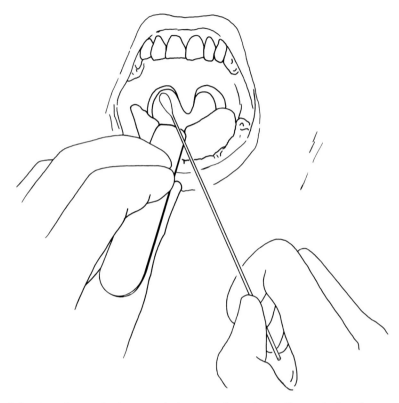

Figure 2.9. In order to obtain a good pharyngeal specimen, the posterior pharyngeal wall as well as the tonsillar crypts are swabbed vigorously.

oculum. A moistened, cotton-tipped application (moist swabs yield a greater percentage of positive cultures than dry swabs) is used to swab the inferior and superior tarsal conjunctiva (Figure 2.10).

Laboratory Diagnosis

Direct Staining

Methylene blue stain is the most rapid method of identification of gonococci. In this stain, bacteria are uniformly blue, and gonococci as well as other flora may look similar. This method is best used only in cases with typical (purulent discharge) gonorrhea and situations in which other methods cannot be applied.

Gram's stain has the value of differentiation between gram-negative and gram-positive bacteria and is the most widely accepted staining technique used to diagnose gonococcal infection. The diagnosis is made by finding gram-negative diplococci of typical uniform shape within polymorphonuclear leukocytes (Figures 2.11 and 2.12). In men, this is diagnostic of gonorrhea. In women, the normal flora, which includes gram-negative species, can be the cause of false positive results. Moreover, staphylococci, which have been ingested by polymorphonuclear

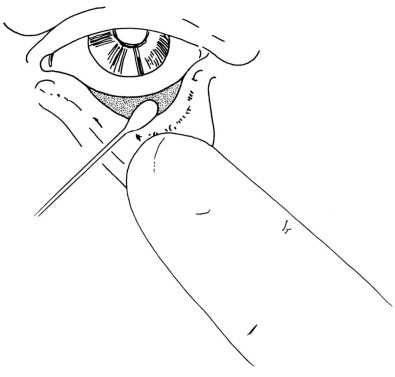

Figure 2.10. A conjunctival specimen is obtained by swabbing both the inferior and superior tarsal conjunctiva.

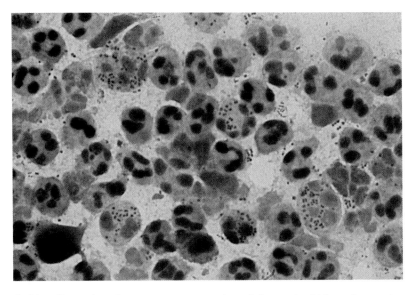

Figure 2.11. Gonorrhea in men: gram-negative diplococci within polymorphonuclear leukocytes.

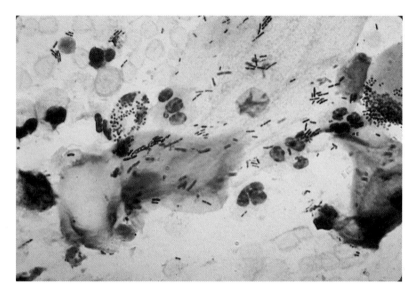

Figure 2.12. Gonorrhea in women: gram-negative diplococci within polymorphonuclear leukocytes.

leukocytes, may lose their gram-positive nature and be the cause of confusion. In case of any uncertainty, a culture should be performed.

Direct fluorescent antibody staining in the diagnosis of gonorrhea is dependent on the specificity of the antisera. Antisera against *N. gonorrhoeae* may cross-react with other *Neisseria* species and have been reported to be negative for some of PPNG strains.[75,76] The method requires the use of a fluorescent microscope and a dark room. The use of this technique is not routine.

Routine Culture Media

Since clinical specimens for the diagnosis of gonorrhea are taken from anatomical sites with abundant normal flora which can easily overgrow gonococci, *N. gonorrhoeae* is best cultured on selective media. For optimal results, specimens should be placed on *both* selective and nonselective media. The most widely used selective medium for the culture of gonococci is the modified Thayer-Martin medium.

All of selective media contain ingredients capable of inhibiting the growth of other bacteria as well as molds and yeasts. However, none of them are perfect: some gonococci may be inhibited by vancomycin, some normal flora may grow, or proteus may overgrow the gonococci.

Transport Media

For clinics or hospitals without a bacteriological service, several media have been developed which enable transportation or transportation and growth of gonococci. The most popular nutrient growth/transport systems are Transgrow and JEMBEC, plus a dozen others. These media perform reasonably well when compared with the use of selective media incubated in a candle jar. Depending on the system, their sensitivity is reported as between 85 and 90 percent.[77]

Gonococci grow the best in a 3–10 percent CO_2 atmosphere and a temperature of 35–37°C. Presumptive identification can be based on colony morphology, Gram's staining, and the oxidase reaction. After 24–48 hours of incubation, the typical colony is small (less than 1 mm in diameter), round, whitish gray, opaque, and glistening.

Gonococci are oxidase positive. After application of the oxidase reagent (1% tetramethyl-*p*-phenylenediamine HCl), gonococcal colonies turn a pink color, which rapidly deepens to purple. Oxidase-positive colonies should be Gram's stained, and the typical kidney bean–shaped gram-negative bacteria should be seen.

Presumptive identification is usually satisfactory in anogenital gonorrhea, but for the specimens obtained from sites where other *Neisseria* may occur, further identification is necessary.

Sugar Fermentation Test

Several methods to test sugar fermentation have been developed and are commercially available: CTA, Columbia agar, Minitek, BACTEC, and NeIDENT. The test sugars include glucose, maltose, fructose, sucrose, and lactose. Gonococci react only with glucose, whereas other members of *Neisseria* produce different fermentation patterns (Table 2.1). The sugar fermentation test should be used to confirm all isolates obtained from sites other than the anus or genitals or in specimens obtained from children. It should be also performed when the diagnosis of gonorrhea is unlikely or when there are special, social, or medicolegal situations.

Coagglutination Method

This coagglutination method (Phadebact) is rapid and can be used on primary isolates. It makes use of the nonspecific I_gG binding by protein A found in the wall of *Staphylococcus aureus*.

TABLE 2.1. Differential characteristic of *Neisseria* spp. and *Branhamella catarrhalis* in sugar fermentation test

	Glucose	Maltose	Lactose	Fructose	Sucrose
N. gonorrhoeae	+	−	−	−	−
N. meningitidis	+	+	−	−	−
N. sicca	+	+	−	+	+
N. lactamica	+	+	+	−	−
Branhamella catarrhalis	−	−	−	−	−
N. subflava	+	+	−	V*	V*
N. mucosa	+	+	−	+	+
N. flavenscens	−	−	−	−	−

*V = fermentation variable.

Direct Fluorescent Antibody Staining

Direct fluorescent antibody staining is a good technique for the diagnosis of gonorrhea and has been described earlier (see Direct Staining, above).

Antigen Detection

The Gonozyme test (Abbott Laboratories) is a solid-phase enzyme immunoassay for detecting gonococcal antigens in urethral and endocervical specimens. The test requires multiple reagents and special equipment (a spectrophotometer). Its sensitivity and specificity vary, depending on the populations studied.[78,79]

Although the most reliable method for the diagnosis of *N. gonorrhoeae* remains culture, antigen detection techniques or methods based on the detection of gonococcal DNA,[80] will probably be the diagnostic approach in the near future.

Differential Diagnosis

Gonococcal Urethritis

Gonococcal urethritis in men should be distinguished from

- *Nongonococcal urethritis (NGU):* Although clinical manifestations of typical NGU are different from those of acute gonorrhea (see Table 1.4), culture on selective medium is necessary for exclusion of gonococcal urethritis. A positive test for *C. trachomatis, Ureaplasma urealyticum,* and *Trichomonas vaginalis* may help to establish diagnosis.
- *Urethritis caused by herpes simplex virus:* Vesicles or erosions are seen in the meatus, and there is a positive Tzanck or other test for HSV as well as a negative culture for *N. gonorrhoeae.* (Recurrences are frequent.)
- *Urethritis caused by intraurethral warts:* Warts may be present in the meatus and there is a negative culture for *N. gonorrhoeae.*
- *Trauma and urethritis caused by repeated ''stripping'' of the penis, a foreign body, or irritating chemicals:* History of trauma or insertion of foreign body or chemicals. There is also a negative culture for *N. gonorrhoeae.*
- *Venerophobia (psychiatric patient):* There is a negative white blood cell (WBC) count (mean number of WBC per field < 4), a negative Gram-stain smear, and a negative culture for *N. gonorrhoeae.*

Gonococcal Cervicitis

Endocervical gonococcal infection in women should be distinguished from

- *Mucopurulent cervicitis caused by C. trachomatis:* There is a postive culture or a positive direct immunofluorescence test for *C. trachomatis* and a negative culture for *N. gonorrhoeae.*
- *Genital herpes:* There is the presence of vesicles or erosions on the cervix or the skin of the vulva or vaginal mucosa, a positive Tzanck test or other test for HVS, and a negative culture for *N. gonorrhoeae.* (Recurrences are frequent).
- *Vaginitis/vulvovaginitis:* There is a negative culture for *N. gonorrhoeae* and a posi-

tive culture for *T. vaginalis, C. albicans, Gardnerella vaginalis*, anaerobes, or other pathogens.

- *Cervical cancer:* There is the characteristic clinical appearance of the cervix, with a positive pap smear.

Gonococcal Proctitis

Gonococcal proctitis should be distinguished from

- *Proctitis caused by other sexually transmitted pathogens* such as *C. trachomatis*, HSV, *Treponema pallidum:* There will be negative culture for *N. gonorrhoeae* and positive cultures for tested pathogens or positive syphilis serology test.
- *Proctitis due to enteric infections:* This is more common in homosexual men. There are positive tests for *Entamoeba histolytica, Giardia lamblia, Shigella, Salmonella* or other enteric pathogen and negative culture for *N. gonorrhoeae.*
- *Hemorrhoids:* There is the presence of varices and a history of bleeding and recurrences. There is also negative culture for *N. gonorrhoeae.*

Gonococcal pharyngitis

Gonococcal pharyngitis is clinically indistinguishable from pharyngitis due to other causes. There will be negative culture for *N. gonorrhoeae* and positive tests for streptococci or other pathogens.

TREATMENT OF UNCOMPLICATED GONORRHEA

Treatment recommendations for gonorrhea are being updated constantly according to the changing pattern of antimicrobial resistance and the development of new antimicrobials. The following recommendations are based on, or in many instances are an exact copy of, "Sexually Transmitted Disease Treatment Guidelines 1989," issued by the U.S. Department of Health and Human Services, Public Health Service, Centers for Disease Control, Atlanta, GA.

Uncomplicated Urethral, Endocervical, or Rectal Infections

General Considerations

Single-dose efficacy is a major consideration in choosing an antibiotic regimen to treat *N. gonorrhoeae.* Another important concern is coexisting chlamydial infection, documented in up to 45% of gonorrhea cases in some populations. Until universal testing for chlamydia with quick, inexpensive, and highly accurate tests becomes available, it is generally more cost effective to treat presumptive chlamydial infections in all persons with gonorrhea. Simultaneous treatment of all gonorrhea infections with antibiotics effective against both *C. trachomatis* and *N. gonorrhoeae* may lessen the possibility of the failure of gonorrhea treatment due to antibiotic resistance.

The recommended regimen is

Ceftriaxone, 250 mg IM once,*
Plus
Doxycycline, 100 mg orally 2 times a day for 7 days.

Alternative Regimens

For patients who cannot take ceftriaxone, the preferred alternative is *spectinomycin*, 2 g IM in a single dose (followed by doxycycline). Other alternatives, for which experience is less extensive, include *ciprofloxacin*,° 500 mg orally once; *norfloxacin*,° 800 mg orally once; *cefuroxime axetil*, 1 g orally once with *probenecid*, 1 g, *cefotaxime*, 1 g IM once; and *ceftizoxime*, 500 mg IM once. All of these regimens are followed by *doxycycline*, 100 mg orally twice daily for 7 days. If infection was acquired from a source proven not to have penicillin-resistant gonorrhea, a penicillin such as *amoxicillin*, 3 g orally, with *probenecid*, 1 g, followed by *doxycycline* may be used for treatment.

Tetracycline may be substituted for doxycycline; however, compliance may be worse since tetracycline must be taken at a dose of 500 mg 4 times a day. For patients who cannot take a tetracycline (e.g., pregnant women), erythromycin may be substituted (erythromycin base or stearate, 500 mg orally 4 times a day for 7 days, or erythromycin ethylsuccinate, 800 mg orally 4 times a day for 7 days).

Special Considerations

All patients diagnosed with gonorrhea should have a serologic test for syphilis and should be offered confidential counseling and testing for HIV infection. The majority of patients with incubating syphilis (those who are seronegative and have no clinical signs of syphilis) may be cured by any of the regimens containing β-lactams (e.g., ceftriaxone) or tetracyclines.

Spectinomycin and the quinolones (ciprofloxacin, norfloxacin) have not been shown to be active against incubating syphilis. Patients treated with these drugs should be followed with a serologic test for syphilis in 1 month. Patients with gonorrhea and documented syphilis and gonorrhea patients who are sex partners of syphilis patients should be treated for syphilis as outlined in Chapter 8 as well as for gonorrhea.

Management of Sex Partners

Persons exposed to gonorrhea within the preceding 30 days should be examined, cultured, and treated presumptively.

Follow-up

Treatment failure following combined ceftriaxone/doxycycline therapy is likely to be rare; therefore, a follow-up culture ("test-of-cure") is not essential.

---

*Some authorities prefer a dose of 125 mg ceftriaxone IM because it is less expensive and can be given in a volume of only 0.5 ml, which is more easily administered in the deltoid muscle. However, the 250 mg dose is recommended because it may delay the emergence of ceftriaxone-resistant strains. At this time, both doses appear highly effective for mucosal gonorrhea at all sites.

°Not recommended in pregnant women and children under 16 years of age.

According to CDC a more cost-effective strategy may be to reexamine with culture 1–2 months after treatment ("rescreening"). This approach should enable the detection of both treatment failures and reinfections. Patients should be advised to return for examination if any symptoms persist at the completion of treatment.

Treatment Failures

Persistent symptoms after treatment should be evaluated by culture for *N. gonorrhoeae*, and any gonococcal isolate should be tested for antibiotic sensitivity. Symptoms of urethritis may also be caused by *C. trachomatis* and other organisms associated with nongonococcal urethritis (see Nongonococcal Urethritis, p. 5). Additional treatment for gonorrhea should be ceftriaxone, 250 mg, followed by doxycycline. Infections occurring after treatment with one of the recommended regimens are commonly due to reinfection rather than treatment failure and indicate a need for improved sex-partner referral and patient education.

Treatment of Pharyngeal Gonococcal Infection

Patients with uncomplicated pharyngeal gonococcal infection should be treated with ceftriaxone, 250 mg IM once. Patients who cannot be treated with ceftriaxone should be treated with ciprofloxacin* 500 mg orally as a single dose. Since experience with this regimen is limited, such patients should be evaluated with repeat culture 3–7 days after treatment.

Treatment of Adult Gonococcal Ophthalmia

Adults and children over 20 kg with nonsepticemic gonococcal ophthalmia should be treated with ceftriaxone, 1 g IM once. Irrigation of the eyes with saline or buffered ophthalmic solutions may be useful adjunctive therapy to eliminate discharge. All patients must have careful ophthalmologic assessment including slit-lamp exam for ocular complications. Topical antibiotics alone are not sufficient therapy and are unnecessary when appropriate systemic therapy is given. Simultaneous ophthalmic infection with *C. trachomatis* has been reported and should be considered in patients who do not respond promptly.

COMPLICATIONS IN MEN

Epididymitis

Epididymitis is a common complication of gonococcal urethritis, especially in men under 35 years of age.[82,83] The pathogenesis of this complication is not clear, but it is believed to be the result of retrograde passage of infected urine from the urethra and then through the vas deferens to the epididymis.

---

*Not recommended in pregnant women and children under 16 years of age.

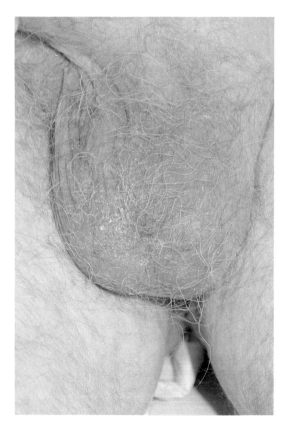

Figure 2.13. Epididymitis caused by gonococci. Left epididymis is affected. Notice erythema of the overlying stitch. Courtesy of Dr. Raju Thomas.

The onset of the disease may be gradual or acute. In the latter, the patient develops a painful swelling on one site of the scrotum. As the condition progresses, the pain becomes more and more intense and may be agonizing. Usually, the lower pole of the epididymis is inflamed and tender, followed by inflammation of the whole epididymis. The condition is usually unilateral, but the other epididymis may be affected later. The patient may have a fever (temperature, 38–40°C [100.4–104°F]) and may complain of malaise and headache.

Enlargement of the testicle due to sympathetic hydrocele or due to orcho-epididymitis has been described, where the adjacent testicle has been secondarily affected.

On examination, the affected site on the scrotum is enlarged and swollen (Figure 2.13). There also may be edema and redness of the overlying skin. On palpation, the whole epididymis or the lower pole of it may be swollen and extremely tender.

On recovery, there may be a residual thickening of the lower pole of the epididymis, and the patient may experience a dull ache for some time. Blockage of the lumen is common, and if the condition is bilateral, the patient may become sterile.

With the development of epididymitis, the urethral discharge (if previously present) may diminish in amount and even cease, temporarily making gonococci difficult to find. However, an attempt should be made to culture *N. gonorrhoeae* from urethral specimens.

Gonococcal epididymitis is to be distinguished from epididymitis due to other causes, such as *C. trachomatis*, coliform bacteria, *Pseudomonas,* and *Mycobacterium tuberculosis.* The non–sexually transmitted pathogens are especially important in men over the age of 35 years and in men who are not sexually active. Preceding purulent urethritis, a recent history of sexual intercourse with a casual or new partner, and a positive test for *N. gonorrhea* will confirm this diagnosis.

Differential Diagnosis

The conditions easily confused with epididymitis include torsion of spermatic cord, testicular infarction, testicular tumor, testicular abscess, traumatic rupture, hernia, orchitis due to mumps, cancer, hydrocele, hematocele, and varicocele. In cases of suspected epididymitis in a prepubertal boy, prompt surgical exploration may be advised, since spermatic cord torsion is common in this age group.

A diagnosis of epididymitis can be confirmed by ultrasound or radionuclide flow scan.[83]

Treatment

Treatment of gonococcal epididymitis should be the same as for gonococcal urethritis, with the extension of doxycycline or tetracycline up to 10–14 days. Nonspecific measures include bed rest, scrotal elevation, and oral administration of nonsteroidal anti-inflammatory drugs and analgesics.

Prostatitis

Acute prostatitis, common in the preantibiotic era, is presently a rare complication of gonococcal urethritis in men. Although occasional hematogenous and lymphatic routes have been reported, the ascending spread of gonococci seems to be the primary route of infection. Acute gonococcal prostatitis should be suspected in any case of gonorrhea in which the patient develops shivering, fever accompanied by pain in the perineum, or suprapubic discomfort. Urinary and rectal symptoms may occur. The patient may complain of urgency, frequency, and hematuria. The two-glass urine test may show haziness in both glasses. Rectal symptoms include constipation and painful defecation. On rectal examination, the prostate is enlarged, warmer than the surrounding tissue, tender and indurated. Patients have raised temperatures of 38–39°C.

The condition usually subsides under treatment. Rarely it may progress to form a prostatic abscess. Diagnosis is confirmed by demonstration of gonococci in urethral discharge or prostatic fluid. (The prostate should not be massaged when acutely inflamed.)

Chronic prostatitis is more likely to occur as a complication of nongonococcal urethritis; however, few patients may suffer from chronic prostatitis due to gonococcal infection. Patients may complain of a dull pain in the perineum, persistent gleet, nocturia, and hematospermia. Some patients experience suprapubic or testicular pain or dysuria.

Since all these symptoms may be attributable to conditions other than prostatitis, demonstration of the causative agent is necessary to prove diagnosis.

Treatment

The patient should be treated with one of several regimens recommended for uncomplicated gonococcal urethritis, but administration of antibiotics should be extended to 10–14 days. Some authors recommend administration of trimethoprim or trimethoprim-sulfamethoxazole,[84] since trimethoprim readily enters the prostate and is active in the acid environment present there.

Acutely sick patients should be hospitalized. Adequate hydration and administration of antipyretics, analgesics, and spasmolytics are recommended. In case of treatment failure or poor response or when prostatic abscess is suspected, cooperation with an experienced urologist is advisable.

Local Complications

Local complications of gonococcal urethritis in men include urethral stricture, periurethral abscess, Tyssonitis (Figure 2.14), Littritis, and Cowperitis. These complications, which were not rare in the preantibiotic era, have practically disappeared as a result of modern methods of treatment.

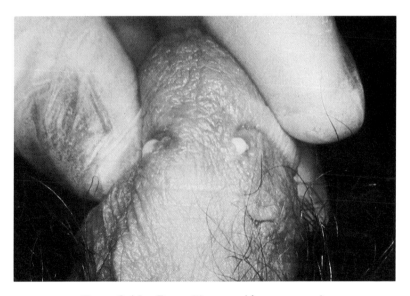

Figure 2.14. Tyssonitis caused by gonococci.

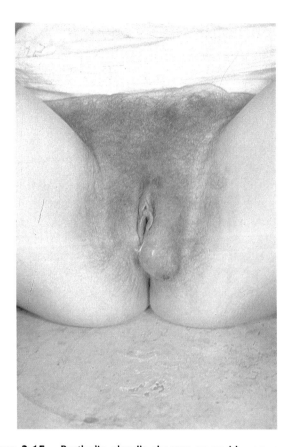

Figure 2.15.   Bartholin gland's abscess caused by gonococci.

COMPLICATIONS IN WOMEN

Gonococcal PID

Pelvic inflammatory disease is the most common complication of gonorrhea in women. For a detailed discussion of PID, the reader is referred to Chapter 3.

Bartholinitis

Involvement of Bartholin's duct is common in women with genital tract gonorrhea but often not diagnosed because of a lack of minimal symptoms. In the case of an abscess of Bartholin's gland, the patient complains of pain in the vulva accompanied by tenderness and swelling and may experience difficulty in walking. On inspection, there is swelling and reddening of the overlaying skin in the lower part of the labium majus (Figure 2.15). Gentle pressure may express a small bead of pus from the duct opening (Figure 2.16). However, this may not be always possi-

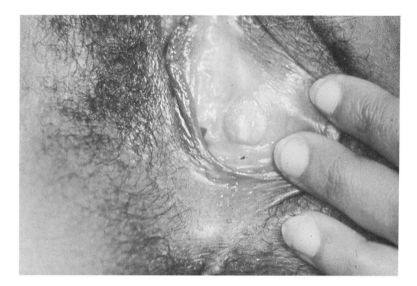

Figure 2.16. Gonococcal Bartholinitis: pus expressed from the opening of Bartholin's gland.

ble, since the duct may be blocked by the inflammation. Diagnosis is confirmed by demonstration of gonococci in the contents of the abscess cavity, or if this is not possible, by demonstration of gonococci from other sites such as the endocervix, urethra, or rectum. Treatment for Bartholinitis is the same as for uncomplicated gonorrhea. In addition, in case of an abscess, incision and drainage are recommended.

Skenitis

Skene's paraurethral glands are located at both sites of the urinary meatus. Occasionally, a small abscess may form in one of these glands, causing pain, discomfort, and difficulties upon urination. On examination, a small indurated mass may be palpable on the site of the urethra. Complications are rare, and treatment is as for uncomplicated genital gonorrhea.

COMPLICATIONS IN BOTH SEXES

Fitz-Hugh-Curtis Syndrome (Perihepatitis)

Fitz-Hugh-Curtis syndrome occurs in 1–10 percent of women with pelvic infection.[85] The most likely pathogenesis of this syndrome is spread of infection from the fallopian tube. The microorganisms may probably reach the liver through the lymphatic system from the pelvis. Besides gonococci,[86] *C. trachomatis* is a common cause of this syndrome.[87,88] Perihepatitis has been also described in men.[89,90] (For symptoms and signs, see p. 78).

Disseminated Gonococcal Infection

Disseminated gonococcal infection (DGI) occurs when, because of the hematogenous spread of gonococci, various extragenital parts of the body become infected. The incidence of DGI appears to vary in different countries, and its prevalence among total gonorrhea cases in the United States ranges from 0.1 to 2 percent.[91-93] This complication has been seen more frequently in women than in men. The sex distribution is probably related to the fact that the majority of men suffering from gonorrhea are symptomatic and receive prompt treatment, whereas gonorrhea in a big proportion of the infected female population is asymptomatic or with minimal or nonspecific symptoms, is underdiagnosed, and is not treated.

DGI occurs commonly in women at the time of or shortly after menstruation. Other risk factors include pregnancy (especially the third trimester) and asymptomatic and pharyngeal infection. About 90% of DGI is caused by the AHU auxotype of *N. gonorrhoeae*.[22] They generally belong to serogroup W-1 and are highly sensitive to penicillin. These strains are also more resistant to the bactericidal action of normal human serum.[94] In addition, specific complement component deficiencies have been found to be associated with an increased risk for DGI.[95,96]

The common manifestations of DGI are arthritis and dermatitis (so-called arthritis-dermatitis syndrome), while the much less frequent but more serious manifestations include endocarditis, meningitis, and osteomyelitis.

Manifestations

Arthritis-Dermatitis.   The clinical course of the arthritis-dermatitis syndrome occurs in two different phases: an early bacteremic phase and a septic joint phase.[91,97,98] The first (bacteremic) phase appears early in the disease and is characterized by fever, chills, malaise, anorexia, polyarthritis, skin lesions, and small joint effusion. Some patients may be without systemic symptoms and fever. In this stage, blood cultures are often positive, while joint fluid cultures are negative. In the second (septic joint) phase, monoarticular, purulent joint effusion is noted, with few systemic signs or symptoms. Blood cultures are usually negative and joint fluid often positive.

The knee, ankles, elbows, and joints of the wrist, hands, and feet are most frequently involved (Figure 2.17). On examination, the affected joints are painful, swollen, hot, and tender. The overlying skin is reddened. Tendon sheats may also be affected, and tenosynovitis may be an important diagnostic sign. If neglected, a septic joint may progress to destructive changes and ankylosis.

The bacteremic stage is associated with skin lesions which are considered to be due to gonococcal embolization and the release of endotoxins following phagocytosis. Skin lesions are the single most common and clinically characteristic manifestations of DGI.[91,98-100] They occur concomitant with arthritis in up to 50 percent of cases[91,93,98,101] and usually start as tiny red macules or papules and progress to vesicular and pustular stages (Figure 2.18). Many of them have a hemorrhagic base and a necrotic center (Figure 2.19). Large hemorrhagic bullae surrounded by an erythematous zone can occur, but they are relatively uncommon.[102] The skin lesions appear during the first few days of symptoms and may occur on any body region but are most frequently present on distal parts of extremities near the periar-

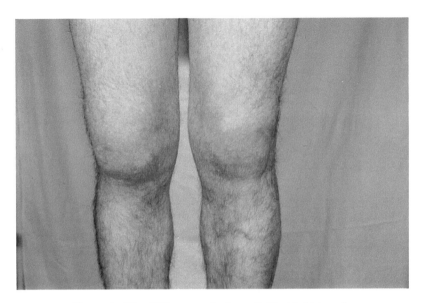

Figure 2.17. DGI: monarticular arthritis (right knee).

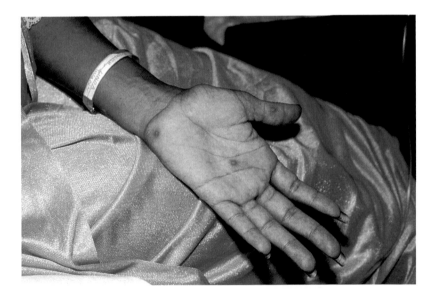

Figure 2.18. DGI: pustular lesions on the palm.

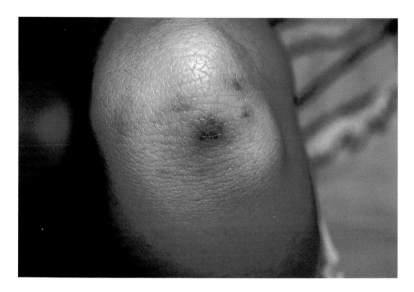

Figure 2.19. DGI: Skin lesion with hemorrhagic base and necrotic center.

ticular regions (Figure 2.20). The number of lesions varies, and they are seen in various stages of development. They resolve spontaneously within a few days without residual scarring. Deep necrotic lesions may persist over a longer period and resolve as eschars. Gonococci may be demonstrated in lesion specimens by Gram's stain, culture, or fluorescent antibody technique, with the latter giving the best results.

Meningitis. Meningitis is an uncommon complication of DGI.[103,104] Clinically, gonococcal meningitis is similar to that caused by meningococci. A definitive diagnosis and differentiation from meningococcal meningitis depends upon cultural isolation of the microorganism from spinal fluid and confirmation of the isolate by sugar fermentation test or fluorescent antibody staining.

Endocarditis, Myocarditis, and Myopericarditis. Currently, the life-threatening complications of the preantibiotic era—endocarditis, myocarditis, and myopericarditis—are seen rather infrequently.[91,104,105] Several abnormalities including heart block may occur,[106] but most patients are asymptomatic for myocardial or pericardial involvement.

Hepatitis. Hepatitis in its mild form, similar to that noted in other bacteremias, may occur in DGI. It is estimated that about half of the patients with gonococcemia may develop this complication.[107] The disease is confirmed by elevation of the serum bilirubin and transaminase levels.

Other Manifestations. Other rare but reported manifestations associated with DGI include pneumonia and osteomyelitis.[108]

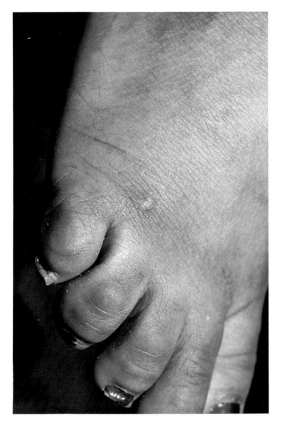

Figure 2.20. DGI: pustular lesion on the dorsal side of the foot (the same patient as in Figure 2.18).

Diagnosis

Apart from the clinical manifestations of arthritis, typical skin lesion, or other symptoms or signs of DGI, the diagnosis of the condition depends on demonstration of *N. gonorrhoeae* in the blood, joint fluid, skin lesions, or cerebrospinal fluid. Isolation of gonococci from primary sites of infection (urethra, endocervix, pharynx, or rectum) with clinical presentation of DGI helps to establish diagnosis.

The differential diagnosis of DGI should include Reiter's syndrome, reactive arthritis caused by enteric infections, rheumatoid arthritis, psoriatic arthritis, secondary syphilis, pyogenic or traumatic arthritis, gout, and carpal tunnel syndrome. Skin conditions that may mimic DGI skin lesions should include septicemias caused by other microorganisms (meningococci, staphylococci, and fungi). A recently published study shows that bacteremia caused by meningococci may produce a picture identical to that of DGI, and the authors suggest that, with the decreasing incidence of gonorrhea in the community along with decreasing prevalence of AHU strains, *N. meningititis* should be considered more frequently in the differential diagnosis of the acute arthritis-dermatitis syndrome.[109]

Treatment

Hospitalization of patients with disseminated gonococcal infection is recommended, especially for those who cannot reliably comply with treatment, have uncertain diagnosis, or have purulent synovial effusions or other complications. Attempts should be made to exclude endocarditis or meningitis.

DGI Inpatient. The recommended regimen is

Ceftriaxone, 1 g IM or IV every 24 hours

Or

Ceftizoxime, 1 g IV every 8 hours

Or

Cefotaxime, 1 g IV every 8 hours

Patients who are allergic to β-lactam drugs should be treated with *spectinomycin*, 2 g IM every 12 hours. When the infecting organism is proven to be penicillin sensitive, parenteral treatment may be switched to *ampicillin*, 1 g every 6 hours (or equivalent).

Reliable patients with uncomplicated disease may be discharged 24–48 hours after all symptoms resolve and complete therapy (for a total of 1 week of antibiotic therapy) with an oral regimen of *cefuroxime axetil*, 500 mg 2 times a day, *or amoxicillin*, 500 mg with clavulanic acid 3 times a day, *or*, if not pregnant, *ciprofloxacin*, 500 mg 2 times a day.

Patients treated for DGI should be tested for genital *C. trachomatis* infection. If chlamydial testing is not available, then patients should be treated empirically for coexisting chlamydial infection.

Meningitis and Endocarditis. Meningitis and endocarditis caused by *N. gonorrhoeae* require high-dose IV therapy with an agent effective against the strain causing the disease, such as *ceftriaxone*, 1–2 g IV every 12 hours. Optimal duration of therapy is unknown, but most authorities treat patients with gonococcal meningitis for 10–14 days and with gonococcal endocarditis for at least 4 weeks. Patients with gonococcal nephritis, endocarditis or meningitis, or recurrent DGI should be evaluated for complement deficiencies. Treatment of complicated DGI should be undertaken in consultation with an expert.

GONOCOCCAL INFECTION IN PREGNANCY

Gonococcal infection in pregnancy creates risk both for maternal, fetal, or neonatal complications.[110-112] As mentioned previously in this chapter, pregnancy is a predisposing factor for DGI. It was suggested that the increased vascularity of the pelvic and genital organs that occurs in pregnant women might at least in part explain this phenomenon.[113] A number of studies have identified an association between untreated endocervical gonorrhea in pregnant women and perinatal complication, including an increased incidence of premature rupture of membranes, preterm delivery, chorioamnionitis, neonatal and maternal postpartum sepsis, as well as intrauterine growth retardation.[110,114-116] Moreover, females undergoing abortions who have untreated endocervical gonococcal infection are at risk for developing postabortion endometritis.[117]

Treatment of Pregnant Women

The recommended regimen is

Ceftriaxone, 250 mg IM once
Plus
Erythromycin base,* 500 mg orally 4 times a day for 7 days

Pregnant women allergic to β-lactams should be treated with *spectinomycin* 2 g IM once (followed by *erythromycin*). Follow-up cervical and rectal cultures for *N. gonorrhoeae* should be obtained 3–7 days after completion of treatment.

Ideally, pregnant women with gonorrhea should be treated for chlamydia on the basis of chlamydial diagnostic studies. If chlamydial diagnostic testing is not available, then treatment for chlamydia should be given. Tetracyclines (including doxycycline) and the quinolones are contraindicated in pregnancy because of the possibility of adverse effects on the fetus. Treatments for pregnant patients with chlamydial infection, acute salpingitis, and disseminated gonorrhea in pregnancy are described in respective chapters.

Treatment of Infants Born to Mothers with Gonococcal Infection

Infants born to mothers with untreated gonorrhea are at high risk of infection (e.g., ophthalmia and DGI) and should be treated with a single injection of *ceftriaxone*, 50 mg/kg IV or IM, not to exceed 125 mg. Ceftriaxone should be given cautiously to hyperbilirubinemic infants, especially premature infants. Topical prophylaxis for neonatal ophthalmia is not adequate treatment for documented infections of the eye or other sites. All pregnant women should have endocervical cultures for *N. gonorrhoeae* and *C. trachomatis* plus serologic test for syphilis at the time of the first visit as an integral part of the prenatal care. A second culture for gonococci as well as tests for *C. trachomatis* and syphilis late in the third trimester should be done on women at high risk of sexually transmitted diseases.

GONORRHEA IN OLDER CHILDREN

Gonococcal Vulvovaginitis

Vulvovaginitis in prepubertal girls caused by *N. gonorrhoeae* can be acquired in three different ways: accidentally in a family with poor hygiene,[118-120] as a result of sexual child abuse,[121,122] or, usually in children over 10 years of age, as a conse-

---

*Erythromycin stearate, 500 mg, or erythromycin ethylsuccinate, 800 mg, or equivalent may be substituted for erythromycin base.

quence of voluntary sexual activity.[123] In prepubertal girls, the vagina is more susceptible to gonococcal infection than that in adults. It has a thin epithelium with poor glycogen content and a relatively alkaline pH, providing an appropriate environment for gonococcal infection.

The incubation period is usually a few days, after which the girl complains of soreness, dysuria, and discharge. On occasion, a physician's advice is sought because the mother has noticed discharge on the child's underclothes or an erythematous, swollen vulva.

On examination, the signs of infection may be minimal or the girl may be found to have purulent vaginitis with secondary vulvitis. Examination should be very gentle, and specimens have to be obtained from the vaginal orifice without the use of a speculum. If necessary, specimens should be taken from the urethra and/or rectum. Cultures of the vaginal specimens are necessary for diagnosis because of the presence of other microorganisms that may mimic gonococcal infection in a Gram-stained smear. Moreover, culture confirmation of the diagnosis is necessary if sexual abuse is a consideration.

Gonococcal Infection in Boys

Boys may acquire urethritis, proctitis, or pharyngitis as a result of sexual abuse or voluntary sexual activity. Infection resulting from poor hygiene is extremely rare, if at all possible. Symptoms and signs do not differ from those that occur in adult men and usually include severe dysuria and purulent discharge. A Gram-stain of urethral exudate will confirm the diagnosis of gonococcal urethritis, but cultures should be done to prove it. Culture is necessary to confirm gonococcal proctitis, and culture plus sugar fermentation test is necessary to confirm pharyngeal infection.

Since a high percentage of children with gonococcal infection have been subjected to sexual abuse, any case with the slightest suspicion of sexual abuse should be reported to the appropriate authorities for investigation.

Treatment

Children who weigh over 45 kg should receive adult regimens. Children who weigh less than 45 kg should be treated as follows. For uncomplicated vulvovaginitis and urethritis, administer Ceftriaxone 125 mg IM in a single dose. Patients who cannot tolerate ceftriaxone may be treated with: Spectinomycin 40 mg/kg IM once.

Children 8 years of age or older should also be given doxycycline 100 mg 2 times a day for 7 days. All patients should be evaluated for coinfection with syphilis and *C. trachomatis*. Bacteremia or arthritis should be treated with ceftriaxone 50 mg/kg (maximum 1 g) once daily for 7 days. For meningitis, the duration of treatment is increased to 10 to 14 days and the maximum dose is 2 g.

Special Consideration

All patients should have follow-up cultures, and the source of infection should be identified, examined, and treated. Child abuse should be carefully considered and evaluated.

GONOCOCCAL INFECTION IN NEONATES

Gonococcal infections in neonates result from transmission of *N. gonorrhoeae* from the mother to the infant during passage through the birth canal. Sporadically, children born by cesarean section may be infected, but this usually follows prolonged rupture of the membranes.[124] The incidence of neonatal gonorrhea depends on the incidence of this infection among pregnant women. Gonococcal infection of the newborn can take several forms, which include ophthalmia, septicemia, arthritis, and meningitis.

Ophthalmia Neonatorum

As a result of silver nitrate prophylaxis, *N. gonorrhoeae* is today one of the least common causes of neonatal conjunctivitis. The risk of transmission of gonococci from an infected mother to her infant in the presence of silver nitrate prophylaxis is probably less than 2 percent.[125] The incubation period of neonatal conjunctivitis is usually 2–4 days. The affected eye becomes red and inflamed. The eyelids can be markedly swollen, and pus may be oozing between the eyelids. On occasion, use of an eyelid retractor may be necessary to examine the eye or to obtain a specimen. The conjunctival reaction may be quite severe with marked hyperemia. The disease can progress with the development of corneal dullness, ulceration, iridocyclitis and subsequent blindness.

In instances where ineffective prophylactic measures have been used, the symptoms and signs may be mild, with minor conjunctival irritation and/or minimal serous discharge.

The diagnosis is made by demonstration of gonococci either by Gram-stained smears or culture.

Gonococcal ophthalmia neonatorum should be distinguished from conjunctivitis caused by: *C. trachomatis*, Herpes simplex virus, other bacteria or viruses (*Staphylococcus, Pseudomonas, Human papova virus, Molluscum contagiosum virus*), and chemicals.

Other Manifestations of Neonatal Gonococcal Infection

Other manifestations result from gonococcal septicemia and include DGI, meningitis, and endocarditis. Unlike disseminated gonococcal infection in adults, arthritis is usually not associated with skin lesions. The diagnosis of neonatal gonococcal infection should be anticipated when a sick infant presents with typical clinical manifestations and Gram-stained specimen that is positive for Gram-negative diplococci. However, positive blood or joint fluid cultures are necessary to confirm diagnosis.

Treatment

Infants with documented gonococcal infections at any site (e.g., eye) should be evaluated for DGI. This evaluation should include a careful physical examination, especially of the joints, as well as blood and CSF cultures. Infants with gonococcal ophthalmia or DGI should be treated for 7 days (10 to 14 days if meningitis is present) with one of the following regimens:

Ceftriaxone 25–50 mg/kg/day IV or IM in a single daily dose

Or

Cefotaxime 25 mg/kg IV or IM 2 times a day.

Alternative Regimen. Limited data suggest that uncomplicated gonococcal ophthalmia in infants may be cured with a single injection of ceftriaxone (50 mg/kg up to 125 mg). A few experts use this regimen in children who have no clinical or laboratory evidence of disseminated disease.

If the gonococcal isolate is proven to be susceptible to penicillin, crystalline penicillin G may be given. The dose is 100,000 units/kg/day given in 2 equal doses (4 equal doses per day for infants more than 1 week old). The dose should be increased to 150,000 units/kg/day for meningitis.

Infants with gonococcal ophthalmia should receive eye irrigations with buffered saline solutions until discharge has cleared. Topical antibiotic therapy alone is inadequate. Simultaneous infection with *C. trachomatis* has been reported and should be considered in patients who do not respond satisfactorily. Therefore, the mother and infant should be tested for chlamydial infection.

Prevention of Ophthalmia Neonatorum

Instillation of a prophylactic agent into the eyes of all newborn infants is recommended to prevent gonococcal ophthalmia neonatorum and is required by law in most states. While all regimens proposed below effectively prevent gonococcal eye disease, their efficacy in preventing chlamydial eye disease is not clear. Furthermore, they do not eliminate nasopharyngeal colonization with *C. trachomatis*. Treatment of gonococcal and chlamydial infections in pregnant women is the best method for preventing neonatal gonococcal and chlamydial disease.

The recommended regimen is

Erythromycin (0.5%) ophthalmic ointment,

Or

Tetracycline (1%) ointment,

Or

Silver nitrate (1%).

One of these should be instilled into the eyes of every neonate as soon as possible after delivery, and definitely within 1 hour after birth. Single-use tubes or ampules are preferable to multiple-use tubes.

The efficacy of tetracycline and erythromycin in the prevention of TRNG and PPNG ophthalmia is unknown. However, because of the high concentrations of drug in these preparations, both are probably effective.

REFERENCES

1. Barnes RC, Homes KK: Epidemiology of gonorrhea: Current perspective. *Epidemiol Rev* 6:1–30, 1984.

2. Rothenberg R, Bross DC, Vernon TM: Reporting of gonorrhea by private physicians: A behavioral study. *Am J Public Health* 70:983–986, 1980.

3. Rice RJ, Aral SO, Blount JH, et al: Gonorrhea in the United States 1975–1984. Is the giant only sleeping? *Sex Transm Dis* 14:83–87, 1987.

4. Morton RS: Control of sexually transmitted diseases today and tomorrow. *Genitourin Med* 63:202–209, 1987.

5. Osoba AO: Sexually transmitted diseases in tropical Africa: A review of the present situation, *Br J Vener Dis* 57:89–94, 1981.

6. Latif AS: Sexually transmitted diseases in clinic patients in Salisbury, Zimbabwe. *Br J Vener Dis* 57:181–183, 1981.

7. Spence MR: Gonorrhea. *Clin Obstet Gynecol* 25:111–124, 1983.

8. Hooper RR, Reynods GH, Jones OG, et al: Cohort study of venereal disease. I: The risk of gonorrhea transmission from infected women to men. *Am J Epidemiol* 108:136–144, 1978.

9. Dans PE: Gonococcal anogenital infection. *Clin Obstet Gynecol* 18:103–119, 1975.

10. Thin RNT, Williams IA, Nicol CS: Direct and delayed methods of immunoflourescent diagnosis of gonorrhea in women. *Br J Vener Dis* 47:27–30, 1971.

11. Osborne NG, Grubin L: Colonization of the pharynx with *Neisseria gonorrhoeae:* Experience in a clinic for sexually transmitted disease. *Sex Transm Dis* 6:253–256, 1979.

12. Kellog DS, Peacock WL, Deacon WE, et al: *Neisseria gonorrhoeae.* I: Virulence genetically linked to clonal variation. *J Bacteriol* 85:1274–1279, 1963.

13. Kellog DS, Cohen IR, Norins LC, et al: *Neisseria gonorrhoeae.* II: Colonial variation and pathogenicity during 35 months in vitro. *J Bacteriol* 96:596–605, 1968.

14. Tramont EC, Wilson C: Variations in buccal cell adhesions of *Neisseria gonorrhoeae.* *Infect Immun* 16:709–711, 1977.

15. Pearce WA, Buchannan TM: Attachment role of gonococcal pili: Optimum conditions and quantitation of adherence of isolated pili to human cell in vitro. *J Clin Invest* 61:931–943, 1978.

16. Thomas DW, Hill JC, Tyeryar FJ: Interaction of gonococci with phagocytic leukocytes from men and mice. *Infect Immun* 8:98–104, 1973.

17. Dilworth JA, Hendley JO, Mandell GL: Attachment and ingestion of gonococci by human neutrophils. *Infect Immun* 11:512–516, 1975.

18. Sparling PF: Genetic transformation of *Neisseria gonorrhoeae* to streptomycin resistance. *J Bacteriol* 92:1364–1371, 1966.

19. Lind I, Reimann K: Indirect hemagglutination test for demonstration of gonococcal antibodies using gonococcal pili as antigen, in Brooks GF, Gotschlish EC, Holmes KK, Sawyer WF, Young FE (eds): *Immunobiology of Neisseria gonorrhoeae.* Washington DC, American Society of Microbiology, 1978, p. 385.

20. Buchanan TM, Swanson J, Holmes KK, et al: Quatitative determination of antibody to gonococcal pili: Changes in antibody levels with gonococcal infection. *J Clin Invest* 52:2896–2909, 1973.

21. Catlin BW: Nutritional requirements and auxotypin, in Roberts R (ed): *The gonococcus,* New York, John Wiley & Sons, 1977 p. 91–109.

22. Knapp JS, Holmes KK: Disseminated gonococcal infections caused by *Neisseria gonorrhoeae* with unique nutritional requirements. *J Infect Dis* 132:204–208, 1975.

23. Knapp JS: Typing gonococci, in Brooks GF, Donegan EA (eds): *Gonococcal Infection.* London, Edward Arnold, 1985, Current Topics in Infection Series, p. 159–167.

24. Sandstrom EG, Danielson D: Serology of *Neisseria gonorrhoeae:* Classification with co-agglutination. *Acta Pathol Microbiol Immunol Scand [B]* 88:27–38, 1980.

25. Sandstrom EG, Knapp JS, Buchanan TM: Serology of *Neisseria gonorrhoeae:* W-antigen serogrouping by coagglutination and protein 1 serotyping by enzyme-linked immuno-sorbent assay both detect protein 1 antigens. *Infect Immun* 35:229–239, 1982.

26. Tam MR, Buchanan TM, Sandstrom EG, et al: Serological classification of *Neisseria gonorrhoeae* with monoclonal antibodies. *Infec Immun* 36:1042–1053, 1982.

27. Buchanan TM, Hildebrandt JF: Antigen-specific serotyping of *Neisseria gonorrhoeae:* Characterization based upon principal outer membrane protein. *Infec Immun* 32:1483–1489, 1981.

28. Centers for Disease Control: Penicillin-resistant gonorrhea—North Carolina. *MMWR* 32:273–275, 1983.

29. Rice RJ, Biddle JW, Jean Louis YA, et al: Chromosomally mediated resistance in *N. gonorrhoeae* in the United States: Results of surveillance and reporting 1983–1984. *J Infect Dis* 153:340–345, 1986.

30. Phillips I: Beta-lactamase-producing, penicillin resistant gonoccus. *Lancet* 2:656–657, 1976.

31. Ashford WA, Golash RG, Hemming VG: Penicillinase-producing *Neisseria gonorrhoeae.* *Lancet* 2:657–658, 1976.

32. Perine PL, Morton RS, Piot P, et al: Epidemiology and treatment of penicillinase-producing *Neisseria gonorrhoeae.* *Sex Transm Dis* 6:152–158, 1979.

33. Rajan VS, Thirumoorthy T, Tan NJ: Epidemiology of penicillinase-producing *Neisseria gonorrhoeae* in Singapore. *Br J Vener Dis* 57:158–161, 1981.

34. McCutchan JA, Adler MW, Barrie JRH: Penicillinase-producing *Neisseria gonorrhoeae* in Great Britain, 1977–1981: Alarming increase incidence and recent development of endemic transmission. *Br Med J* 285:337–340, 1982.

35. Notifiable diseases summary. *Canada Dis Weekly Rep* 136:11–31, 1985.

36. *Sexually Transmitted Disease Statistics, 1984.* Washington, DC, US Department of Health and Human Services, 1985, PHS, CDC No. 134, p. 6.

37. Elwell LP, Roberts M, Mayer LW, et al: Plasmid mediated beta-lactamase production in *Neisseria gonorrhoeae.* *Antimicrob Agents Chemother* 11:528–533, 1977.

38. Perine PL, Thorsberry C, Schalla W, et al: Evidence for two distinct types of penicillin-ase-producing *Neisseria gonorrhoeae.* *Lancet* 2:993–995, 1977.

39. Embden JDA van, Dessens-Kroon M, Klingeren B van: A new betalactamase plasmid in *Neisseria gonorrhoeae.* *J Antimicrob Chemother* 15:247–258, 1985.

40. Dillon JR, Pauze M, Yeung K-H: Molecular and epidemiological analysis of penicillin-ase producing strains of *Neisseria gonorrhoeae* isolated in Canada 1976–1984: Evolution of new auxotypes and beta lactamase encoding plasmids. *Genitourin Med* 62:151–157, 1986.

41. Ison CA, Gedney J, Harris JRW, et al: Penicillinase producing gonococci: A spent force? *Genitourin Med* 62:302–307, 1986.

42. Kohl PK, Knapp JS, Hofmann H, et al: Epidemiological analysis of *Neisseria gonorrhoeae* in the Federal Republic of Germany by auxotyping and serological classification using monoclonal antibodies. *Genitourin Med* 62:145–150, 1986.

43. Dillon JR, Bygdeman SM, Sandstrom EG: Serological ecology of *Neisseria gonorrhoeae* (PPNG and non-PPNG) strains: Canadian perspective. *Genitourin Med* 63:160–168, 1987.

44. Swanson J, Sparks E, Young D, et al: Studies on gonococcus infection X. Pili and

leukocyte association factor as mediators of interactions between gonococci and eukaryotic cells in vitro, *Infect Immun* 11:1352–1361, 1975.

45. Ramstedt KM, Halhagen GJ, Bydeman SM, et al: Serologic classification and contact-tracing in the control of microepidemic of betalactamase-producing *Neisseria gonorrhoeae. Sex Transm Dis* 12:209–214, 1985.

46. King GJ, Swanson J: Studies on gonococcus infection XV, Identification of surface proteins of *Neisseria gonorrhoeae* correlated with leukocyte association. *Infect Immun* 21:575–584, 1978.

47. Sugasawara RJ, Cannon JG, Black WJ, et al: Inhibition of *Neisseria gonorrhoeae* attachment to HeLa cells with monoclonal antibody directed against protein II. *Infect Immun* 42:980–985, 1983.

48. Handsfield HH, Lipman TO, Harnish JP, et al: Asymptomatic gonorrhea in men. *N Engl J Med* 290:117–123, 1974.

49. McCormack MW: Clinical spectrum of infection with *Neisseria gonorrhoeae. Sex Transm Dis* 8:305–307, 1981.

50. Wiesner PJ: Gonorrhea. *Cutis* 27:249–254, 1981.

51. Curran JW, Rendtorff RC, Chandler RW, et al: Female gonorrhea: Its relation to abnormal uterine bleeding, urinary tract symptoms and cervicitis. *Obstet Gynecol* 45:195–198, 1975.

52. Schmale JD, Martin JE, Domescik G: Observation on the culture diagnosis of gonorrhea in women. *JAMA* 210:312–314, 1969.

53. Mroczkowski TF, Martin DH: Unpublished data.

54. Caldwell JG, Price EV, Pazin GJ, et al: Sensitivity and reproducibility of Thayer-Martin culture medium in diagnosing gonorrhea in women. *Am J Obstet Gynecol* 109:463–468, 1971.

55. Dans PE: Gonococcal anogenital infection. *Clin Obstet Gynecol* 18:103–119, 1975.

56. Klein EJ, Fisher LS, Chow AW, et al: Anorectal gonococcal infection. *Ann Intern Med* 86:340–346, 1977.

57. Kilpatrick ZM: Gonorrheal proctitis. *N Engl J Med* 287:967–969, 1972.

58. Lebedeff DA, Hochman EB: Rectal gonorrhea in men: Diagnosis and treatment. *Ann Int Med* 92:463–466, 1980.

59. Fluker JL, Deherogoda P, Platt DJ, et al: Rectal gonorrhea in male homosexuals: Presentation and therapy. *Br J Vener Dis* 56:397–399, 1980.

60. Quinn TC, Goodel SE, Mkrtichian E, et al: *Chlamydia trachomatis* proctitis. *New Engl J Med* 305:195–200, 1981.

61. Quinn TC, Correy L, Chaffee RG, et al: The etiology of anorectal infections in homosexual men. *Am J Med* 71:395–406, 1981.

62. Wiesner PJ, Tronca E, Bonin P, et al: Clinical spectrum of pharyngeal gonococcal infection. *New Engl J Med* 288:181–185, 1973.

63. Osborne NG, Grubin L: Colonization of the pharynx with *Neisseria gonorrhoeae*: Experience in a clinic for sexually transmitted disease. *Sex Transm Dis* 6:253–256, 1979.

64. Fiumara NJ, Wise HH, Many M: Gonorrheal pharyngitis. *N Engl J Med* 276:1248–1250, 1967.

65. Tice AW, Rodriguez VL: Pharyngeal gonorrhea. *JAMA* 246:2717–2719, 1981.

66. Hutt DM, Judson FN: Epidemiology and treatment of oropharyngeal gonorrhea. *Ann Intern Med* 104:655–658, 1986.

67. Wallin J, Siegel MS: Pharyngeal *Neisseria gonorrhoeae*: Colonizer of pathogen? *Brit Med J* 1:1462–1463, 1979.

68. Stoltz E, Schuller J: Gonococcal oro- and naso-pharyngeal infection. *Br J Vener Dis* 50:104–108, 1974.

69. Nobel RC, Cooper RM, Miller BR: Pharyngeal colonization by *Neisseria gonorrhoeae* and *Neisseria meningitis* in black and white patients attending a venereal disease clinic. *Br J Vener Dis* 55:14–19, 1979.

70. Bro-Jorgensen A, Jensen T, Gonococcal pharyngeal infection: Report of 110 cases. *Br J Vener Dis* 49:491–499, 1973.

71. Wiesner PJ: Gonococcal pharyngeal infection. *Clin Obstet Gynecol* 18:121–129, 1975.

72. Handsfield HH: Disseminated gonococcal infection. *Clin Obstet Gynecol* 18:131–142, 1975.

73. Buchta RM: Hemorrhagic *Neisseria gonorrhoeae* conjunctivitis in an adolescent female. *J Adolesc Health Care* 1:60–61, 1986.

74. Sng E-H, Rajan VS, Yeo K-L, et al: The recovery of *Neisseria gonorrhoeae* from clinical specimens: Effects of different temperatures, transport times and media. *Sex Transm Dis* 9:74–78, 1982.

75. Lind I: Methodologic aspects of routine procedures for identification of *Neisseria gonorrhoeae* by immunofluorescence. *Ann NY Acad Sci* 254:400–406, 1975.

76. Waitkins SA: A review of techniques for the identification of *Neisseria gonorrhoeae* and of new developments in Facklam R, Laurell G, Lind I (eds): *Recent Developments in Laboratory Identification Techniques*. Amsterdam, Excerpta Medica 1980, pp. 34–43.

77. Lewis JS: New test systems for the identification of *Neisseria gonorrhoeae*, in Facklam R, Laurell G, Lind I (eds): *Recent Developments in Laboratory Identification Techniques*. Amsterdam, Excerpta Medica 1980, pp. 69–72.

78. Thomas E, Scott SD, Grefkees I, et al: Validity and cost-effectiveness of the Gonozyme test in the diagnosis of gonorrhea. *Can Med Ass J* 134:121–124, 1986.

79. Skeels MR, Matsuda B, Horton H, et al: Evaluation of a modified enzyme immunoassay for *Neisseria gonorrhoeae* in high and low risk females. *Can J Microbiol* 31:893–895, 1985.

80. Jaffe HW, Kraus SJ, Edwards TA, et al: Diagnosis of gonorrhoea using a genetic transformation test on mailed clinical specimens. *Infect Dis* 146:275–279, 1982.

81. Judson FN: Treatment of uncomplicated gonorrhea with ceftriaxone: A review. *Sex Transm Dis* (Suppl) 13(3):199–202, 1986.

82. Berger RE: Acute epididymitis. *Sex Transm Dis* 8:286–289, 1981.

83. Ireton RC, Berger RE: Prostatitis and epididymitis. *Urol Clin North Am* 11:38–93, 1984.

84. Pfau A, Prostatitis: A continuing enigma. *Urol Clin North Am* 13:695–714, 1986.

85. Eschenbach DA, Holmes KK: Acute pelvic inflammatory disease: Current concepts of pathogenesis, etiology and management. *Clin Obstet Gynecol* 18:35–56, 1975.

86. Fitz-Hugh T: Acute gonococcic peritonitis of the right upper quadrant in women. *JAMA* 102:2094–2096, 1934.

87. Wang S-P, Eschenbach DA, Holmes KK, et al: *Chlamydia trachomatis* infection in Fitz-Hugh-Curtis syndrome. *Am J Obstet Gynecol* 138:1034–1038, 1980.

88. Paavonen J, Valtonen VV: *Chlamydia trachomatis* as a possible cause of peritonitis and perihepatitis in a young woman. *Br J Vener Dis* 56:341–343, 1980.

89. Kimball MW, Knee S: Gonococcal perihepatitis in a male: The Fitz-Hugh-Curtis syndrome. *N Engl J Med* 282:1082–1084, 1970.

90. Francis TI, Osoba AO: Gonococcal hepatitis (Fitz-Hugh-Curtis) syndrome in a male patient. *Br J Vener Dis* 48:187–188, 1972.

91. Holmes KK, Counts GW, Beaty HN: Disseminated gonococcal infection. *Ann Intern Med* 74:979–993, 1971.

92. Felman YM, Nikitas JA: Disseminated gonococcal infection. *Cutis* 27:140–154, 1981.

93. Suleiman SA, Grimes EM, Jones HS: Disseminated gonococcal infections. *Obstet Gynecol* 61:48–51, 1983.

94. Schoolnick GK, Buchanan TM, Holmes KK: Gonococci causing disseminated gonococcal infection are resistant to the bactericidal action of normal human sera. *J Clin Invest* 58:1163–1173, 1976.

95. Peterson BH, Lee TJ, Snyderman R, et al: *Neisseria meningitidis* and *Neisseria gonorrhoeae* bacteremia associated with C_6 C_7 C_8 deficiency. *Ann Intern Med* 90:917–920, 1979.

96. Forster GE, Pinching AJ, Ison CA, et al: New microbial and host factors in disseminated gonococcal infection: Case report. *Genitourin Med* 63:169–171, 1987.

97. Gelfand SG, Masi AT, Garcia-Kutzbach A: Spectrum of gonococcal arthritis. Evidence for sequential stages and clinical subgroups. *J Rheum* 2:83–90, 1975.

98. Keiser H, Ruben FL, Wolinsky E, et al: Clinical forms of gonococcal arthritis. *N Engl J Med* 279:234–240, 1968.

99. Svanbom M, Bengtsson E, Strandell T, et al: Benign gonococcemia with skin lesions and arthritis. *Scan J Infect Dis* 2:191–200, 1970.

100. Barr J, Danielsson D: Septic gonococcal dermatitis. *Br Med J* 1:482–485, 1971.

101. Chapman DR, Fernandez-Rocha L: Gonococcal arthritis in pregnancy. *S Afr Med J* 68:1333–1336, 1975.

102. Ackerman AB: Hemorrhagic bullae in gonococcemia. *N Engl J Med* 282:793–794, 1970.

103. Centers for Disease Control: Disseminated gonococcal infection and meningitis, Pennsylvania (CDC). *MMWR*. 12:158, 1984.

104. Felman YM, Nikitas JA: Some aspects of gonococcal dissemination, especially as related to meningitis. *Cutis* 34:128–130, 1984.

105. Vietzke WM: Gonococcal arthritis with pericarditis. *Arch Int Med* 117:270–272, 1966.

106. Gann D, Narula OS, Kaplan S, et al: Complete heart block with gonococcal septicemia. *Ann Int Med* 86:749–750, 1977.

107. Brooks GF: Disseminated gonococcal infection, in Brooks GF, Donegan AE (eds): *Gonococcal Infection.* London, Edward Arnold, 1985, p. 121.

108. Masi AT, Eisenstein BI: Disseminated gonococcal infection (DGI) and gonococcal arthritis (GCA). II. Clinical manifestations, diagnosis, complications, treatment and prevention. *Semin Arthritis Rheum* 10:173–197, 1981.

109. Rompalo AM, Hook EW, Roberts RP, et al: The acute arthritis-dermatitis syndrome: The changing importance of *Neisseria gonorrhoeae* and *Neisseria meningitidis. Arch Intern Med* 147:281–283, 1987.

110. Handsfield HH, Hodson A, Holmes KK: Neonatal gonococcal infection. I: Orogastric contamination with *Neisseria gonorrhoeae. JAMA* 225:6977–6701, 1973.

111. Israel KS, Rissing KB, Brooks GF: Neonatal and childhood gonococcal infections. *Clin Obstet Gynecol* 18:143–151, 1975.

112. Amstey MS, Steadman KT: Asymptomatic gonorrhea and pregnancy. *Sex Transm Dis* 3:14–16, 1976.

113. Zbella EA, Deppe G, Elrad H: Gonococcal arthritis in pregnancy (review). *Obstet Gynecol Surv* 39:8–11, 1984.

114. Sarrel PM, Pruett KA: Symptomatic gonorrhea during pregnancy. *Obstet Gynecol* 32:670–673, 1968.

115. Edwards LE, Barrada MI, Hamann AA, et al: Gonorrhea in pregnancy. *Am J Obstet Gynecol* 132:637–641, 1978.

116. Yvert F, Frost E, Walter P, et al: Prepartal infection of the placenta with *Neisseria gonorrhoeae. Genitourin Med* 61:103–105, 1985.

117. Burkman RT, Tonascia JA, Atienza MF, et al: Untreated endocervical gonorrhea and endometritis following abortion. *Am J Obstet Gynecol* 126:648–651, 1976.

118. Michalowski B: Difficulties in diagnosis and treatment of gonorrhea in young girls. *Br J Vener Dis* 37:142–144, 1961.

119. Shore WB, Winkelstein JA: Nonvenereal transmission of gonococcal infections in children. *J Pediatr* 79:661–663, 1971.

120. Tunnessen WW, Jastremski M: Prepubescent gonococcal vulvovaginitis. *Clin Pediatr* 13:675–676, 1974.

121. Tilelli JA, Turek D, Jaffe AC: Sexual abuse of children: Clinical findings and implications for management. *N Engl J Med* 302:319–323, 1980.

122. Kramer DG, Jason J: Sexually abused children and sexually transmitted diseases. *Rev Infect Dis* 4:S883–S889, 1982.

123. Wald ER, Woodward CL, Marston G, et al: Gonorrheal disease among children in a university hospital. *Sex Transm Dis* 7:41–43, 1980.

124. Strand CL, Arango VA: Gonococcal opthalmia neonatarum after delivery by caesarean section: Report of a case. *Sex Transm Dis* 6:77–78, 1979.

125. Rein MF: Epidemiology of gonococcal infection, in Roberts RB (ed): *The Gonococcus.* New York, John Wiley & Sons, 1977, pp. 12–31.

3

PELVIC INFLAMMATORY DISEASE

Pelvic inflammatory disease (PID) is a clinical syndrome resulting from the ascending spread of microorganisms from the vagina and endocervix to the endometrium, endosalpinx, ovaries, and perimetrial and adjacent tissues. Synonyms for PID are *salpingitis, endometritis-salpingitis-peritonitis,* and *salpingo-oophoritis.*

EPIDEMIOLOGY

PID is a health care problem with worldwide distribution. The prevalence of the syndrome is unknown, and any estimates made will vary depending upon the population studied.

In the United States, an estimated 1 million women experience an episode of acute PID every year.[1] Over 2.5 million physician visits occur annually for PID, and an estimated 150,000 surgical procedures are performed each year for complications of acute salpingitis.[1,2] The syndrome is a significant problem with regard to its economic impact, and it is estimated that the annual cost resulting from PID and its sequelae is approximately $2.7 billion.[3,4] PID has long been known as one of the major causes of female infertility and increases a woman's risk for chronic abdominal pain, ectopic pregnancy, and recurrent pelvic inflammatory disease.[5] In the United States, an estimated 25,000 ectopic pregnancies and 90,000 cases of chronic abdominal pain are attributed to PID each year.[6]

Numerous risk factors are thought to be important in the development of PID. The disease has been found to be more common among young adolescent females. In one study, nearly 70% of patients with acute salpingitis were younger than 25 years of age, and 33% of them experienced a first infection before the age of 19.[6] Single and nulliparous females are more likely to develop PID than married women,[6-8] possibly because single, nulliparous patients are more likely to have multiple sex partners. Women with multiple sex partners have a 4.6-fold greater risk of developing acute PID compared with women in a monogamous relationship.[9]

Patients who use intrauterine contraceptive devices (IUD) are at increased risk of developing PID.[7-10] It has been estimated that IUD users have a threefold to fivefold greater risk of developing acute salpingitis, and the risk progressively increases in proportion to the duration of the use (and the brand name) of the product.[10-12] On the other hand, the use of oral contraceptives decreased the risk of developing PID as compared with patients using IUDs or no contraceptive method.[7,10,13,14] The barrier forms of contraceptive (condom, diaphragm, spermicidal foams, or jellies) also decreased the risk for developing PID, probably by preventing microorganismal spread from the vagina to the upper genital tract and, indirectly, by reducing the overall risk of acquiring sexually transmitted disease.[14,15]

Females who have had previous episodes of gonococcal PID are more likely to develop it again.[9,16] This may perhaps be attributed to tubal damage done by the toxin produced by gonococci[17] and changes in the normal fallopian tube endothelial architecture, mucosal hyperplasia, and focal necrosis observed following acute salpingitis.[18]

Moreover, asymptomatic gonococcal infection in either sexual partner is another risk factor for developing PID, and male sexual partners of women with PID are more likely to have asymptomatic gonococcal urethritis than other men with gonorrhea.[19]

ETIOLOGY

Inaccessibility of the infected organs is a major problem in determining the microbial etiology of PID. Endocervical cultures do not reliably reveal the microorganisms that cause the syndrome, and when laparoscopy or culdocentesis is performed, the microorganisms from the fallopian tubes or the cul-de-sac do not always correspond to those cultured from the endocervix or vagina.[20,21] For practical purposes, PID is categorized as either gonococcal or nongonococcal, based primarily on endocervical isolates.

Based on cervical isolates, gonococcal PID accounts for 40–80 percent of PID in the United States, but the isolation rate of gonococci from the fallopian tubes or peritoneal cavity was only 22–33 percent.[20,21]

Nongonococcal PID is caused primarily by *Chlamydia trachomatis*, a frequently sexually transmitted pathogen.[22,23] In the United States and Canada, 20–50 percent of women with PID had cervical chlamydial infection.[24,25] Similar results (22–47 percent) were presented from Scandinavia.[26-29] Even more important for the etiology of PID are the results obtained from women undergoing laparoscopy where *C. trachomatis* was isolated in 9–30 percent of women with PID in Scandinavia[26,27] and 24–50 percent in women from the United States.[30,31]

Besides *C. trachomatis*, a variety of microorganisms has been recovered from women with nongonococcal PID, and some of them have been implicated as the causative agents of the disease. These include *Mycoplasma hominis, Ureaplasma urealyticum,* and anaerobic and aerobic bacteria.[24,32,33] A polymicrobial infection is the usual result when anaerobes are involved.

SYMPTOMS AND SIGNS

The clinical diagnosis of pelvic inflammatory disease is difficult, inaccurate, and often uncertain. The syndrome presents with a broad spectrum of clinical manifestations, including lower abdominal pain, purulent or mucopurulent cervical discharge, cervical motion tenderness, adnexal tenderness, moderate fever, and leukocytosis. Other findings attributed to PID include adnexal mass and displacement of the cervix. Some patients may complain of recent abnormal uterine bleeding and painful coitus. However, these traditionally accepted symptoms and signs were based upon unconfirmed clinical observations and may occur in many other diseases. Laparoscopy has shown that the diagnosis of PID, based on these clinically accepted criteria, is often inaccurate and unsatisfactory.[34]

Recognizing that laparoscopy is currently the most reliable way to make a diagnosis of PID, it is nevertheless impractical and uneconomical to recommend it for all patients suspected of having the disease. The clinical criteria proposed in Table 3.1 should help to establish the diagnosis of PID based on clinical grounds. All patients should have the initial three findings (A). However, because these are all subjective, one of the six additional findings (B), characteristic for acute inflammation, should also be present.

Although acute PID presents the same signs and symptoms regardless of the etiology, certain clinical and epidemiological differences have been observed between gonococcal and nongonococcal PID. In nongonococcal PID in which *C. trachomatis* is the most common cause, the symptoms and signs are usually milder, the patient is often afebrile with minimum tenderness, and pain often is not associated with menses. Foul-smelling vaginal discharge, uterine bleeding, and cramplike abdominal pain preceding the onset of the disease, and with gradual response to therapy, is more characteristic of nongonococcal forms of PID. The acute onset of pain that usually occurs at the time of menstruation is more characteristic for gonococcal infection. In gonococcal PID, the discharge is usually purulent, and the disease responds to therapy more dramatically. If the patient is black and has a history of abdominal pain of short duration, she is more likely to have gonococcal PID, whereas a white woman with a previous history of gonococcal infection is

---

TABLE 3.1. Criteria for the Diagnosis of Acute Salpingitis

A. Three of the following signs and symptoms must be present:
  1. Lower abdominal pain and tenderness, with or without rebound tenderness
  2. Cervical motion tenderness
  3. Adnexal tenderness

B. In addition, one or more of the following conditions must be present:
  1. Fever ≥ 38°C
  2. Leukocytosis ≥ 10,800 WBC/mm³
  3. Presence of an inflammatory mass noted on pelvic examination or sonography.
  4. A culdocentesis which yields peritoneal fluid containing white blood cells and bacteria.
  5. Elevated ESR.
  6. Endocervical material positive for *N. gonorrhoeae* and/or *C. trachomatis*

Source: Adapted from Hager WD, Eschanbach DA, Spencer MR, Sweet RL: Criteria for diagnosis and grading of salpingitis. *Obstet Gynecol* 61:113–114, 1983.

TABLE 3.2. Conditions Frequently Misdiagnosed as PID

Acute appendicitis
Ectopic pregnancy
Twisted or ruptured ovarian cyst
Septic abortion
Acute pyelonephritis
Ureteral stone
Acute cholecystitis
Mesenteric lymphadenitis
Endometriosis
Pain with ovulation

more likely to have nongonococcal PID.[35] However, in a recently published study of PID among adolescents, no significant differences were found between the two groups, except that vaginal bleeding, current usage of oral contraception, and an elevated erythrocyte sedimentation rate were more often related to the presence of *C. trachomatis* in the endocervix.[36]

DIAGNOSIS

Patients who fulfill the criteria cited in Table 3.1 can be diagnosed as having PID. However, many serious conditions that can present in a similar manner should be ruled out; some of them are listed in Table 3.2.

Patients who do not have all of the first three diagnostic critria (see Table 3.1), or have the first three without one of the subsequent six, could still have PID. This may occur when they are seen very early in the course of their illness or have been inadequately treated before. Even though Gram-stained smear and direct immunofluorescence (IF) are reliable tests for *Neisseria gonorrhoeae* and *C. trachomatis*, cultures of the endocervix and anal canal for *N. gonorrhoeae* and cultures of the endocervix and urethra for *C. trachomatis* should be performed wherever possible. Endocervical cultures for other organisms are not indicated, since the opportunistic microorganisms involved in PID are often found in the lower genital tract of healthy women.

Laparoscopy is the most accurate of the diagnostic methods and is indicated for diagnostically difficult cases. The aspirates obtained should be cultured not only for *N. gonorrhoeae* and *C. trachomatis* but also for mycoplasmas and aerobic and anaerobic bacteria.

DIFFERENTIAL DIAGNOSIS

Pelvic inflammatory disease can be confused with numerous pathologic conditions affecting the lower abdomen in women (Table 3.2):

- *Acute appendicitis:* The pain is most often localized only in the right lower abdominal quadrant and is unilateral (whereas it is usually bilateral in PID). Direct abdominal tenderness, rebound tenderness, and marked muscle spasm are frequently present. The patient feels nauseated and may vomit. Leukocytosis is elevated.

- *Ectopic pregnancy:* Unilateral pain without fever is present unless rupture has occurred. A history of recent menstrual irregularity can be elicited. The uterus is enlarged. The exudate obtained by culdocentesis in ruptured ectopic pregnancy contains nonclotting blood. In PID it is purulent.
- *Twisted or ruptured ovarian cyst:* Unilateral lower abdominal pain is present without fever.
- *Septic abortion:* History and/or evidence of intrauterine manipulation or evidence of the product of conception is usually present. The cervix is dilated.
- *Acute pyelonephritis:* Flank pain, nausea and vomiting, and costovertebral angle tenderness on the infected site are present or elicitable. Bladder irritation may result in increased frequency and urgency of urination.

SEQUELAE

- *Infertility:* PID has been recognized as one of the most common causes of infertility among women.[37] It has been proved that the infertility rate increases with each subsequent bout of the disease. Approximately 10 percent of patients may become infertile after one episode of PID. This increases to about 30 percent after two episodes and to almost 75 percent after three or more.[5] Infertility as a consequence of PID is more often seen in the nongonococcal than in the gonococcal form of the disease.
- *Ectopic pregnancy:* Tubal damage (occlusion, scarring, adhesions) due to PID is one of the most common factors in ectopic pregnancy. It has been well documented that women with previous salpingitis have a several-fold increased risk for ectopic pregnancy as compared with women who have never had the disease.[5,38,39]
- *Tubo-ovarian abscess, pyosalpinx, hydrosalpinx:* These are the common complications of PID. They are more likely to occur in women who have already had one or more prior episodes of PID. The major threat of a tubo-ovarian abscess is its rupture, which can be the cause of death from PID if prompt operative intervention is not undertaken. Abscess formation has been observed more often in nongonococcal forms of PID.
- *Fitz-Hugh-Curtis syndrome (perihepatitis):* This occurs in both forms of PID. It used to occur in 1–10 percent of gonococcal PID[40,41] and has also been found in association with PID caused by *C. trachomatis*.[42-44] Recent studies suggest that most cases of perihepatitis are now associated with chlamydial infections.[45] This syndrome is characterized by the presence of acute right upper quadrant pain and tenderness with or without clinical evidence of PID. Patients may be febrile and have nausea or vomit.[46] A "friction rub" can be heard over the liver, and so-called "violin strings" adhesions may form between the abdominal wall and the liver capsule.
- *Chronic abdominal pain:* A significant proportion of women with PID suffer from

chronic abdominal pain lasting more than 6 months. Such pain has been associated with multiple infections and is more common in women with a history of infertility.

TREATMENT

Treatment of PID should depend upon the etiologic agents causing the infection, and accurate data as to which microorganisms is responsible can be established by direct examination of the intraabdominal site by culdoscopic or laparoscopic procedures. These, however, are often inappropriate or not feasible, and the choice of treatment, in most instances, depends on clinical assessment to decide which microorganisms are the most likely cause. Early administration of appropriate antibiotics is crucial to the preservation of fertility and prevention of the chronic residue of infection. Table 3.3 presents the latest treatment schedule for PID recommended by the CDC. In general, these recommendations attempt to provide treatment regimens that are active against the broad range of possible pathogens that

TABLE 3.3. Treatment Schedules for Acute Pelvic Inflammatory Disease as Recommended by the U.S. Centers for Disease Control, 1989

Ambulatory Management of PID
  Recommended Regimen
    Cefoxitin, 2 g IM, *plus* probenecid, 1 g orally concurrently *or* equivalent
      cephalosporin, *or* ceftriaxone, 250 mg IM
    Plus
    Doxycycline, 100 mg orally 2 times a day for 10–14 days
  Alternative Regimen for Patients Who Do Not Tolerate Doxycycline
    Erythromycin, 500 mg orally 4 times a day for 10–14 days
In-patient Management of PID (one of the following)
  Recommended Regimen A
    Cefoxitin, 2 g IV every 6 hours, *or* cefotetan* IV, 2 g every 12 hours
    Plus
    Doxycycline, 100 mg every 12 hours orally or IV
  The above regimens are given for at least 48 hours after the patient clinically
    improves.
  After discharge from hospital, continue
    Doxycycline orally, 100 mg 2 times a day for 10–14 days total
  Recommended Regimen B
    Clindamycin IV, 900 mg every 8 hours
    Plus
    Gentamicin loading dose IM or IV (2 mg/kg) followed by a maintenance dose (1.5
      mg/kg) every 8 hours
  The above regimens are given for at least 48 hours after the patient improves. After
    discharge from hospital, continue
    Doxycycline, 100 mg orally 2 times a day for 10–14 days total

---

*Other cephalosporins such as ceftizoxime, cefotaxime, and ceftriaxone which provide adequate gonococcal, other facultative gram-negative aerobic, and anaerobic coverage may be utilized in appropriate doses.

TABLE 3.4. Criteria for Hospitalization of Patients
with Acute Pelvic Inflammatory Disease

1. Suspected pelvic or tubo-ovarian abscess
2. Pregnancy
3. Surgical emergencies such as appendicitis and ectopic pregnancy cannot be
   excluded
4. Uncertain diagnosis
5. Nausea and vomiting precluding oral medications
6. Upper peritoneal signs
7. Failure to respond to outpatient therapy
8. Adolescent patients
9. Clinical follow-up within 72 hrs. of starting antibiotic treatment cannot be arranged
10. Patient is unable to follow or tolerate an outpatient regimen

can be associated with PID, including *N. gonorrhoeae, C. trachomatis,* anaerobic
bacteria, and *M. hominis.* Single drug therapy is not adequate for the treatment of
polymicrobial PID, and the major emphasis has been to use combinations of agents
to cover the multitude of microorganisms involved.

Many women with acute PID can be treated on an ambulatory basis: however,
there are several indications for hospitalization[47] (see Table 3.4). Some experts
recommend that all patients with PID be hospitalized for treatment.

Follow-Up

Every patient treated for PID as an outpatient should return 2–3 days after
initiation of therapy for evaluation of progress and for a test of cure and again 4–6
days after completing therapy.

PREVENTION AND MANAGEMENT
OF SEX PARTNERS

The strategies for preventing PID are the same as those aimed at preventing the
acquisition of sexually transmitted disease caused by *C. trachomatis* and *N. gonorrhoeae.* These include education of the public regarding sexually transmitted diseases and their consequences, promoting the use of condoms, and encouraging the
patients to seek medical attention in the very early stage of the disease. It is very
important to identify and treat all male sexual partners of women with PID, since
many of them may be asymptomatic and yet could be sources of reinfection.

Physicians working at STD clinics or emergency rooms should maintain a high
index of suspicion for PID so that an early diagnosis can be made and treatment
undertaken. This is particularly important since mild cases of PID, which often
present themselves at STD clinics, may be easily missed.

REFERENCES

1. Washington A, Cates W, Zaidi AA: Hospitalization for pelvic inflammatory disease: Epidemiology and trends in the United States, 1975 to 1981. *JAMA* 251:2529–2533, 1984.

2. Jones OB, Zaidi AA, St. John RK: Frequency and distribution of salpingitis and pelvic inflammatory disease in short stay hospitals in the United States. *Am J Obstet Gynecol* 138:905–908, 1980.

3. Curran J: Economic consequences of pelvic inflammatory disease in the United States. *Am J Obstet Gynecol* 138:848–851, 1980.

4. Washington A, Arno P: Economic cost of pelvic inflammatory disease: Including associated ectopic pregnancy and infertility. *JAMA* 255:1735–1738, 1986.

5. Westrom L: Effect of acute pelvic inflammatory disease on fertility. *Am J Obstet Gynecol* 121:707–713, 1975.

6. Westrom L: Incidence, prevalence and trends of acute pelvic inflammatory disease and its consequences in industrialized countries. *Am J Obstet Gynecol* 138:880–892, 1980.

7. Eschenbach DA, Harnish JP, Holmes KK: Pathogenesis of acute pelvic inflammatory disease: Role of contraception and other risk factors. *Am J Obstet Gynecol* 128:838–850, 1977.

8. Westrom L, Bengtsson LP, Mardh P-A: The risk of pelvic inflammatory disease in women using intrauterine contraceptive devices as compared to non-user. *Lancet* 2:221–224, 1976.

9. Eschenbach DA: Epidemiology and diagnosis of acute pelvic inflammatory disease. *Obstet Gynecol* 55:142S–152S, 1980.

10. Lee NC, Rubin GL, Ory AW, et al: Type of intrauterine device and the risk of pelvic inflammatory disease. *Obstet Gynecol* 62:1–3, 1983.

11. Sparks RA, Purrier BG, Watt PJ, et al: Bacteriological colonization of uterine cavity: Role of tailed intrauterine contraceptive devices. *Br Med J* 282:1189–1191, 1981.

12. Skangolis M, Mahoney CJ, O'Leary WM: Microbial presence in the uterine cavity as affected by varieties of intrauterine contraceptive devices. *Fertil Steril* 37:263–269, 1982.

13. Osser S, Gullberg B, Liedholm P, et al: Risk of pelvic inflammatory disease among intrauterine device users irrespective of previous pregnancy. *Lancet* 1:386–388, 1980.

14. Senanayake P, Kramer DG: Contraception and pelvic inflammatory disease. *Sex Transm Dis* 8:89–91, 1981.

15. Keith L, Berger GS, Moss W: Cervical gonorrhoea in women using different methods of contraception. *J Am Vener Dis Assoc* 3:17–19, 1976.

16. Eschenbach DA, Holmes KK: Acute pelvic inflammatory disease: Current concepts of pathogenesis, etiology and management. *Clin Obstet Gynecol* 18:35–56, 1975.

17. Gregg CR, Melly MA, McGee ZA: Gonococcal lipopolysaccharide: A toxin for human fallopian tube mucosa. *Am J Obstet Gynecol* 138:981–984, 1980.

18. Draper DL, Donegan EA, James JF, et al: In vitro modeling of acute salpingitis caused by *Neisseria gonorrhoeae*. *Am J Obstet Gynecol* 138:996–1002, 1980.

19. Handsfield HH, Lipman TO, Harnish JP, et al: Asymptomatic gonorrhea in men: Diagnosis, natural course, prevalence and significance. *N Engl J Med* 290:117–123, 1974.

20. Thompson SE, Hager WD, Wong K-H, et al: The microbiology and therapy of acute pelvic inflammatory disease in hospitalized patients. *Am J Obstet Gynecol* 136:179–186, 1980.

21. Sweet RL, Draper DL, Shachter J, et al: Microbiology and pathogenesis of acute salpingitis as determined by laparoscopy: What is the appropriate site to sample? *Am J Obstet Gynecol* 138:985–989, 1980.

22. Mardh P-A, Ripa T, Svensson L, et al: Role of *Chlamydia trachomatis* infection in acute salpingitis. *N Engl J Med* 296:1377–1379, 1977.

23. Holmes KK, Eschenbach DA, Knapp JS: Salpingitis, overview of etiology and epidemiology. *Am J Obstet Gynecol* 138:893–900, 1980.

24. Eschenbach DA, Buchanan TM, Pollock HM, et al: Polymicrobial etiology of acute pelvic inflammatory disease. *N Engl J Med* 293:166–171, 1975.

25. Bowie WR, Jones H: Acute inflammatory disease in outpatients: Association with *Chlamydia trachomatis* and *Neisseria gonorrhoea. Ann Intern Med* 95:686–688, 1981.

26. Mardh P-A, Ripa T, Svensson L, et al: *Chlamydia trachomatis* infection in patients with acute salpingitis. *N Engl J Med* 296:1377–1379, 1977.

27. Paavonen J: *Chlamydia trachomatis* in acute salpingitis. *Am J Obstet Gynecol* 138:957–959, 1980.

28. Gjonnaess H, Dalaker K, Anestad G, et al: Pelvic inflammatory disease: Etiological studies with emphasis on chlamydial infection. *Obstet Gynecol* 59:550–555, 1982.

29. Eilard ET, Brorsson J-E, Hamark B, et al: Isolation of chlamydia in acute salpingitis. *Scand J Infect Dis* 9(Suppl):82–84, 1976.

30. Sweet RL, Schachter J, Robbie MO: Failure of beta-lactam antibiotics to eradicate *Chlamydia trachomatis* in the endometrium despite apparent clinical cure of acute salpingitis. *JAMA* 250:2641–2645, 1983.

31. Wasserheit JN, Bell TA, Kiviat NB, et al: Microbial causes of proven pelvic inflammatory disease and efficacy of clindamycin and tobramycin. *Ann Intern Med* 104:187–193, 1986.

32. Mardh P-A, Westrom L: Tubal and cervical cultures in acute salpingitis with special reference to *Mycoplasma hominis* and T-strain mycoplasms. *Br J Vener Dis* 46:179–186, 1970.

33. Kinghorn GR, Duerden BI, Hafiz S: Clinical and microbiological investigation of women with acute salpingitis and their consorts. *Br J Obstet Gynecol* 93:869–880, 1986.

34. Jacobson L, Westrom L: Objectivized diagnosis of acute pelvic inflammatory disease. *Am J Obstet Gynecol* 105:1088–1098, 1969.

35. Tavelli BG, Judson FN: Comparison of the clinical and epidemiologic characteristics of gonococcal and non-gonococcal pelvic inflammatory disease seen in a clinic for sexually transmitted diseases 1978–79. *Sex Transm Dis* 13:119–122, 1986.

36. Cromer BA, Heald FP: Pelvic inflammatory disease associated with *Neisseria gonorrhoeae* and *Chlamydia trachomatis:* Clinical correlates. *Sex Transm Dis* 14:125–129, 1987.

37. Thompson SE, Washington A: Epidemiology of sexually transmitted *Chlamydia trachomatis* infections. *Epidemiol Rev* 5:96–123, 1983.

38. Urquhart J: Effect of the venereal disease epidemic on the incidence of ectopic pregnancy—implications for evaluation of contraceptives. *Contraception* 19:455–480, 1979.

39. Westrom L, Bengtsson LPh, Mardh P-A: Incidence, trends and risks of ectopic pregnancy in a population of women. *Br Med J* 282:15–18, 1981.

40. Fitz-Hugh T: Acute gonococcic peritonitis of the right upper quadrant in women. *JAMA* 102:2094–2096, 1934.

41. Stanley MM: Gonococcic peritonitis of the upper part of the abdomen in young women. *Arch Intern Med* 78:1–13, 1946.

42. Wang S, Eschenbach DA, Holmes KK, et al: *Chlamydia trachomatis* infection in Fitz-Hugh-Curtis syndrome. *Am J Obstet Gynecol* 138:1034–1038, 1980.

43. Paavonen J, Valtonen VV: *Chlamydia trachomatis* as a possible cause of peritonitis and perihepatitis in a young woman. *Br J Vener Dis* 56:341–343, 1980.

44. Darougar S, Forsey T, Wood JJ, et al: Chlamydia and the Fitz-Hugh-Curtis syndrome. *Br J Vener Dis* 57:391–394, 1981.

45. Shanahan D, Gau D: Chlamydial Fitz-Hugh-Curtis syndrome (letter). *Lancet* 1:1216, 1986.

46. Paavonen J, Saikku P, von Knorring J: Association of infection with *Chlamydia trachomatis* with Fitz-Hugh-Curtis Syndrome. *J Infect Dis* 144:176, 1981.

47. Sweet RL: Pelvic inflammatory disease. *Sex Transm Dis* (suppl) 13(3):192–198, 1986.

4

VAGINITIS/ VULVOVAGINITIS

Vaginitis and vulvovaginitis are very common syndromes among women seeking treatment for sexually transmitted diseases,[1] and in general practice, vaginal discharge is a common and important problem.

Vaginal discharge can be physiologic:[2] caused by secretions from the upper genital tract, the cervical glands, the vagina, and the vestibular glands and the periurethral, sebaceous, and apocrine glands of the vulva. (Table 4.1) In newborn girls, there may be a noticeable vaginal discharge resulting from transplacental transfer of maternal estrogens. In prepubertal girls, a white vaginal discharge may be noted before the onset of menarche, and in women of reproductive age increased vaginal secretion can be caused by use of oral contraceptives, frequent erotic stimulation, anxiety, cervical ectropion, or frequent vaginal douching. Vaginal discharge may be also associated with the use of deodorants containing chemical irritants, the presence of retained foreign bodies such as tampons[3] or cervical caps, and the instillation of chemicals, including antiseptics.

Other diseases and conditions that can cause vaginal discharge/vulvovaginitis include tumors, cervical polyps, vulvar cancer, or medical conditions such as contact dermatitis, Stevens Johnsons syndrome, fixed drug eruptions, and pemphigus.[4] In postmenopausal women, atrophic changes of the vagina epithelium resulting from a reduction in estrogen production may cause vaginal discharge and other symptoms of vaginitis.[5]

From the STD point of view, the most important condition is vaginitis or vulvovaginitis caused by microorganisms that can be sexually transmitted[6] (Table 4.2). The three most common types of vaginal infections are trichomoniasis, vaginal candidosis, and bacterial vaginosis.

TRICHOMONIASIS

Trichomoniasis is a common sexually transmitted disease caused by the protozoa *Trichomonas vaginalis*. In women *T. vaginalis* causes primarily vaginitis whereas in men it causes urethritis. The synonym for trichomoniasis is *trick*.

TABLE 4.1. Characteristics of Physiologic Vaginal Discharge

Whitish gray, may leave grayish brown stain
Nonhomogeneous, floccular
Nonadherent
Odor nonoffensive
High viscosity
Nonpruritic
Unaccompanied by vulvar soreness
Contain few or no polymorphonuclear leukocytes

Etiology

Humans are host to three *Trichomonas* species: *T. vaginalis, T. hominis, and T. tenax. Trichomonas vaginalis* is found in the vagina and urethra and is thought to be the only species in humans that causes disease. The remaining two are believed to be saprophytic organisms resident in the intestine and in the mouth.

Trichomonas vaginalis is a unicellular organism with an ellipsoidal, pear-shaped body approximately $7 \times 10\mu m$ in diameter. There are four anterior flagella and an undulating membrane. The motion of the membrane and the flagella assist in the identification of this parasite.

Different strains of *Trichomonas* appear to differ in intrinsic virulence as demonstrated in animal models and tissue culture.[7,8] Differences in biologic properties,[9] cytotoxicity,[10] and hemolytic activity[8] have been suggested in an attempt to explain the variable clinical expression of the disease. Moreover, the antigenic variations of *T. vaginalis* were demonstrated in reference to its epidemiology and virulence.[11]

Epidemiology

Trichomonas vaginalis is a major cause of vaginitis in women.[12-14] It has also been found to be the cause of urethritis in men.[15-17] The microorganism is responsi-

TABLE 4.2. Microorganisms Commonly Associated with Vaginal Discharge in Adult Women

Microorganism	Primary Site of Infection
Trichomonas vaginalis	Vagina
Candida albicans	Vagina, vulva
Gardnerella vaginalis and anaerobic bacteria	Vagina
Neisseria gonorrhoeae	Cervix, urethra, rectum*
Chlamydia trachomatis	Cervix, urethra, rectum*
Herpes simplex virus	Vulva, vagina, cervix
Human papilloma virus	Vulva, vagina, cervix

*Although *N. gonorrhoeae* and *C. trachomatis* can produce vulvovaginitis in prepubertal girls, the vagina of adult women is not infected with these organisms, and vaginal discharge is secondary to cervicitis.

ble for approximately a quarter of all causes of clinially evident vaginal infections.[12] As many as 50 percent of infected women may be asymptomatic carriers.[18]

In the United States, *T. vaginalis* is found in about 10 percent of healthy women and nearly 50 percent of STD clinic patients. There is an approximate annual incidence of 180 million infections world-wide and 2.5–3 million infections in the United States.[19-21] The peak incidence occurs between the ages of 16 and 35, and the peak prevalence occurs between the ages of 35 and 45.[13,22,23] Having multiple sex partners was mentioned as an important risk factor;[11] there is a prevalence among prostitutes of 50–75 percent.[14]

Trichmonas vaginalis is transmitted primarily by sexual intercourse, and a small portion of transmission occurs indirectly from bath or toilet articles or after communal bathing.[8] The organism can survive for 24 hours in urine and nearly as long on sponges, tampons, or wet clothes.[22,23] Infants may occasionally acquire *Trichomonas* from infected mothers while receiving routine infant care.[22,23] The female partners of infected males almost always harbor *T. vaginalis*,[24] whereas male partners of infected women harbor the microorganism less frequently.[19] There are, however, technical difficulties in detecting the parasite in the male urethra, where, due to anatomical conditions, they are present in small numbers.

Clinical Manifestations

The incubation time is up to 3 weeks, averaging 7 days. Many women with *Trichmonas* infection (25 percent of women seen at STD clinics) may be asymptomatic. Among those with symptoms, the vaginal discharge is usually copious, homogenous, and malodorous. A frothy, gray-green discharge is often cited as the typical finding, but it has not been confirmed by all investigators.[18] In some patients, speculum examination may reveal an erythematous vagina with punctuate red areas that bleed easily. Punctuate mucosal hemorrhages of the cervix, the so-called "strawberry" or "flea-bitten" cervix, may be seen infrequently (Figure 4.1). There may be also inguinal lymphadenopathy with enlarged and somewhat tender nodes, but this is rather a rare finding. Many women with trichomoniasis complain of vaginal and vulvar pruritus which may involve the inner thighs, especially when erythema and maceration extend to the genitofemoral areas. However, pronounced itching is more suggestive of an infection with *Candida albicans* rather than *T. vaginalis*. Other symptoms can include mild lower abdominal pain and infrequently dysmenorrhea or menorrhagia. Dysuria and dyspareunia are not uncommon.

The onset or recrudescence of symptoms in women with trichomonal vaginitis is frequently coincident with menstruation, with increased vaginal pH providing the optimal environmental condition for the growth of *T. vaginalis*.

For many years, *T. vaginalis* was considered to be a harmless resident that caused no serious disease or a benign "nuisance" of the lower genital tract of women.[22] Nevertheless, in addition to the vaginal discomfort and sometimes unbearable symptoms, occasionally serious consequences have been recognized in association with vaginal trichomoniasis:

1.   There is an increased rate of sterility among women with trichomoniasis that is ascribed to the decreased motility of sperm caused by toxic products of *T. vaginalis* or to salpingitis caused by the protozoan.[22,23,25,26]

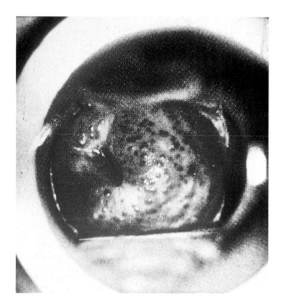

Figure 4.1. Punctate hemorrhages on the cervix ("strawberry cervix") may accompany vaginal trichomoniasis.

2. *Trichomonas vaginalis* was found in PID in women[27] and can serve as a vector for the spread of other pathogens.[28]
3. This organism may cause bartholinitis, skenitis, urethritis and cystitis.
4. The infection can spread to sex partners as well as to offsprings, causing on occasion serious illness.
5. Chronic infection was associated with cellular atypia or cervical erosion.[22,23,29]
6. Trichomoniasis may interfere with the diagnosis of other STDs: for example, gonorrhoea.[22,23,30]

Diagnosis

Because of the variations in signs and symptoms, one can not rely upon a "typical" clinical picture of trichomoniasis. Under most circumstances the clinical diagnosis can be confirmed by the following:

1. *Wet mount:* Mix a drop of vaginal secretion (which for optimal results is taken from the posterior fornix) with a few drops of saline on a slide. Trichomonads are best recognized by their twitching motility. Because trichomoniasis may produce a heavy polymorphonuclear infiltrate, it is easy to miss the protozoa. The specimen should be examined in an area with relatively few white blood cells. Gentle warming of the slide prior to examination may improve the motility of *T. vaginalis.* Trichomonads can be located under low-power magnification, and a switch to high-power magnification allows positive identification (Figure 4.2). Phase or dark-field microscopy is superior when available.

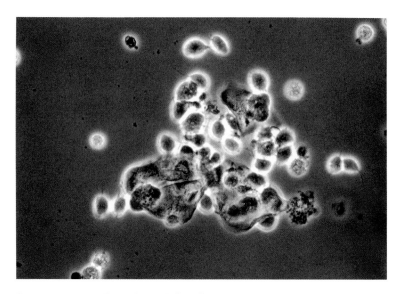

Figure 4.2. Wet-mount: Pear shaped, flagellated trichomonads which are slightly larger than PMN. Motility is the most characteristic diagnostic feature.

2. *Stained smears:* A variety of staining techniques including the Giemsa stain and Papanicolaou's stain test have been described,[31] but none has an advantage over the wet mount.

3. *Fluorescent microscopy:* Two staining techniques are available that require the use of a fluorescent microscope. The *Trichomonas* Direct Specimen test contains a mixture of three fluorescein-labeled murine monoclonal antibodies specific to trichomonads.[32] The test is very reliable and much more sensitive and specific than wet-mount or stained smears[33] but is relatively expensive. Acridine orange staining is also more sensitive then the wet mount or Pap smear.[34]

4. *Cultures:* Culture techniques are the most sensitive diagnostic measures, and several media are available, including some culture kits for office or even field setting use.[35] The most commonly used is modified Diamond's medium;[36] its disadvantages include its relatively high cost and the long time necessary for incubation (2–3 days for positive cases and up to 6–7 days in negative cases).

5. *Serologic tests:* The indirect hemagglutination test[37] and enzyme-linked immunosorbent assay (ELISA)[38] have seen limited use. Both lack sensitivity and specificity.

Differential Diagnosis

- *Vaginal candidosis and bacterial vaginosis:* see Table 4.4.
- *Gonorrhea:* purulent cervical discharge; Gram's stained smear positive for *N. gonorrhoeae;* positive culture.
- *Mucopurulent cervicitis* due to *C. trachomatis* infection: mucopurulent cervical discharge; positive culture or other tests.

- *Foreign body vaginitis:* Identification of foreign body in vagina and its removal establishes diagnosis.
- *Postmenopausal vaginitis* (diagnosis is made by exclusion): negative culture for common vaginal pathogens (*C. albicans, T. vaginalis, Gardnerella vaginalis,* etc.; paucity of the large superficial squamous cells on vaginal smear.
- *Vulval lesions of genital herpes:* grouped vesicles and/or erosions; positive Tzanck test; positive culture and other tests.

Since mixed infections are quite common among women with trichomoniasis, cultures for *N. gonorrhoeae, C. trachomatis, G. vaginalis,* and *C. albicans* as well as serologic tests for syphilis should be performed.

Treatment

Patients should receive *metronidazole,* 2.0 g by mouth in a single dose or 250 mg by mouth 3 times daily for 7 days or *metronidazole* 500 mg twice daily for 7 days. Patients undergoing this therapy should be instructed not to drink alcohol (because of an antabuselike effect) and either to refrain from sex or use condoms for at least 24 hours after she and all her sex partners have completed therapy. Treatment failure may be due to inactivation of metronidazole by vaginal bacteria, drug interference (e.g., phenobarbital) or *Trichomonas* resistance to metronidazole.[39-41]

In pregnant women, the use of metronidazole is contraindicated during the first trimester.[42,43] Alternative regimens include 100 mg of clotrimazole intravaginally each night for 7 days or the use of Betadine or vinegar douches. Some authors are of the opinion that if the patient remains symptomatic late in pregnancy, despite alternative therapy, the standard single oral dose of 2.0 g of metronidazole is justified in order to prevent perinatal complications in the mother and infant.[44-46] Lactating women treated with a single 2.0 g oral dose of metronidazole should stop breast feeding for at least 24 hours.

Management of Sex Partners

All male consorts of women with trichomoniasis should be treated with a single 2.0 g oral dose of metronidazole[43] or one of the 7-day metronidazole regimens.

VAGINAL CANDIDOSIS

Candida albicans has been identified as the cause of several diseases, of which candidal vaginitis and vulvovaginitis in women and balanitis or balanoposthitis in men may be considered sexually acquired infections. Synonyms for vaginal candidosis are *vaginal candidiasis, moniliasis,* and *thrush.*

Etiology

Vaginal candidosis results from infections by *Candida* species, which belong to the family Cryptococcaceae, Fungi Imperfecti. There are at least seven species of

Candida and two of *Torulopsis* that are of medical importance. Two of them are of significance as sexually transmitted agents: *C. albicans* and *T. glabrata*, of which *C. albicans* is overwhelmingly the most frequent vaginal yeast pathogen.[47-49]

The yeasts have a predilection for mucous membranes and moist skin surfaces and have frequently been isolated from the mouth, throat, large intestine, vagina, and skin in "healthy" individuals.[47] The question of whether *C. albicans* can be a genital commensal in some cases, i.e., present without producing the symptoms, or whether it should always be considered a pathogen still remains unanswered. However, more and more investigators agree that detection of *C. albicans* on the genitalia indicates a disease-like state that should be treated.[50]

Generally, a genital yeast infection is a minor condition in both sexes, but its high incidence and frequent recurrences, especially in women, along with the discomfort experienced by the infected patient make the disease of special concern.

Epidemiology

According to gynecologists *C. albicans* is currently the most common actual or potential pathogen in the female genital tract.[51] Among women attending family planning clinics, the incidence of vaginal candidosis was 21 percent[52] as opposed to 37 percent found at sexually transmitted disease clinics.[49] Other studies reported similar isolation rates in STD clinic and non-STD clinic populations.[53,54]

It is estimated that about one-half million women attending clinics for sexually transmitted disease in the United States have vaginal candidosis.[55] The peak incidence of vaginal candidosis in women occurs between ages of 16 and 30, corresponding to the ages of high sexual activity.[50] Vaginal candidosis is probably not, strictly speaking, a sexually transmitted disease, and sexual acquisition of candidosis by women is probably rare, whereas men commonly acquire it from women with vaginal candidosis.[56,57] Male contacts of infected women often have positive urine culture and/or urethritis, and about 10 percent may have symptoms of balanoposthitis.[50,56-58] Some authors have presented evidence that yeast infections are spread sexually in up to 40 percent of genital candidosis.[59] A relationship between oral sex and genital candidosis has also been reported.[60-62] The latter route of infection is supported by the isolation of the same strain of *C. albicans* from the oral cavities of women and from the genitalia of their sexual partners.[60] Infants born to mothers suffering from genital candidosis are at risk of acquiring oral thrush. The incidence of neonatal oral candidosis is several times higher among babies born to women with genital candidosis than among babies born to uninfected mothers.[63,64]

Vaginal candidosis has been also observed in sexually inactive women. The intestinal tract is a possible source of infection for these patients, as genital infection is often associated with the presence of the same strain of yeast in the digestive tract.[60,65,66]

Pathogenesis and Predisposing Factors

The mechanisms by which *C. albicans* and other yeasts causes infection is not entirely understood. There is little doubt that vaginal *Candida* may remain in some

TABLE 4.3. Factors Predisposing to Genital Candidosis

Pregnancy	Endocrine disorders
Menstruation	Diabetes mellitus
Medications	Hypothyroidism
Broad-spectrum antibiotics	Hypoparathyroidism
Immunosupressants	Hypoadrenalism
Corticosteroids	Malignancies
Oral contraceptives	Lymphosarcoma
Metronidazole	Hodgkin's disease
Environmental factors	Other diseases
Poor hygiene	AIDS
Excessive warmth and moisture due to wearing of	Severe anemia
synthetic fiber undergarments	Agammaglobulinemia
Trauma, abrasion, and breaks in the skin and mucous	Malnutrition
membranes	Pancreatitis
	Obesity

women without causing recognizable symptoms or signs. In others, periods of asymptomatic colonization follow episodes of mild to acute exacerbations. In some patients candidosis is a chronic, unremitting disease. It seems that the basis for these differences is very complex, since a great number of factors may play a role. Among these factors are microbial virulence expressed both by the ability of the yeast to multiply and to produce toxic metabolites, hydrolytic enzymes, etc., and by host resistance, which can be altered by the so-called predisposing factors commonly obsesrved among patients with genital candidosis (Table 4.3).

Predisposing host factors in genital and other forms of candidosis include endocrine disorders (of which diabetes mellitus seems to be the most important), certain malignancies, AIDS, and other diseases. Pregnancy and menstruation seem to aggravate candidosis, as does prolonged use of antibiotics, steroids, or immunosuppressive drugs. The role of oral contraceptives is not entirely clear, although the overwhelming majority of studies point out an increased risk of genital candidosis in women using them. Among environmental factors, the increased warmth and moisture attributed to the wearing of synthetic fiber undergarments have been implicated.[67] Moreover, any trauma, skin breaks, or mucous membrane abrasions disturbing the mechanical barriers provided by the skin and ciliated epithelial surfaces provide an opportunity for *Candida* to invade the tissue.[68]

The pathogenic mechanisms through which predisposing factors contribute to development or exacerbation of the disease are again complex and not completely understood. There is little doubt, however, that humoral and cell-mediated immunities play a very important role.[47,69-71] The increased prevalence of oral and vaginal thrush in women, and oral and penile thrush in male patients with AIDS, points out the role of T helper lymphocytes in the pathogenesis of candidosis. It is probable that the same mechanism plays a role in patients with lymphosarcoma and Hodgkin's disease. Frequent candidal infections in malnourished patients and in persons with agammaglobulinemias may suggest a role of gammaglobulins in candidosis.

The high incidence of vaginal candidosis in pregnancy can be explained by the changes in the hormonal status of pregnant women, which results in an increase in glycogen stores in the vaginal epithelium, as well as by the depressed cellular immunity observed in pregnancy.[72] The incidence increases during the course of gestation. Syptomatic candidal vulvovaginitis was observed in about 10 percent of pregnant women during the first trimester and in 23–55 percent of women during the third trimester.[63,73-75] An even higher incidence of candidal vulvovaginitis (up to 90 percent) was observed in pregnant women who had been vaginal carriers of C. albicans.[47,48,54,75]

It is generally accepted that candidal infections (including genital infections) are more prevalent in diabetics than in the general population.[76-79] and recurrent episodes of genital candidosis may sometimes be the first noticeable manifestation of this serious disease. Even so, some authors claim that the incidence of candidosis in diabetics is not increased when the disease is well controlled.[78,79] Vulvovaginal candidosis is common in girls suffering from diabetes, and 77 percent of them cultured for C. albicans yield positive results. Almost 100 percent of cultures taken from girls with symptoms and signs of vulvovaginitis grew C. albicans. In two thirds of the patients, the same yeast flora was cultured from the anus as well as the vulva.[77] It has been observed that a decrease in glycosuria is associated with remission of signs and cessation of symptoms.[78]

The role of oral contraceptives in vaginal candidosis is controversial. It has been suggested that birth control pills encourage yeast growth, based on the findings that a significantly higher percentage of infected than uninfected women use oral contraceptives.[80] Other reports, however, have claimed that the incidence of candidosis in women using birth control pills is no higher than in women using other forms of contraception.[51,58] It is probable that oral contraceptives may predispose women to vaginal carriage but that other factors may be necessasry for the development of vulvovaginitis.

Many patients develop genital candidosis during the course of treatment with broad-spectrum antimicrobials.[81,82] It was demonstrated that vaginal fluid aspirated from randomly selected healthy women could serve as a culture medium for C. albicans, but the addition of broad-spectrum antibiotics significantly enhanced its growth-promoting activity.[83] This might at least partly explain the phenomenon of frequent development of genital candidosis in patients treated with antibiotics.

Clinical Manifestations

About 30 percent of women may be asymptomatic;[49] others may complain of minimal to severe symptoms. Symptoms of vulvovaginal candidosis are of abrupt onset, usually prior to menstruation. The most common manifestation is vulvar pruritis present in 81–90 percent of symptomatic women.[84,85] About three-fourths of these women complain of vulvar soreness;[79] some complain of burning, especially during and after intercourse, and of pruritus and burning around the anus. Dysuria may also occur if the urine comes in contact with the inflamed vulva.

Physical examination reveals an erythematous, somewhat edematous vulva, frequently with excoriations, although none of these findings are constant. In one prospective study, vulvar redness was observed in 54.5 percent of patients with symptomatic candidosis.[84] The vagina may be erythematous and may demonstrate

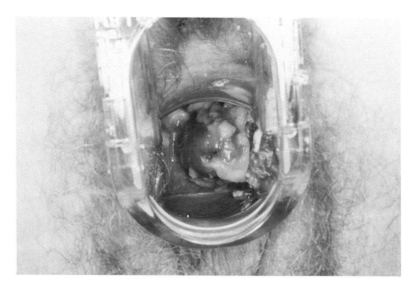

Figure 4.3. Vaginal candidosis: white cottage cheese—like discharge adheres to the vaginal wall and cervix.

a thick, cottage-cheese—like discharge which adheres to the vaginal wall and forms white, curdy patches (Figure 4.3). These patches are more common in pregnant women.[68] On rare occasions the discharge may be thin and watery, producing a white sheen on the vagina and vulva. Vulvar candidosis may extend to the adjacent skin (Figure 4.4) and concomitant perianal involvement as a papulopustular dermatitis may accompany vaginal lesions. Remote satellite lesions may be seen on

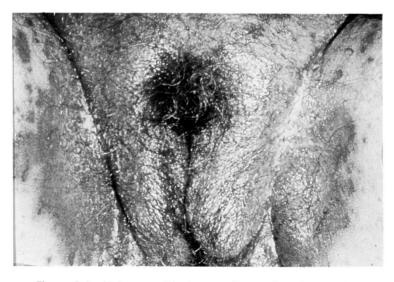

Figure 4.4. Vulvar candidosis extending to the adjacent skin.

the labia, inner thighs, or perineum. As in healthy women, the pH of vaginal secretion is less than 4.5, and the odor of vaginal fluid mixed with KOH is normal.

The clinical spectrum of candidal vulvovaginitis ranges from the typical presentation just described to minimal pruritus experienced by some patients prior to menstruation.

Complications

A rare complication of candidosis which may occur in immunocompromised patients is disseminated candidosis. The clinical triad of fever, rash, and muscle tenderness in immunocompromised patients receiving broad-spectrum antibiotics should alert the physician to possible disseminated candidosis. Immediate antifungal therapy should be considered since the complication is frequently fatal.[86]

There is a possibility that C. albicans may inhibit N. gonorrhoeae, impairing detection and confirmation of gonorrhea.[87,88] Failure to culture gonococci from women suspected of having gonorrhea should be considered a possible false-negative result if genital candidosis is present.

Diagnosis

Diagnosis of genital candidosis is established by clinical findings, laboratory tests, and exclusion of other causes of vulvovaginitis. Even though the clinical picture may be very suggestive for candidosis, the diagnosis on clinical grounds alone is generally unreliable and should be confirmed by demonstration of the pathogenic microorganism by laboratory tests.

Microscopic Examination

Potassium Hydroxide Preparation. Microscopic examination of vaginal discharge in wet mounts with 10 percent KOH allows the visualization of yeast forms and pseudohyphae (Figure 4.5). Potassium hydroxide dissolves epithelial and inflammatory cells, leaving behind fungal elements and making them easy to observe. The KOH solution destroys other elements and thus cannot be used for the diagnosis of conditions other than fungal infection.

Gram-stained smears. Candida may be visualized on Gram's staining where it appears as dense, gram-positive, ovoid bodies (Figure 4.6). Pseudohyphae can be seen as long, gram-positive tubes of the same diameter as the spores. The sensitivity of the Gram's stain is probably higher than that of the KOH test, but the latter method is more popular, especially among gynecologists, for rapid diagnosis of vaginal candidosis in the office. Gram-stained smears may also detect "clue cells" and N. gonorrhoeae but are not useful for detection of another frequent cause of vulvovaginitis—T. vaginalis.

Culture

Culture is the most sensitive and reliable method for identification of C. albicans both in symptomatic and asymptomatic women. It has been suggested that 40–60 percent of yeast infections in women would be missed if microscopic exami-

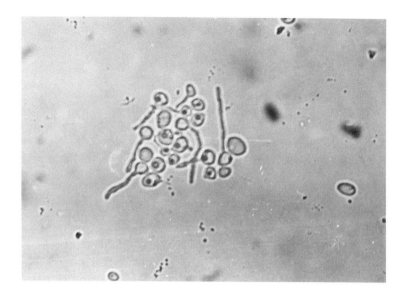

Figure 4.5. KOH preparation: *Candida* appears as oval cells with buds and pseudo-hyphae.

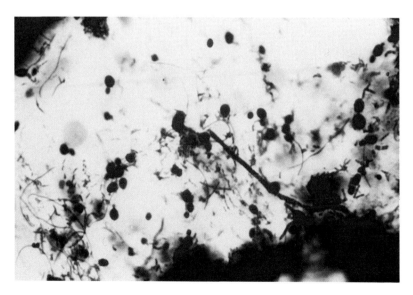

Figure 4.6. *Candida* in Gram-stained smear showing gram-positive oval cells, some of them budding.

nations alone were used.[89,90] The most reliable identification and differentiation of *Candida* species are provided by Sabouraud's dextrose agar and Neckerson's medium.[91] Culture does, however, have disadvantages: it is relatively expensive, and several days are needed to obtain the results. Other methods available but not routinely applied are

- Fluorescent antibody stains and enzyme-linked immunosorbent assay (ELISA).
- Latex agglutination test: This is a simple and rapid method and seems to be superior to microscopy for immediate diagnosis; it detects soluble cell wall antigens of *Candida* spp.[92]
- Serologic tests.
- Biopsy: This is taken mainly for scientific purposes, since *C. albicans* usually does not invade layers underneath the epithelium.

Differential Diagnosis

Even positive microscopic and culture results for *C. albicans* do not mean that *C. albicans* is the only cause of the disease. Other causes of vulvovaginitis or vaginal discharge should be ruled out (Table 4.4); these include trichomoniasis, bacterial vaginosis, and other bacterial genital infections such as gonococcal or chlamydial cervicitis. Secondary syphilis, genital herpes, and genital warts may be the cause of vaginal discharge or vulvitis as well. Other conditions that should be considered in the differential diagnosis include postmenopausal vaginitis and vaginal discharge due to foreign bodies, chemical irritants, douches, or deodorants.

TABLE 4.4. Helpful Diagnostic Features in the Differential Diagnosis of Vaginal Discharge

	Candida	Trichomonas	Bacterial	N. gonorrhoeae* and C. trachomatis*
Itching	+ + + +	+ / −	+ / −	+ / −
Vulvar sore, vaginal discomfort	+ + +	+ + + +	+ +	+
Odor	+	+ +	+ + + +	+
Dyspareunia	+ + +	+ + + +	+	+ / −
Relationship to menstrual cycle	+ + + +	−	−	−
Recent new sex partner	+	+ / −	−	+ + + +
Onset of symptoms related to systemic antibiotic use	+ + + +	−	−	−

Note: Presence of symptoms ranges from occasionally (+) to nearly always (+ + + +); − = no symptoms.
*Vaginal discharge secondary to cervicitis.

Treatment

The following are possible management regimens:

- *Miconazole nitrate:* 2 percent vaginal cream or 100 mg vaginal suppositories intravaginally once daily at bedtime for 7 days
- *Miconazole nitrate:* 200 mg suppositories intravaginally once daily at bedtime for 3 days
- *Clotrimazole:* 1 percent vaginal cream or 100 mg vaginal tablets intravaginally once daily at bedtime for 7–14 days
- *Clotrimazole:* 2 percent vaginal cream or 200 mg vaginal tablets intravaginally once daily at bedtime for 3 days
- *Terconazole* 80 mg vaginal suppository or 0.4% vaginal cream, intravaginally at bedtime for 3 days;
- *Butoconazole* nitrate 2% vaginal cream, intravaginally at bedtime for 3 days
- *Ketoconazole:* 200 mg (1 tablet) orally once daily for 7–14 days

Other regimens are available.[93-95]

Recurrences have been observed frequently in apparently adequately treated women. In these cases elimination of predisposing factors (control of diabetes mellitus, discontinuation of oral antibiotics or oral contraceptives[78,94] should be considered. Some authors recommend simultaneous treatment of male sexual partners[51] or oral administration of antifungals to prevent reinfection from the gastrointestinal tract.[95]

BACTERIAL VAGINOSIS

The term "bacterial vaginosis" (BV) is being used to designate a condition characterized by a gray, homogenous, odorous discharge with pH $\geq$ 5.0 from which neither *T. vaginalis* nor *C. albicans* can be recovered. The disease is characterized by an increased concentration of *G. vaginalis* and/or anaerobic bacteria as well as suppression of some components of the normal vaginal flora such as *Lactobacillus* species. Synonyms for bacterial vaginosis are nonspecific vaginosis, nonspecific vaginitis, Gardnerella vaginitis, Haemophilus vaginitis, and Corynebacterium vaginitis.

Etiology

The role of *G. vaginalis* as a primary or sole cause of BV is still controversial, although the microorganism (previously known as *Haemophilus vaginalis* or *Corynebacterium vaginale*) has been isolated from a high proportion of women with vaginitis[96-98] and has been found to be a predominant microorganism in women with bacterial vaginosis.[99-101]

Experimental intravaginal inoculation with vaginal material containing *G. vaginalis* resulted in clinical disease in 73 percent of cases and vaginal colonization in 100 percent of cases.[102] On the other hand, *G. vaginalis* has been recovered from healthy women with no evidence of vaginitis.[103-105] Many reports have suggested that anaerobic bacteria may play an important, if not predominant, role in the etiology of BV.[98,99,106] *Gardnerella vaginalis,* presumed to be sexually transmissible, may really constitute part of the normal flora of the reproductive tract,[107] and its association with the anaerobes might be the cause of BV.[98,99,108,109] The anaerobes might increase the pathogenic potential of *G. vaginalis* by interfering with phagocytic activity.[110] This seems likely and is a helpful explanation for the lack of one-to-one correlation of *G. vaginalis* with BV. Finally, recent reports suggest variations between strains of *G. vaginalis* as measured by the McCoy cell adherence test and indicate a possible role for adherent strains of *G. vaginalis* in the pathogenesis of BV.[111]

Whatever the relationship between *G. vaginalis* and abnormal vaginal discharge, it is clear that a syndrome associated with the microooorganism does exist. Further investigation will hopefully determine whether *G. vaginalis* acts as a marker indicating the presence of abnormal vaginal anaerobes, alters vaginal condition to enhance anaerobic growth, acts as a sole pathogen (perhaps only certain strains), or acts as a copathogen with other microorganisms.

Epidemiology

Bacterial vaginosis is not a reportable disease in the United States, but it seems that it is the common cause of abnormal discharge in women in this country.[2] *Gardnerella vaginalis* vaginosis is rarely seen in prepubertal girls[105,112] but frequently seen in adolescent women.[73,113,114] The reported incidence is higher in blacks,[103,113,115] in women of lower socioeconomic classes,[116] and in women who have multiple sex partners or an unstable martial situation.[113,116] The use of oral contraceptives[103,113] and the presence of other sexually transmitted diseases have been reported as risk factors too.[117,118] Sexual transmission of BV is a matter of controversy,[103] but a high prevalence of *G. vaginalis* among male partners of infected women has been reported.[98,102]

Clinical Manifestations

The incubation period is probably less than 7 days.[102,119] The chief symptom is odorous vaginal discharge, although a large proportion of women with BV may be asymptomatic.[120,121] Physical examination usually reveals homogeneous grayish discharge frequently adherent to the vaginal walls. The pH of vaginal fluid is elevated above normal range and is usually between 5.0 and 6.0. When the specimen of a discharge is mixed with 10 percent KOH a characteristic fishy odor is produced. It is thought that the diamines, putrescine and cadaverine are most responsible for this phenomenon.[106] Microscopic examination of a vaginal specimen mixed with saline shows characteristic "clue" cells. These are the epithelial cells that appear to be stippled or granular. The stippling or granularity is secondary to the adherence of *G. vaginalis* to the surface of the cell. Small, pleomorphic coccobacilli make up the predominant bacterial flora in the specimen. The paucity of polymorphonuclear leukocytes is one of the characteristic features of BV.

Bacterial vaginosis, although highly prevalent, is considered a minor disease.

However, the condition was associated with preterm, premature rupture of the membranes, preterm labor, and amniotic fluid infection.[122] Several severe infections associated with *G. vaginalis* have been also described, including puerperal fever and sepsis,[123,124] endometritis,[125,126] amniotic fluid infections,[125-127] and neonatal sepsis.[128] Anaerobes associated with vaginosis in pregnant females may also be significant in preterm, premature rupture of the membranes[129] and spontaneous preterm labor.[130]

Diagnosis

The diagnosis of BV is based on the presence of at least three of the following signs:

1. Odorous homogeneous, gray-white, adherent discharge
2. Vaginal fluid pH > 4.5
3. Amine (fishy) odor with KOH
4. Clue cells

True clue cells are epithelial cells which are so heavily stippled with bacteria that their borders are obscured. Cells with few bacteria and clear borders should not be identified as clue cells.

Clinical criteria may not be sufficient to establish diagnosis, and the following laboratory procedures have been used to support it:

1. Gram-stained smears: may reveal gram-negative small bacilli stippling epithelial cells; paucity of polymorphonuclears.
2. Wet-mount: may reveal paucity of polymorphonuclears and the presence of clue cells.
3. Papanicolaou's smear: may demonstrate *G. vaginalis*, but false positive results have been noted.[131]
4. Gas-liquid chromatography:[99,122,132] identifies microbial organic acid metabolites.
5. Culture: Casman's blood agar and other variations of blood agars and broths have been employed for the identification of *G. vaginalis*.[104,33] Since the genital tract is highly colonized with microorganisms, colistin, nalidixic acid, and amphotericin are usually added to the media to preclude growth of concomitant microorganisms. Since *G. vaginalis* is a facultative anaerobe, its isolation is enhanced by incubation in either a candle jar or a gas-pack system.[134]

Differential Diagnosis

Bacterial vaginosis should be distinguished from other diseases associated with vaginal discharge (Table 4.4, p. 96); these include vaginitis caused by *C. albicans* and *T. vaginalis* as well as postmenopausal vaginitis and vaginal discharge due to the presence of foreign bodies, chemical irritants, or douches.

TABLE 4.5. Comparison between Physiological Vaginal Secretion and Discharge Caused by BV

	Physiological Secretion	*BV*
Volume	Minimal	Moderate
Odor	Nonoffensive	Malodorous
Color	Whitish gray	Grayish
Consistency	Nonhomogeneous, floccular	Homogeneous
Adherence	Nonadherent	Adherent
Viscosity	High	Low
pH	≤4.5	≥5.0
"Clue" cells	Absent	Present
Lactobacillus spp.	Predominant	Absent or decreased
KOH test	Negative	Amine odor
Relationship to ovulation, menstruation, and pregnancy	Yes	No
Vulvar soreness	No	May occur

The following are common differential diagnoses:

- Vaginal discharge secondary to *cervical infection* with *N. gonorrhoeae* and *C. trachomatis* can be confirmed by Gram's stain cervical smears, cultures, or immunofluorescent techniques.
- Vaginal discharge secondary to *genital herpes* or *genital warts* can be distinguished by the presence of skin or mucosal lesions as well as positive Tzanck test and culture or DNA hybridization as well as histopathology.
- *Primary* and *secondary syphilis* may produce cervical or intravaginal lesions causing secondary discharge; serologic test may be positive; darkfield examination may reveal spirochetes.
- Normal vaginal secretions. With increased public interest in sexually transmitted diseases caused by the AIDS epidemic, one should anticipate an increased number of cases of *venerophobia*. Table 4.5 may be helpful in distinguishing BV from normal vaginal secretions.

Treatment

Patients should be treated with *metronidazole,* either 500 mg orally twice daily for 7 days or 2 g orally in a single dose. An alternative regimen for individuals for whom metronidazole is contraindicated (e.g., early pregnancy) is *clindamycin* 300 mg orally, 2 times a day for 7 days.

Management of Sex Partners

No clinical counterpart of BV is recognized in the male, and treatment of the male sexual partner has not been shown to be beneficial for the patient or the male partner.

REFERENCES

1. CDC, Nonreported sexually transmitted disease. *MMWR* 28:61, 1979.

2. Eschenbach DA: Vaginal infection. *Clin Obstet Gynecol* 26:186–202, 1983.

3. Freidrich EG, Siegesmund KA: Tampon-associated vaginal ulcerations. *Obstet Gynecol* 55:149–156, 1980.

4. Naseman T, Sauerbrey W, Burgdorf WHC: Fundamentals of dermatology. New York, Springer-Verlag, 1983, p. 156.

5. Ledger WJ: *Infection in the Female.* Philadelphia, Lea & Febiger, 1986, p. 139.

6. McMillan A: Vaginal discharge. *Br Med J* 293:1357–1360, 1986.

7. Honigberg BM: Comparative pathogenicity of *Trichomoniasis vaginalis and Trichomonas gallinae* to mice. I. Gross Pathology, quantitative evaluation of virulence and some factors affecting pathogenicity. *J Parasitol* 47:545–571, 1961.

8. Krieger JN, Poisson MA, Rein MF: Beta-hemolytic activity of *Trichomonas vaginalis* correlates with virulence. *Infect Immun* 41:1291–1295, 1983.

9. Keieger JN, Rein MF: Zinc sensitivity of *Trichomonas vaginalis:* In vitro studies and clinical implications. *J Infect Dis* 146:341–345, 1982.

10. Rasmussen SE, Nielsen MH, Lind I, et al: Morphological studies of the cytotoxicity of *Trichomonas vaginalis* to normal vaginal epithelial cells in vitro. *Genitourin Med* 62:240–246, 1986.

11. Krieger JN, Holmes KK, Spencer MR, et al: Geographic variation among isolates of *Trichomonas vaginalis:* Demonstration of antigenic heterogeneity by using monoclonal antibodies and the indirect immunofluorescence technique. *J Infect Dis* 152:979–984, 1985.

12. Osborne NG, Grubin L, Pratson L: Vaginitis in sexually active women: Relationship to nine sexually transmitted organisms. *Am J Obstet Gynecol* 142:962–967, 1982.

13. Feo LG: The incidence of *Trichomonas vaginalis* in the various age groups. *Am J Trop Med Hyg* 5:786–790, 1956.

14. Rein MF, Chapel TA: Trichomoniasis, candidiasis and the minor venereal disease. *Clin Obstet Gynecol* 18:73–88, 1975.

15. Krieger JN: Urologic aspects of trichomoniasis. *Invest Urol* 18:411–417, 1981.

16. Latif AS, Mason PR, Marowa E: Urethral trichomoniasis in men. *Sex Transm Dis* 14:9–11, 1987.

17. Mroczkowski TF: Post-gonococcal urethritis in men. II. Etiology and treatment. *Przegl Dermatol* 2:173–179, 1976.

18. McLellan R, Spence MR, Brockman M, et al: The clinical diagnosis of trichomoniasis. *Obstet Gynecol* 60:30–34, 1982.

19. Lossick JG: Treatment of *Trichomonas vaginalis* infections. *Rev Infect Dis* 4(Suppl):801–818, 1982.

20. Catterall RD: Trichomonal infections of the genital tract. *Med Clin North Am* 56:1203–1209, 1972.

21. Wiesner PJ: Magnitude of the problem of sexually transmitted diseases in the United States, in: *Sexually Transmitted Disease, 1980 Status Report,* Washington DC, NIAID Study Group, 1981, p. 21.

22. Honinberg BM: Trichomonads of importance in human medicine, in Krieger JP (ed): *Parasitic Protozoa,* New York, Academic Press, 1978, Vol. 2.

23. Jirovec O, Petru M: *Trichomonas vaginalis* and trichomoniasis. *Adv Parasitol* 6:117–118, 1968.

24. Catterall RD, Nicol CS: Is trichomonal infestation a venereal disease? *Br Med J* 1:1177–1179, 1960.

25. Paulson J, Leto S, Asmar P: *Trichomonas vaginalis* in human reproduction, in Keith LK, Berger GS, Edelman DA (eds): *Infections in Reproductive Health, Vol. 1, Common Infections.* Lancaster, England, MTP Press, 1985, p. 137.

26. Sherman K, Daling JR, Weiss NS; Sexually transmitted diseases and tubal infertility. *Sex Transm Dis* 14:12–16, 1987.

27. Mardh P-A, Westrom L: Tubal and cervical cultures in acute salpingitis with special reference to *Mycoplasma hominis* and T. strain mycoplasmas. *Br J Vener Dis* 46:179–186, 1970.

28. Keith LG, Friberg J, Fullan N, et al: The possible role of *Trichomonas vaginalis* as a "vector" for the spread of other pathogens. *Int J Fertil* 31:272–277, 1986.

29. Frost JK; *Trichomonas vaginalis* and cervical epithelial changes. *Ann NY Acad Sci* 97:792–799, 1962.

30. Ovcinnikow NM, Delektorskij VV, Turanova EN, et al: Further studies of *Trichomonas vaginalis* with transmission and scanning electron microscopy. *Br J Vener Dis* 51:357–375, 1975.

31. Spence MR, Hollander DH, Smith J, et al: The clinical and laboratory diagnosis of *Trichomonas vaginalis* infection. *Sex Transm Dis* 7:168–171, 1980.

32. Chang TH, Tsing SY, Tzeng S: Monclonal antibodies against *Trichomonas vaginalis*. *Hybridoma* 5:43–51, 1986.

33. Krieger JN, Tam MR, Stevens CE, et al: Diagnosis of trichomoniasis. Comparison of conventional wet-mount examination with cytologic studies, culture and monoclonal antibody staining of direct specimens. *JAMA* 259:1223–1227, 1988.

34. Hipp SS, Kirkwood MW, Gaafar HA: Screening for *Trichomonas vaginalis* infection by use of acridine orange fluorescent microscopy. *Sex Transm Dis* 6:235–238, 1979.

35. Brady KW, Paine DD, Frye LP, et al: Evaluation of new plastic envelope microbiology (PEM) methods of adjuncts in the diagnosis of *Candida albicans* and *Trichomonas vaginalis* vaginitis. *Milit Med* 151:478–480, 1986.

36. Diamond LS: The establishment of various trichomonads of animals and man in axenic cultures. *J Parasitol* 43:488–490, 1957.

37. Kuberski T: Evaluation of the indirect hemagglutination technique for study of *Trichomonas vaginalis* infections, particularly in men. *Sex Transm Dis* 5:97–102, 1978.

38. Street DA, Taylor-Robinson D, Ackers JP: Evaluation of an enzyme-linked immunosorbent assay for detection of antibody to *Trichomonas vaginalis* sera and vaginal secretions. *Br J Vener Dis* 58:330–333, 1982.

39. Sweet RL, Gibbs RS: Infectious vulvovaginitis, in: *Infectious Disease of the Female Genital Tract.* Baltimore, Williams & Wilkins, 1985, Chap. 6, p. 89.

40. Ray DK, Tendulkar JS, Shrivastova VB, et al: A metronidazole-resistant strain of *Trichomonas vaginalis* and its sensitivity to Go 10213. *J Antimicrob Chemother* 14:423–426, 1984.

41. Krajden S, Lossick JG, Wilk E, et al: Persistent *Trichomonas vaginalis* infection due to a metronidazole-resistant strain. *Can Med Assoc J* 134:1373–1374, 1986.

42. Rein MF; Current therapy of vulvovaginitis. *Sex Transm Dis* 8:316–320, 1981.

43. U.S. Public Health Service CDC: STD treatment guidelines. 1985. Atlanta, pp 25–26.

44. Rodin P, Hass G: Metronidazole and pregnancy. *Br J Vener Dis* 42:210–212, 1966.

45. McCormack WM: Management of sexually transmittable infections during pregnancy. *Clin Obstet Gynecol* 18:57–71, 1975.

46. Felman YM, Nikitas JA: Trichomoniasis, Candidiasis and *Corynebacterium vaginale* vaginitis. *NY State J Med* 79:1563–1566, 1979.

47. Odds FC: *Candida and Vaginal Candidosis.* Baltimore, University Park Press, 1979.

48. Hurley R, Leask B, Faktor JA, et al: Incidence and distribution of yeast species and of *Trichomonas vaginalis* in the vagina of pregnant women. *J Obstet Gynaecol Br Com W,* 80:252–257, 1973.

49. Willmott FE: Genital yeasts in female patients attending a VD clinic. *Br J Vener Dis* 51:119–122, 1975.

50. Oriel JD, Patridge BM, Denny MJ, et al: Genital yeast infections. *Br Med J* 4:761–764, 1972.

51. Merkus JM, Bisschop MP, Stolte LAM: The proper nature of vaginal candidosis and the problem of recurrence. *Obstet Gynecol Surv* 40:493–504, 1985.

52. Goldacre MJ, Watt B, Loudon N, et al: Vaginal microbial flora in normal young women. *Br Med J* 1:1450–1453, 1979.

53. Thin RN, Rendell P, Wadsworth J: How often are gonorrhea and genital yeast infection sexually transmitted? *Br J Vener Dis* 55:278–280, 1979.

54. Persson K, Persson K, Hansson H, et al: Prevalence of nine different microorganisms in the female genital tract: A comparison between women from a venereal disease clinic and from a health control department. *Br J Vener Dis* 55:429–433, 1979.

55. NIAID Study Group: *Sexually Transmitted Diseases: 1980 Status Report.* Washington DC, U.S. Government Printing Office, 1981, pp. 181–193 and 249–254.

56. Masteron G, Sengupta SM, Schofield CBS: Natamycin in genital candidosis in men. *Br J Vener Dis* 51:210–212, 1975.

57. Rodin P, Kolator B: Carriage of yeasts on the penis. *Br Med J* 1:1123–1124, 1976.

58. Diddle AW, Gardner WH, Williamson PJ, et al: Oral contraceptives, medications and vulvovaginal candidiasis. *Obstet Gynecol* 34:373–377, 1969.

59. Thin RN, Leighton M, Dixon MJ: How often is genital yeast infection sexually transmitted? *Br Med J* 2:93–94, 1977.

60. Warnock DW, Speller DCE, Milne JD, et al: Epidemiological investigation of patients with vulvovaginal candidiasis. *Br J Vener Dis* 55:357–361, 1979.

61. White W, Spencer-Phillips PJ: Recurrent vaginitis and oral sex. *Lancet* 1:621, 1979.

62. Oates JK: Recurrent vaginitis and oral sex. *Lancet* 1:785, 1979.

63. Morton RS, Rashid S: Cadidal vaginitis: Natural history, predisposing factors and prevention. *Proc Med* 70(Suppl 4):3–13, 1977.

64. Hurley R, deLouvois J: *Candida* vaginitis. *Postgrad Med J* 55:645–647, 1979.

65. Miles RM, Olsen L, Rogers A: Recurrent vaginal candidiasis: Importance of an intestinal reservoir. *JAMA* 238:1036–1037, 1977.

66. Hilton AL, Warnock DW: Vaginal candidiasis and the role of the digestive tract as a source of infection. *Br J Obstet Gynecol* 82:922–926, 1975.

67. Elegbe IA, Botu M: A preliminary study on dressing patterns and incidence of candidiasis. *Am J Public Health* 72:176–177, 1982.

68. Felman YM, Nikitas JA: Genital candidiasis. *Cutis* 31:369–382, 1983.

69. Dwyer JM: Chronic mucocutaneous candidiasis. *Ann Rev Med* 32:491–497, 1981.

70. Syverson RE, Buckley H, Givian J, et al: Cellular and humoral immune status in women with chronic *Candida* vaginitis. *Am J Obstet Gynecol* 134:624–627, 1979.

71. Mathur SM, Virella G, Koistinen J, et al: Humoral immunity in vaginal candidiasis. *Infect Immunol* 15:287–294, 1980.

72. Brunham RC, Martin DH, Hubbard TW, et al: Depression of the lymphocyte transformation response to microbial antigens and to phytohemagglutinin during pregnancy. *J Clin Invest* 72:1629–1638, 1983.

73. Paavonen J, Heinonen PK, Aine R, et al: Prevalence of nonspecific vaginitis and other cervicovaginal infections during the third trimester of pregnancy. *Sex Transm Dis* 12:5–8, 1986.

74. Carrol CJ, Hurley R, Stanley VC: Criteria for diagnosis of *Candida* vulvovaginitis in pregnant women. *J Obstet Gynaecol Br Com W* 80:258–263, 1973.

75. Hopsu-Havu VK, Gronroos M, Punnonen R: Vaginal yeasts in parturients and infestation of the newborns. *Acta Obstet Gynecol Scand* 59:73–77, 1980.

76. Gilgor RS: Cutaneous infections in diabetes mellitus, in Jelinek JE (ed): *The Skin in Diabetes*. Philadelphia, Lea & Febiger, 1986, pp. 111–132.

77. Sonck CE, Semersalo O: The yeast flora of the anogenital region in diabetic girls. *Arch Dermatol* 88:846–852, 1963.

78. Vallance-Owen J: Diabetes mellitus. *Br J Dermatol* 81(Suppl 2):9–13, 1969.

79. Bagdade JD: Infection in diabetes. *Postgrad Med* 59:160–164, 1976.

80. Bramley M, Kinghorn G: Do oral contraceptives inhibit *Trichomonas vaginalis*. *Sex Transm Dis* 6:261–263, 1979.

81. Oriel JD, Waterwarth PM; Effect of minocycline and tetracycline on the vaginal yeast flora. *J Clin Pathol* 218:403–406, 1975.

82. Caruso LJ: Vaginal moniliasis after tetracycline therapy. *Am J Obstet Gynecol* 90:374–378, 1964.

83. Bisschop MP, Merkus MJ, Van Cutsem J: The influence of antibiotics on the growth of *Candida albicans* in the vagina: An experiment with vaginal fluid. *Eur J Obstet Gynecol Reprod Biol* 20:113–119, 1985.

84. Gough PM, Warnock DW, Turner A, et al: Candidosis in the genital tract in nonpregnant women. *Eur J Obstet Gynecol Reprod Biol* 19:237–246, 1985.

85. Gardner HL, Kaufman RH: Candidiasis, in *Benign Diseases of the Vulva and Vagina*. Boston, G.K. Hall Medical Publishers, 1981, chap. 12.

86. Jacobs MI, Magid MS, Jarowski CI: Disseminated candidiasis. *Arch Dermatol* 116:1277–1279, 1980.

87. Hipp SS, Lawton WD, Chen NC, et al: Inhibition of *Neisseria gonorrhoeae* by factor produced by *Candida albicans*. *Appl Microbiol* 27:192–196, 1974.

88. Wallin J, Gnarpe H: Possible inhibition on *N. gonorrhoeae* by *C. albicans*. *Br J Vener Dis* 51:174–175, 1975.

89. Burgess SG, Manusco PG, Kalish PE, et al: Clinical and laboratory study on vaginitis. Evaluation of diagnostic methods and results of treatment. *NY State J Med* 15:2086–2091, 1970.

90. O'Connor BH, Adler MW: Current approaches to the diagnosis, treatment and reporting of trichomoniasis and candidiasis. *Br J Vener Dis* 55:52–57, 1979.

91. Martius J, Hartman AA: Untersuchungen zur Nachweissicherheit und Haufigkeit genitaler Mykosen bei Schwangeren. *Z Geburtshife Perinatol* 187:121–123, 1983.

92. Rajakumar R, Lacey CJN, Evans EGV, et al: Use of slide latex agglutination test for rapid diagnosis of vaginal candidosis, *Genitourin Med* 63:192–195, 1987.

93. Fregoso-Duenas F: Ketoconazole in vulvovaginal candidosis. *Rev Infect Dis* 2:620–622, 1980.

94. Sobel JD: Management of recurrent vulvovaginal candidiasis with intermittent ketoconazole prophylaxis. *Obstet Gynecol* 65:435–440, 1985.

95. Ledger WJ: *Infection in the Female.* Philadelphia, Lea & Febiger, 1986, p. 127.

96. Gardner HL, Dampeer TK, Dukes CD: The prevalence of vaginitis: A study in incidence. *Am J Obstet Gynecol* 73:1080–1087, 1957.

97. Akerlund M, Mardh P-A: Isolation and identification of *Corynebacterium vaginale* (*Haemophilus vaginalis*) in women with infections of the lower genital tract. *Acta Obstet Gynecol Scand* 53:85–90, 1974.

98. Pfeifer TA, Forsyth PS, Durfee MA, et al: Nonspecific vaginitis: Role of *Haemophilus vaginalis* and treatment with metronidazole. *N Engl J Med* 298:1429–1434, 1978.

99. Spiegel CA, Amsel R, Eschenbach D, et al: Anaerobic bacteria in nonspecific vaginitis. *N Engl J Med* 303:601–607, 1980.

100. Eschenbach DA, Critchlow CW, Watkins H, et al: A dose-duration study of metronidazole for the treatment of nonspecific vaginosis. *Scand J Infect Dis* 40(Suppl):73–80, 1983.

101. Blackwell AI, Fox AR, Phillips I, et al: Anaerobic vaginosis (non-specific vaginitis): Clinical, microbiological and therapeutic findings. *Lancet* 2:1379–1383, 1983.

102. Gardner HL, Dukes CD: *Haemophilus vaginalis* vaginitis: A newly defined specific infection previously classified "nonspecific" vaginitis. *Am J Obstet Gynecol* 69:962–976, 1955.

103. McCormack WM, Hayes CH, Rosner B, Vaginal colonization with *Corynebacterium vaginale* (*Haemophilus vaginalis*). *J Infect Dis* 136:740–745, 1977.

104. Dunkelberg WE: *Corynebacterium vaginale. Sex Transm Dis* 4:69–75, 1977.

105. Gardner HL: *Haemophilus vaginalis* vaginitis after twenty-five years. *Am J Obstet Gynecol* 137:385–391, 1980.

106. Chen KCS, Forsyth PS, Buchanan TM, et al: Amine content of vaginal fluid from untreated and treated patients with non-specific vaginitis. *J Clin Invest* 63:828–835, 1979.

107. Tashjian JH, Coulam CB, Washington JA: Vaginal flora in asymptomatic women. *Mayo Clin Prac* 51:557–561, 1976.

108. Taylor E, Barlow D, Blackwell AL, et al: *Gardnerella vaginalis,* anaerobes and vaginal discharge. *Lancet* 1:1376–1379, 1982.

109. Hill LVH: Anaerobes and *Gardnerella vaginalis* in non-specific vaginitis. *Genitourin Med* 61:114–119, 1985.

110. Ingham HR, Tharagonnet D, Sisson PR, et al: Inhibition of phagocytosis in vitro by obligate anaerobes. *Lancet* 2:1252–1254, 1977.

111. Scott TG, Smyth CJ, Keane CT: In vitro adhesiveness and biotype of *Gardnerella vaginalis* strains in relation to the occurrence of clue cells in vaginal discharges. *Genitourin Med* 63:47–53, 1987.

112. Hammerschlag MR, Alpert S, Rosner I, et al: Microbiology of the vagina in children: Normal and potentially pathogenic organisms. *Pediatrics* 62:57–62, 1978.

113. Josey WE, Lambe DW Jr: Epidemiologic characteristics of women infected with *Corynebacterium vaginale* (*Haemophilus vaginalis*). *J Am Vener Dis Assoc* 3:9–13, 1976.

114. Rodgers HA, Hesse FE, Pulley HC, et al: *Haemophilus vaginalis* (*Corynebacterium vaginale*) vaginitis in women attending public health clinics: Response to treatment with ampicillin. *Sex Transm Dis* 5:18–21, 1978.

115. Lewis JF, O'Brien SM: Incidence of *Haemophilus vaginalis. Am J Obstet Gynecol* 103:843–846, 1969.

116. Felamn YM, Nikitas JA: *Gardnerella vaginalis* vaginitis. Newsletter, New York City Bureau of Disease Control. *Sex Transm Dis* 5:1, 1982.

117. Dunkelberg WE, Skaggs R, Kellogg DS, et al: Relative incidence of *Corynebacterium vaginale (Haemophilus vaginalis), Neisseria gonorrhoeae* and *Trichomonas* spp. among women attending a venereal disease clinic. *Br J Vener Dis* 46:187–190, 1970.

118. Mohanty KC, Deighton R: Comparison of two different metronidazole regimens in the treatment of *Gardnerella vaginalis* infection with or without trichomoniasis. *J Antimicrob Chemother* 16:799–803, 1985.

119. Criswell BS, Ladwig CHL, Gardner HL, et al: *Haemophilus vaginalis:* Vaginitis by inoculation from culture. *Obstet Gynecol* 33:195–199, 1969.

120. Amsel R, Totten PA, Spiegel CA, et al: Nonspecific vaginitis: Diagnostic critieria and microbial and epidemiological associations. *Am J Med* 74:14–22, 1983.

121. Embree J, Caliando JJ, McCormack WM: Nonspecific vaginitis among women attending a sexually transmitted disease clinic. *Sex Transm Dis* 11:81–84, 1984.

122. Gravett MG, Nelson HP, DeRouen T, et al: Independent association of bacterial vaginosis and *Chlamydia trachomatis* infection with adverse pregnancy outcome. *JAMA* 256:1899–1903, 1986.

123. Edmunds PN: Haemophilus vaginalis: Its association with puerperal pyrexia and leukorrhea. *J Obstet Gynaec Brit Emp* 66:917–926, 1959.

124. Regamey C, Schoenknecht FD: Puerperal fever with *Haemophilus vaginalis* septicemia. *JAMA* 225:1621–1623, 1973.

125. Platt MS: Neonatal *Haemophilus vaginalis (Corynebacterium vaginalis)* infection. *Clin Pediatr* 10:513–516, 1971.

126. Eschenbach DA, Gravett MG, Chen KCS, et al: Bacterial vaginosis during pregnancy: An association with prematurity and postpartum complications, in Mardh P-A, Taylor-Robinson D (eds): *Bacterial Vaginosis.* Stockholm, Almqvist and Wiksell International, 1984, p. 214.

127. Gravett MG, Eschenbach DA, Spiegel-Brown CA, et al: Rapid diagnosis of amniotic-fluid infection by gas-liquid chromatography. *N Engl J Med* 306:725–728, 1982.

128. Chow AW, Leake RD, Yamauchi T, et al: The significance of anaerobes in neonatal bacteremia: Analysis of 23 cases and review of the literature. *Pediatrics* 54:736–745, 1974.

129. Minkoff H, Grunebaum AN, Schwartz RH: Risk factors of prematurity and premature rupture of membranes: A prospective study of vaginal flora in pregnancy. *Am J Obstet Gynecol* 150:965–972, 1984.

130. Wahbeh CJ, Hale GB, Eden RD, et al: Intra-amniotic bacterial colonization in premature labor. *Am J Obstet Gynecol* 148:739–742, 1984.

131. Smith RF, Rodgers HA, Hines PA, et al: Comparison between direct microscopic and cultural methods for recognition of *Corynebacterium vaginale* in women with vaginitis. *J Clin Microbiol* 5:268–272, 1977.

132. Jokipii AMM, Jokipii L, Vesterinen E, et al: Volatile fatty acid findings in vaginal fluid compared with symptoms, signs, other laboratory results and susceptibility to tinidazole of malodorous vaginal discharges. *Genitourin Med* 62:102–106, 1986.

133. Totten PA, Amsel R, Hale J, et al: Selective differential human blood bilayer media for isolation of *Gardnerella (Haemophilus) vaginalis. J Clin Microbiol* 15:141–147, 1982.

134. Malone BH, Schreiber M, Schneider NJ, et al: Obligately anaerobic strains of *Corynebacterium vaginale (Haemophilus vaginalis). J Clin Microbiol* 2:272–275, 1975.

5

GENITAL HERPES

Genital herpes is a sexually transmitted disease caused by herpes simplex virus type 2 (HSV-2) and, less often, type 1 (HSV-1). Initial exposure to the virus usually produces acute disease characterized by eruption of grouped small vesicles on an erythematous base, but it may also be asymptomatic. After initial infection, the virus becomes latent and the patient is at risk for recurrence of the disease. Pregnant females may transmit the virus to the newborn usually during the passage through the contaminated birth canal.

ETIOLOGY

Herpes simplex virus occurs as two distinct but antigenically related serotypes, HSV-1 and HSV-2. Their genomes have approximately 50 percent DNA homology, and they are much more closely related to each other than any other herpesviruses, but also they are sufficiently different to endow each type with unique biological properties and to allow their differentiation by serologic, immunologic, and biochemical means. HSV is a member of the family *Herpesviridae*, which includes type 1 and 2 HSV, the varicella-zoster virus, the cytomegalovirus, the Epstein-Barr virus, and recently discovered human herpes virus 6 (HHV-6) and simian herpes B virus (Table 5.1). These viruses are large and contain double-stranded linear DNA. Their structure consists of a DNA core surrounded by a capsid consisting of a series of protein layers (capsomers), a fibrillous tegument, and a membranous envelope with protein spikes (Figure 5.1).

Restriction enzyme analysis of HSV-1 and HSV-2 has shown that there is an enormous strain variation and that there are different strains of each type. It has been also found that one patient may be infected at similar sites with more than one type of HSV and/or with more than one strain and may experience periodic recurrences from each of them separately.[1-3]

EPIDEMIOLOGY

Genital herpes is not a reportable disease in the United States and there are no accurate data on incidence. Estimates from the CDC demonstrate that, from 1966

107

TABLE 5.1. Members of the Herpesviridae Family Pathogenic to Humans

Herpes simplex virus types 1 and 2
Varicella-zoster virus
Cytomegalovirus
Epstein-Barr virus
Human herpes virus-6
Simian herpes B virus

to 1984, there was over a 15-fold increase to 450,000 private physician visits resulting from genital herpes in 1984 and a slight decrease in the following years (Figure 5.2).[4] Data from different countries indicate that genital herpes has been increasing in prevalence over the last decade.[5-8] This phenomenon is probably not only due to the real increase in prevalence but also to increasing recognition of the disease.

Genital herpes has been found in all socioeconomic groups, with highest prevalence in the 15–29-year-old age group. It is frequently associated with other sexually transmitted diseases (STDs); it is slightly more prevalent among whites than blacks and among married than single people; and it is frequently seen in middle- and upper-class young adults.[9-13] These variations, however, may change with the time period and population studied.

Genital herpes is transmitted primarily by sexual intercourse. However, investigators documented the survival of the virus in a moist environment.[14] They have suggested that fomites might serve as a source for nonvenereal transmission of HSV, but whether this finding is of any epidemiological importance is not known at this time.

Genital herpes may be caused by either type of herpes simplex virus, but HSV-2 has been found more frequently in genital lesions, whereas HSV-1 has been isolated mainly from oral-facial lesions. Determination of the HSV type in genital infection may have prognostic as well as epidemiologic value. Genital herpes is a recurrent disease, and the frequency of recurrences has been observed more often (threefold to fourfold) with HSV-2 infections than with HSV-1 infections.[13,15,16]

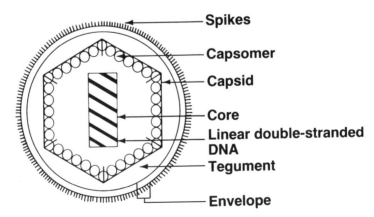

Figure 5.1. Schematic model of herpes simplex virus.

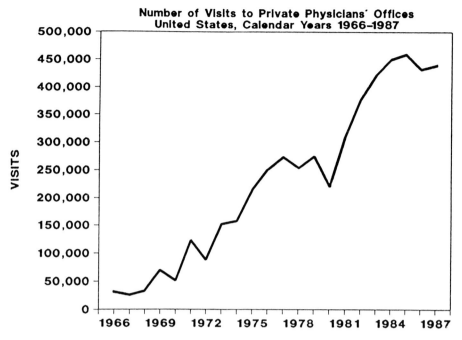

Figure 5.2. Incidence of genital herpes simplex virus infections.

One explanation for this could be the fact that the primary first episode is caused more often by HSV-1, which might indicate the protective effect of prior HSV-1 labial infection.[17]

Immunology

The epidemiology of HSV infection is also influenced by a number of immune factors, and both humoral and cell-mediated immunity is involved. The antibody response is similar to that observed in other viral infections, where persons infected with the virus develop IgM antibodies followed by IgG and IgA. The role of antibodies in resolving the infection or in control of the frequencies of recurrences is rather insignificant, and it seems that the cell-mediated immunity plays a much more important role in the pathogenesis of herpetic infections. Persons with congenital, acquired, or iatrogenically induced cellular immunodeficiencies have more severe and more prolonged infections and more frequent recurrences.[17-20] Periodic deficiencies of cell-mediated immunity have been associated with recurrent herpes in otherwise healthy individuals,[21] and administration of immunosuppressive drugs in patients with organ transplants made them more susceptible to herpes virus infections.[22]

Even though cell-mediated immunity can limit infection, it does not prevent the development of latency and has little effect on subsequent reactivation of the virus.

Many other factors have been investigated, including natural killer cell activities, antibody dependent and independent cytotoxicity, leukocyte migration inhibitory factors, and the role of interferons.[21,23-25] Unfortunately, the pathogenic importance of these observations is still unclear.

CLINICAL FEATURES

The clinical manifestation of genital herpes occurs as three distinct syndromes: (1) first episode, primary; (2) first episode, nonprimary; and (3) recurrent.

First Episode, Primary Genital Herpes

The first episode, primary is the initial infection with HSV in a patient without circulating antibodies to either HSV-1 or HSV-2. The incubation period for both HSV-1 and HSV-2 is 2–7 days, and the first episode, primary is usually associated with systemic and local symptoms. Systemic symptoms include chills and low-grade fever, nausea, malaise, headache, and generalized myalgias. These symptoms are probably related to the transient viremia and introduction of the virus to the central nervous system or to the toxic metabolites, of viral infection; however, the cause is not absolutely understood. Local symptoms include a burning sensation or mild paresthesias and rarely pain at the site of inoculation. As the disease develops, grouped, multiple, small vesicles appear on an erythematous base which after 3–5 days develop into painful shallow ulcers that subsequently crust. In moist areas, for example, on the glans of the penis, on the inner aspect of the prepuce of uncircumcized men, or on the labia minora in women, the vesicles erode faster (within 1–2 days), whereas in drier places of the skin they may persist longer. Occasionally, lesions coalesce to form larger bullae or more irregular ulcerations which involve extensive areas of the skin or mucous membranes.

With the appearance of the vesicles, pain and tenderness become more prominent, and the severity of local symptoms reaches its peak between 8 and 10 days, gradually receding over the second week of illness. In some patients, especially women, where vulvar lesion may be associated with considerable erythema and edema, walking may be difficult, and women with such involvement often walk with a straddling gait. Because of the spread of the virus to lymphatic nodes, they become enlarged and tender, and about half of the patients complain of inguinal pain. Pelvic pain has been reported with the involvement of pelvic lymph nodes. Adenopathy appears usually during the second week of disease and may be the last manifestation to resolve.

The lesions of the first primary episode are generally present for 2–4 weeks. During this time, new vesicles may appear after the initial crop of vesicles. In some patients, the true primary infection may cause extensive cutaneous vesiculation that may involve the entire penis or vulva as well as adjacent areas of the skin in groins and thighs. In most instances, the lesions heal without scarring within 4 weeks, and if they persist longer, one must think of secondary infection or underlying immunosuppression.

In men, the lesions of genital herpes are found most frequently on the prepuce, glans, and shaft of the penis (Figures 5.3 and 5.4). Herpetic balanitis, balanoposthitis, as well as urethritis are not uncommon. Herpetic vesicles and erosions may occur in the urinary meatus and cause severe dysuria. Urethritis is infrequently seen in initial genital infections, and the symptoms may precede by 2–4 days the onset of genital lesions. Severe dysuria, out of proportion to the urethral discharge which is usually scanty and mucoid, is characteristic for urethritis caused by HSV. Etiology of urethritis can be confirmed by the isolation of the virus from urethral

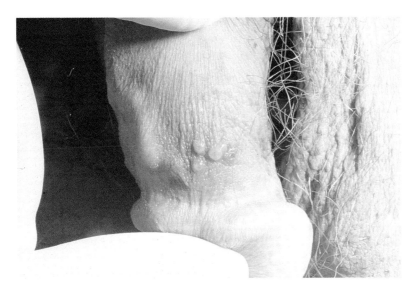

Figure 5.3. Genital herpes: vesicle on the skin of the penis.

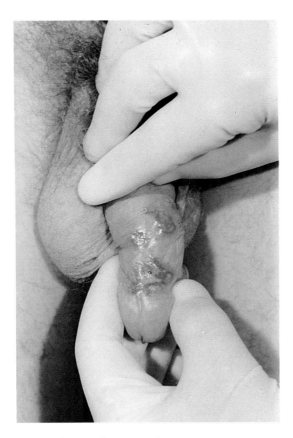

Figure 5.4. Erosive lesion on the penis caused by HSV-2.

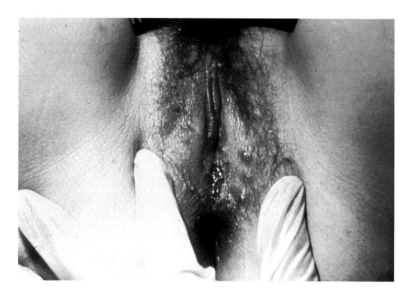

Figure 5.5. Vesicular lesion caused by HSV-2 in woman.

specimens. HSV has also been isolated from the prostate and seminal vesicles, which may indicate ascending infection, which originated in the urethra.[26]

In homosexual men, herpetic infection may affect the anus and perianal area. In most instances of anal herpes, there is a history of anal intercourse. This statement applies to both homosexual men as well as to heterosexual women. Anorectal herpes is characterized by anal vesicles and/or erosions. Rectal itching, pain, difficulty with bowel movement, and sacral paresthesias have been reported. Proctitis is usually associated with anal pain, and tenesmus and may be accompanied by purulent anal discharge.[27,28]

In women, the first episode of primary herpes infection causes severe vulvovaginitis. The lesions usually involve the labia majora, labia minora, cervix, and rarely the vagina (Figure 5.5). Disease is characterized by intense genital edema with extensive vesiculation and/or erosions (Figure 5.6). Women seem to have more discomfort than men, probably because of the larger surface area of involvement with coalesced lesions and possible involvement of the vagina and cervix. Some women complain of extremely painful urination. Paresis of the bladder and urinary retention may occur.[29] Lesions on the cervix may present as diffuse or focal erythema and friability, superficial erosions, or sometimes extensive necrotic cervicitis. A variant, seen mostly in women, is lumbosacral herpes, in which lesions appear on the low back, buttocks, or thighs (Figure 5.7). It seems that these lesions develop by autoinoculation rather than viremic spread or as a primary site of infection; however, it is not entirely clear. Other extragenital lesions may occur on fingers, arms, eyes, and rarely on the other parts of the body.

HSV can cause pharyngitis, especially in individuals practicing orogenital intercourse and regardless of their sex or sexual orientation. The clinical picture of such pharyngitis is similar to that seen in streptococcal infection. Patients develop sore throat with fever, malaise, and muscle aches. Vesicles, ulcerations, plus tender cervical lymphadenopathy may be present. Herpetic pharyngitis may occur as a

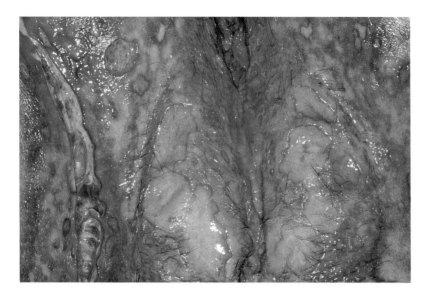

Figure 5.6. Extensive lesions in the vulva caused by HSV infection.

sole infection or may accompany genital lesions. Isolation of HSV from the posterior pharynx confirms the diagnosis.[13]

Asymptomatic primary infection has been documented, but the incidence is difficult to determine.[13,17,30,31] Certain groups of patients with their first episode of genital herpes have serologic evidence suggesting previous, probably asymptomatic infection either with HSV-1 or HSV-2. Asymptomatic infection can be also documented by the isolation of the virus from asymptomatic carriers, mostly women.[13,32]

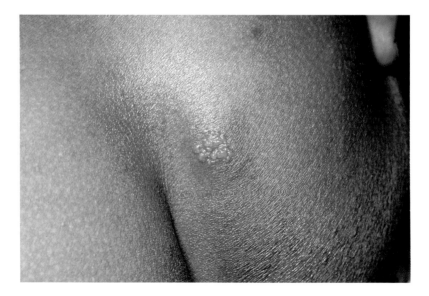

Figure 5.7. Herpetic lesions on the buttock.

First Episode, Nonprimary Genital Herpes

First episode, nonprimary genital herpes occurs in patients with circulating antibodies to HSV. The clinical course of the disease is similar to that seen in recurrent genital herpes. Patients with a nonprimary first episode usually do not develop constitutional symptoms and have fewer complications, but the rate of recurrences seems to be the same.[13]

Recurrent Genital Herpes

Primary HSV infection is often followed by latency of the virus. Animal experiments indicate that, after inoculation of the epithelium HSV spreads along the sensory nerves to the regional sensory ganglia. In the case of genital herpes, the spread is usually, but not always, to the sacral ganglia (S_2 to S_4) (Figure 5.8). This latent infection persists in the presence of humoral antibodies and sensitized lymphocytes. It is not clear why some individuals reactivate the virus and others do not. Most recurrences appear to be due to endogenous reactivation of the virus. At the present time, there are two main theories for the viral reactivation and recrudescences of the disease.[33] The "ganglionic trigger" theory suggests that a

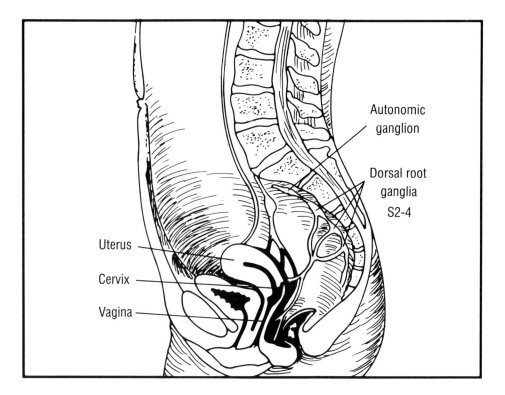

Figure 5.8. Sacral ganglia and autonomic ganglion are probably the most common reservoirs of latent HSV-2 infection.

TABLE 5.2.   Factors Precipitating Recurrent Herpes

Systemic
  Menstruation
  Fatigue
  Emotional stress
  Bacterial or viral disease
  Immunosuppressive drugs
  Malignancies
Local
  Skin trauma
  Chemical burn or irritation
  Sunburn
  Epilation
  Dermabrasion
  Ganglion manipulation
  Application of retinoic acid
  Application of prostaglandin E_2

stimulus (hormonal, physical, immunologic, etc.) affects the interaction between the host's ganglion cell and the virus and reactivates it (unknown mechanism), making the virus travel down the peripheral nerve to the epidermal cell, where it produces characteristic skin lesions. The "skin trigger theory" proposes that a small amount of virus is being produced continuously in the ganglion and reaches the skin cell via nerves, where it establishes microfoci of infection eliminated by a host defense mechanism. Temporary suppression of the local defense mechanism precipitates the reappearance of the skin lesions (Table 5.2). There is evidence supporting and contradicting both theories, and the problem is still unsolved. Since many of the agents "reactivating" latency produce an increased level of prostaglandins in the skin, it was suggested that the prostaglandins may be the important factor in reactivating HSV infection;[34,35] but whether they act by local immunosuppression or affect the virus in the ganglions is unknown as yet.[36,37]

Recurrent disease caused by HSV-2 occurs in about two thirds of cases following the first episode. The frequency of recurrent genital herpes is higher shortly after the primary infection, and the episodes of recurrences decrease in severity and frequency with time. A patient who has recurrences of the disease at 1-month intervals during the first year may have episodes at 3- and 6-month intervals during the second and third years. However, the course of recurrent herpes is, frankly speaking, unpredictable. A patient who had 3 or 4 recurrences at 2-week intervals may be symptom-free for the next several months or years before the next episode. Nevertheless, the natural course of the disease is rather encouraging in many patients, although it may take many years of recurrences before their frequency diminishes to a relatively insignificant number.

In general, manifestations of recurrent genital herpes resemble the lesions of the primary infection, except that they tend to be more localized, there are fewer of them, and they are usually unilateral. The clinical appearance and the evolution of skin lesions are basically the same as in the primary infection (vesicles–erosions–pustules–healing without scarring), but there is a shorter duration of viral shedding and a shorter time to complete healing. The constitutional symptoms are rare and, if present, are milder. Lymphadenopathy is reported only in about 10 percent of cases, with the swollen inguinal nodes on the site where the lesions are located. Prodromal symptoms occur in more than half of the patients and last from a few hours to 2 days before the appearance of vesicles. The prodromes include localized paresthesias, itching, burning, or hypersensitive skin at the site of subsequent lesions. Prodromal neuralgia (radiating pain into the buttocks or knee or sacral dermatomal neuralgia) has been reported. It subsides shortly after the appearance of lesions. As a result of involvement of sensory nerves, some patients experience severe pruritus, which may be limited not only to the affected area but may involve larger, contiguous parts of the skin. This can be the only prodromal symptom which precedes the onset of local lesions or may show up after the lesion disappears.[38]

Unlike in first primary episode, recurrent genital herpes in women is more likely to be confined to the vulva without simultaneous cervicitis, and even if the cervix is involved, the infection is usually asymptomatic or not apparent to the patient. Numerous studies confirmed viral shedding from the cervix in women with a history of genital herpes but who, at the time of isolation, had no symptoms or signs of infection.[39-42] The evidence of asymptomatic viral shedding in males is less convincing. The virus was occasionally cultured from the urethra, prostatic fluid, and vas deferens in asymptomatic men.[26] However, several investigators were unable to isolate HSV from men between recurrences,[43,44] or it was isolated infrequently.[13]

OTHER CLINICAL SYNDROMES ASSOCIATED WITH GENITAL HSV INFECTION

Infection of Cervix

Herpes simplex infection may involve the cervix alone without other skin or mucosal lesions (Figure 5.9). Infection of the cervix may, as described before, produce cervicitis with clinically apparent symptoms and signs or may be asymptomatic. Asymptomatic viral shedding from the cervix during episodes of genital lesions, as well as between recurrences, has been well documented.[39-41,45] The pattern of viral shedding from the cervix is intermittent and the frequency unpredictable.[46]

HSV Pharyngitis

Herpes simplex pharyngitis can be caused either by HSV-1 or HSV-2.[13] In the latter, it frequently follows orogenital contact and frequently is associated with genital lesions. Patients with herpes pharyngitis complain of sore throat, fever, malaise, headache, and myalgia. Clinical signs vary from erythema and tonsillar exudate to a diffuse ulcerative pharyngitis. Many patients have palpable, tender cervical nodes. This form of pharyngitis has been frequently misdiagnosed as streptococcal throat infection or infectious mononucleosis.

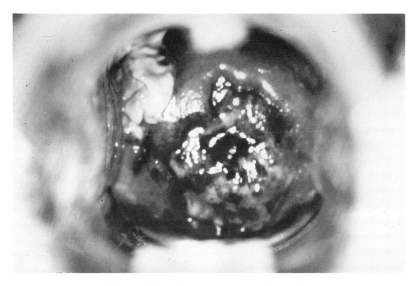

Figure 5.9.   Cervicitis caused by HSV.

HSV Urethritis

Herpes simplex urethritis may be associated with herpetic lesions elsewhere or may occur as the sole symptomatic manifestation of genital herpes. HSV has been isolated from the urethra, urine, prostatic fluid, and semen in men with urethritis[13] and from the urethra and urine in women.[13,47,48] A small percent of women with acute urethral syndrome had positive culture for HSV.[48]

In men, urethritis due to HSV infection is characterized by severe dysuria associated with scanty, white, nonpurulent discharge, and, as mentioned before, the symptoms are out of proportion to the clinical signs. Women with HSV urethritis frequently complain of severe dysuria with minimal discharge present. At times, urination may be exceedingly painful, causing urinary retention.

Anorectal HSV Infection

Both HSV-1 and HSV-2 can cause anorectal infection.[49,50] Herpes of this distribution is more frequently diagnosed among homosexuals and women than heterosexual men. In most instances, there is a history of anal intercourse. Patients with anorectal herpes infection may present with vesicular or ulcerative lesions in the anus or symptoms and signs of proctitis. In one study on homosexual men who presented to a VD clinic with complaints of rectal discharge and pain, HSV was found in 23 percent of cases.[50] Patients with HSV proctitis may have constitutional symptoms frequently observed in the first primary episode of infection. Severe rectal pain often of acute onset, tenesmus, constipation, and bloody and mucoid discharge are usually present. Fever, myalgia, and urinary retention may occur, especially in primary infection. Anoscopic examination generally reveals a friable mucosa and/or ulcerations. Herpetic ulcers above the level of the anal ring may produce marked inflammation and induration which may resemble rectal carcinoma. Biopsy is necessary to rule out such a possibility.

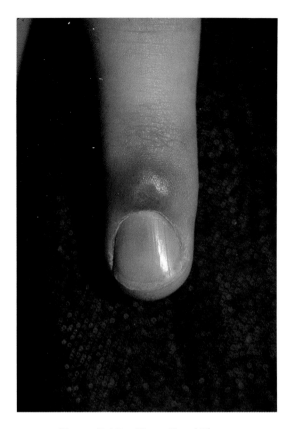

Figure 5.10. Herpetic whitlow.

Extragenital Herpes

Extragenital lesions in areas adjacent to a genital lesion and on the fingers suggest autoinoculation rather than spread via the bloodstream. These lesions are frequently located in the buttocks, in groins or thighs, in the eyes, and on the fingers (herpetic whitlow) (Figure 5.10). The latter location frequently occurs among dentists and may be the primary site of infection.

COMPLICATIONS

Aseptic Meningitis

Aseptic meningitis may occur in primary herpes and seems to be more common in women than men.[13] Patients present with symptoms of a stiff neck, headache, and photophobia with or without fever. In a majority of cases, these symptoms resolve over a period of several days without any sequelae. Some patients, however, may develop more serious disease with nuchal rigidity and positive Kernig's and Brudzinski's signs. Lymphocytic pleocytosis is common, and HSV can be isolated from cerebrospinal fluid.[51] Other findings include highly elevated opening pressure and glucose values usually more than 50% of the blood glucose levels. Symptoms and signs resolve gradually, and neurologic residua are rare. Recurrent aseptic meningitis in association with genital herpes has been reported, but this complication is infrequent and occurs mainly in primary HSV infection.

Disseminated HSV Infection

Blood-borne dissemination of HSV infection occurs mainly in immunosuppressed patients. Individuals with T-cell abnormalities, either congenital or acquired, or those receiving immunosuppressive therapy for other reasons are predisposed to cutaneous or visceral dissemination.[52-55] Pregnancy was reported to be a factor predisposing to dissemination,[56,57] especially in primary HSV infection, and severe mucocutaneous dissemination was reported in association with atopic dermatitis and AIDS.[58,59]

Cutaneous dissemination often occurs in association with aseptic meningitis, hepatitis, and pneumonitis.[60,61] Other complications include monoarticular arthritis[62] and thrombocytopenia.[63] Mortality is high, especially in pregnant women and immunocompromised patients.

Dysfunction of Autonomic Nervous System

Autonomic nervous system dysfunctions have been reported in women and homosexual men (constipation and impotence).[64,65] Those dysfunctions are transient, and symptoms usually resolve over a period of days or weeks.

Eczema Herpeticum (Eruptio Varicelliformis Kaposi)

Eczema herpeticum is an uncommon complication which can be caused either by HSV-1 or HSV-2. Varicella-zoster virus can cause the disease as well. Eczema herpeticum results from the cutaneous spread of the virus [59,65-67] (see Disseminated HSV Infection above) and is a potentially serious disease which can be fatal. Atopic dermatitis patients are at high risk for this problem, particularly during flares, but other skin conditions like Darier's disease, seborrheic dermatitis, and pemphigus have been associated with eczema herpeticum as well.[59]

This complication is characterized by a sudden onset of fever, usually 5–7 days after exposure to HSV, and the development of vesicles that appear in crops. The lesions are commonly found within "atopic skin," but in severe cases, normal skin may be also affected. The lesions undergo typical evolution from vesicles through erosions and progress to pustular and crusted phases. The disease ranges from a mild transient disorder to severe and fatal. Involvement of the central nervous system, secondary cutaneous infection, or pneumonia may lead to death. In fulminant cases, prognosis is poor, but it can be improved by aggressive therapy with various antiviral agents.[68,69]

Erythema Multiforme

Erythema multiforme (EM) has been observed in individuals following infection with genital herpes and may recur following recurrences of the disease. Erythema multiforme is believed to be an allergic reaction to the virus; however, the particles of HSV have been found in the skin lesions. HSV may be the most common trigger of EM in adults.

NEONATAL HERPES

Neonatal herpes simplex virus infection is not a reportable disease in the United States, and the estimated frequency is about 500 cases annually.[13] Herpes in newborns is almost always acquired from the mother's infected birth canal either as an ascending infection through ruptured membranes or during birth.[70,71] Primary genital herpes appears to cause a greater frequency of transmission of HSV to the infant than recurrent disease, and the majority of neonatal herpes acquired during delivery is caused by HSV-2.[72] The risk of neonatal infection among infants delivered vaginally by mothers with genital herpes present at term is approximately 50 percent.[73,74] Neonatal herpes may occur not only among infants born to mothers with clinically evident lesions but also to mothers with recurrent or asymptomatic disease.[75] Possible determinants of whether an infant will develop infection include the time of a primary infection of the mother, the extent of maternal viral shedding, the duration of the rupture of membranes, local environmental and immune factors, neonatal cellular responsiveness, and the titer of maternal antibodies.[13,76] The use of fetal monitoring devices has also been mentioned as a source of infection of the neonate.[77] Occasionally, an infant may become infected postnatally by a person with facial or, rarely, genital lesions handling the newborns or as a nosocomial infection.[78,79]

Infection acquired during birth may be present in two patterns: localized or disseminated. In the first form the infection may be limited to skin, eyes, mouth, or the central nervous system. In the disseminated form of neonatal herpes the central nervous system, the liver, the lungs, and the bone marrow are the organs which are particularly affected.

Skin lesions occur in 50–70 percent of neonates infected with HSV and are similar to those seen in adults (clusters of grouped vesicles on an erythematous base or bullae) (Figure 5.11). These may appear anywhere on the skin, especially on the scalp in vertex presentations and in the perianal area in breech presentations. The appearance of first lesions is usually not associated with symptoms of generalized infection for the first few days; however, more than half of infected newborns, if untreated, will subsequently develop disseminated infection with characteristic signs of central nervous involvement.[80] Mortality is high, and aggressive antiviral treatment is strongly recommended.[81,82]

Few cases of transplacental infection of the fetus have been described,[83-85] and it is clear that HSV acquired in utero is capable of causing severe developmental abnormalities.[80,83-85] Most congenital infections, however, result in fetal death rather than birth defects.[86]

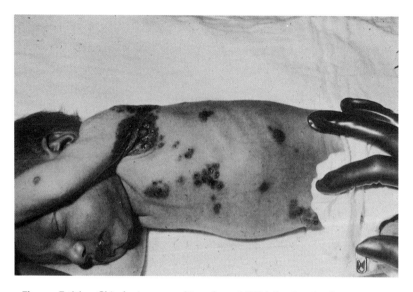

Figure 5.11. Skin lesions resulting from HSV infection in the neonate.

Since transplacental infection with HSV is fortunately rare and most cases of neonatal herpes are acquired upon delivery, special precautions should be undertaken to assure safe delivery of a mother with known genital herpes. Severity of neonatal disease and the lack of satisfactory therapy should justify applying necessary measures.

Women with a history of proven genital herpes or suspected of genital herpes and the sex partners of men with genital herpes should be monitored by viral cultures beginning after 32–36 weeks of gestation and weekly thereafter. It is a general consensus that positive culture or clinically evident lesions near or at the time of delivery should justify cesarean section. Abdominal delivery should be performed preferably before the rupture of the membranes. If the membranes have been ruptured for more than 4–6 hours, the protection of cesarean section is probably lost.[87-90] Some authors, however, reported cases of abdominal deliveries performed more than 6 hours after the rupture of the membranes in which no neonatal herpes was found.[91]

Infants born to mothers considered infectious at delivery should be placed in isolation, and viral cultures, liver function tests, and cerebral spinal fluid (CSF) examination, if necessary, should be obtained during the first 7–12 days of life. Ophthalmoscopic examination should be included as routine. The infants should be carefully watched, and appearance of clinical signs resembling those of bacterial sepsis, convulsions, or other encephalitic signs should alert the physician to possible neonatal herpes and should prompt the initiation of appropriate procedures. Symptomless newborns should be observed for the next 3–4 weeks, assuming a longer incubation period. If the parents are reliable, it is not necessary to delay the infant's discharge. However, they should be informed of signs and symptoms of neonatal herpes and contacted by phone for 3–4 weeks after delivery.

GENITAL HERPES AND CERVICAL CANCER

A number of earlier multidisciplinary studies have shown that HSV-2 infection is a significant risk factor for the development of cervical dysplasia and carcinoma of the cervix.[92-96] Epidemiologic studies demonstrated that the frequency of previous HSV-2 infections is significantly higher in patients with cervical cancer than in controls.[92-97] The risk of developing cervical cancer is also higher among HSV-2-infected women than uninfected women.[98,99] Frequently, HSV-2 infection precedes development of cervical carcinoma.[100] Further evidence for the oncogenic role of HSV-2 in cervical neoplasia is provided by the clinical and biologic characteristics of HSV-2.[101] Cervical herpes infection commonly appears at the squamocolumnar junction, where most cervical dysplasias arise,[102] and HSV-2 has been found to be oncogenic in experimental animals.[103-105] Moreover, several viral proteins and genes involved in cell transformation and oncogenicity were found in cervical cancer cells.[106-109] Some other malignancies (squamous cell carcinoma of the vulva[110] and cancer of the bladder and prostate[111]) have also been implicated in HSV-2 infections, but the association of those malignancies and HSV-2 is not as strong as in the case of cervical cancer.

The hypothesis of a cancerogenic role of HSV-2 in the development of cervical neoplasis is not a new one. Recently, another virus (human papiloma virus [HPV]) that can be sexually transmitted has been associated with cervical cancer as a sole factor or as a cofactor of HSV-2 infection.[112] Frequent isolation of HPV DNA sequences (mainly types 16, 18, 31, 33) in cervical cancer specimens support the theory that HPV rather than HSV may play a more important role in cancerogenesis.[113] Nevertheless, despite the evidence of the association between HSV-2 and cervical carcinoma, it is clear that HSV alone, regardless of other factors, cannot cause cervical cancer. However, the link is apparent, and every woman who has had genital herpes should have a regular (every 6 months) Papanicolaou's smear examination. The 5-year cure rate of carcinoma in situ approaching 100% should justify the inconvenience associated with frequent "Pap smear" examination.[114]

DIAGNOSIS

The diagnosis of genital herpes is usually made on the basis of a characteristic clinical picture, but, wherever possible, it should be confirmed by the isolation of the virus from lesions.

Culture

Cell culture is the most sensitive and reliable method. The optimal yield of the virus is found in early vesicular fluid, and, although the virus titer rapidly declines to very low levels after 2–5 days, it can be occasionally found in crusted lesions.[46] Vesicular fluid may be collected with a cotton swab or by means of a small needle and syringe. Freshly collected material can be inoculated directly into cell culture, if possible, or placed in a viral transport medium and promptly transported to the laboratory. If a delay of 1 or 2 hours is anticipated, the specimen should be stored in a refrigerator at 4°C. For longer delays, specimens should be frozen at −70°C or on

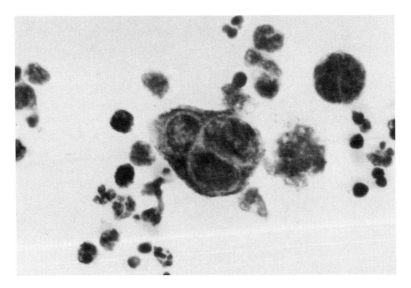

Figure 5.12. Tzanck test: multinucleate giant cells.

dry ice. False-negative results can be due to improper collection or transportation of specimens. Tentative diagnosis can be made within 1–3 days, based on the typical cytopathic effect induced by HSV in cell culture.[115] In doubtful cases, serologic confirmation of isolated HSV is necessary. The major disadvantage of culture is related to the time and the cost incurred.

Tzanck Smear

The Tzanck smear is a much more available but less sensitive method than culture. It is performed by smearing scrapings of the base and margins of vesicles or early erosions, fixing for 1 minute in absolute alcohol, and staining with Giemsa or Wright's stains for 3 minutes. The smear is examined under a light microscope for the presence of multinucleated giant cells (Figure 5.12).

As much exudate as possible should be obtained by vigorous scraping of the floor and roof of chosen vesicles, erosions, pustules, or crusts. However, chances for positive results in material collected from older lesions are slim.[116] Greater sensitivity (70–80 percent) was found in the vesicular stage, as compared with the erosive stage (25–40 percent).[117] Sampling more than one lesion is advisable.[118] The sensitivity and specificity of the test are generally rather low, and the test does not differentiate HSV from varicella-zoster (V-Z) virus. However, the use of monoclonal antibodies tagged with immunofluorescent markers significantly improves the specificity and sensitivity of this test.[119]

Papanicolaou's Smear

Papanicolaou's smear, which is routinely used in gynecologic practice, can reveal multinucleated giant cells in lesion scrapings or cervical smears. The method is less sensitive than culture but more sensitive than the Tzanck smear. It allows the detection of multinucleated giant cells as well as intracellular inclusions. Positive results were obtained from material obtained from asymptomatic individuals.[115]

Electron Microscopy

Demonstration of the virus by direct electron microscopic examination of vesicular fluid is a very attractive method because the results can be obtained rapidly (1–2 hours).[115] Unfortunately, the sensitivity is variable, and this method does not distinguish HSV from V-Z virus. Moreover, most medical centers lack the equipment and expertise to undertake electron microscopic examination.

Other Methods

Numerous new techniques that have been introduced recently provide convenient and rapid diagnosis of HSV infections. These include immunofluorescent microscopic examination[120,121] and immunoperoxidase staining.[122] Although these tests appear to be simple to perform and give rapid results, caution must be exercised, since nonspecific reactions often have been encountered.[115] A variety of other immunologic techniques has been introduced, most of which allow distinguishing between HSV-1 and HSV-2: monoclonal antibody techniques,[123,124] enzyme-linked immunosorbent assay,[125] indirect hemagglutination,[126] and others. Many nonimmunologic techniques have been used to identify HSV: for example, restriction endonuclease analysis,[127,128] nucleic acid hybridization,[109,129] and type-specific enzyme analysis.[130] The latter methods, however, are not routinely applied in clinical practice and are used mainly for research purposes.

Serodiagnosis of HSV Infection

Antibodies to HSV-1 or HSV-2 can be detected by several methods including complement fixation test, enzyme-linked immunosorbent assay, indirect immunofluorescence test, and indirect hemagglutination inhibition. Serologic diagnosis is useful in confirming a primary infection which is indicated by a fourfold rise in serum antibody titer. Recurrences or reinfections cannot be identified serologically, since antibody levels fluctuate without much relation to the presence of skin lesions. Thus, antibody assays are useful primarily for seroepidemiologic studies and not for the diagnosis of HSV infection.[115]

Differential Diagnosis

- *Primary syphilis:* nontender, indurated ulceration; painless lymphadenopathy; positive dark-field examination for *Treponema pallidum;* positive serology (mixed infection with HSV and *T. pallidum* is possible).
- *Chancroid:* (frequently mistaken for herpes) genital ulcer or ulcerations, less numerous than in herpes, usually accompanied by fluctuant adenopathy; positive culture for *Haemophilus ducreyi* or other tests; negative culture for HSV.

- *Lymphogranuloma venereum:* transient, nonrecurrent genital lesion; fluctuant adenopathy-bubo; positive culture or other tests for *Chlamydia trachomatis;* negative HSV culture.
- *Donovanosis:* chronic and progressive granular lesions; recent travel to endemic areas; Donovan bodies in the smear; negative culture for HSV.
- *Scabies:* itchy nodules in the genitalia and pruritic papules in other typical distribution; pruritus worse at night; positive ink test or mite demonstrated in scrapings of the lesions.
- *Erythema multiforme:* characteristic, annular, or iris lesion; history of recent herpes or drug intake (barbiturates, phenothiazines, or antibiotics); negative culture for HSV.
- *Behçet's syndrome:* recurrent aphthae and iritis, besides the genital lesions; other findings include arthritis, renal disease, arteritis, thrombophlebitis; negative culture for HSV.
- *Other conditions:* Stevens-Johnson syndrome, trauma, zoster, adverse drug eruptions.

TREATMENT

Genital herpes is a self-limiting disease and skin and mucous membrane lesion hill unless secondarily infected. Symptomatic treatment includes genital hygiene, loose-fitting undergarments, and compresses with 0.9% saline or cool tap water. Analgesia during a primary attack is indicated with aspirin, codeine, or acetaminophen. Aspirin is preferred because, in addition to its analgesic effect, it also has antiprostaglandin action. Topical 2% lidocaine jelly reduces local pain. The lesions should be kept dry, and topical application of antiseptic drying agents may be of some benefit. Various other topical therapies have been applied, but none have been shown conclusively to be more effective than placebo.

Acyclovir

Acyclovir (Zovirax), a guanosine analog, is the first antiviral agent approved for treatment of HSV infection in the United States. It is the first antiviral drug with demonstrable efficacy in the treatment of genital herpes.[131-133] It is recommended for treatment of the first clinical episode and for treatment of immunocompromised patients.

The recommended regimen for the first clinical episode of genital herpes is 200 mg by mouth 5 times daily for 7–10 days or until clinical resolution occurs. If initiated within 6 days of onset of lesions, acyclovir is believed to shorten the duration of the primary episode by several days and to reduce systemic symptoms. Topical acyclovir has also been shown to have effect in the treatment of the first episode of primary genital herpes,[134,135] but there is a general agreement that this form of treatment is less effective than therapy with the oral drug.

Recommended regimen for the first clinical episode of herpes proctitis is acyclovir, 400 mg orally 5 times a day for 10 days or until clinical resolution occurs.

For hospitalized patients who have severe symptoms or who developed complications, the treatment should be acyclovir IV, 5 mg/kg body weight every 8 hours for 5–7 days, or until clinical resolution occurs. This treatment may shorten the course of the primary episode of herpes by approximately 7 days.

Since the effect of acyclovir for recurrent herpes is minimal, its administration should be limited to patients with severe symptoms, and administration of the drug should be initiated at the beginning of the prodrome or within 2 days of the onset of lesions. The recommended regimen is 200 mg by mouth 5 times a day for 5 days, or 800 mg by mouth 2 times a day for 5 days.

Suppression of Recurrent Genital Herpes

Continuous treatment with acyclovir, 200 mg by mouth 2–5 times daily, or 400 mg by mouth 2 times a day, may reduce the frequency of recurrences of genital herpes.[136] The dose of acyclovir should be individualized for each patient, and cessation of treatment may result in the recurrence of clinical episodes at the pretreatment frequency. Safety and efficacy have been documented among persons receiving daily therapy for up to 3 years.

Acyclovir-resistant strains of HSV have been isolated from persons receiving suppressive therapy, but have not been associated with treatment failure among immunocompetent patients. After 1 year of continuous daily suppressive therapy, acyclovir should be discontinued to reassess the patient's recurrence rate.

Acyclovir in Pregnant Patients

The safety of systemic acyclovir therapy in pregnant women has not been established, and its use should be restricted to life-threatening maternal HSV infection only. In pregnant women without life-threatening disease, systemic acyclovir treatment should not be used to treat recurrent genital herpes or as a suppressive therapy to prevent reactivation near term.

Interferon

Various interferon preparations have been used in clinical trials in the treatment of HSV infections. Most of them showed a significant reduction in viral shedding and duration of symptoms.[137,138] Several new preparations as well as vaccines are being investigated. The results are promising, although further testing is necessary to evaluate its efficacy.

PREVENTION

Although development of an HSV vaccine may be the only effective means for complete prophylaxis of infection at present, the best way of preventing the spread of genital herpes is abstention or the use of barrier methods. The first method should be applied in situations in which one of the sex partners has active lesions. For asymptomatic patients with a history of recurrent genital herpes, spermicidal foams (in women) and condoms are recommended. Similar to contraceptive efficacy, these methods decrease the risk of infection but not completely.

Women who desire to get pregnant should avoid sexual encounters when active lesions are present. They should be informed that childbearing can proceed without or with minimal complications if the proper precautions are undertaken.

Even though cervical cancer occurs only in a minority of female patients with genital herpes, they should be advised of the necessity of regular Pap smears to identify changes in cervical cytology as early as possible.

Genital herpes, and other diseases causing genital ulcers, have been associated with an increased risk of acquiring HIV infections. Therefore, the use of condoms should be encouraged during all sexual exposures.

REFERENCES

1. Buchman TG, Roizman B, Nahmias AJ: Demonstration of exogenous genital reinfection with herpes simplex virus type 2 by restriction endonuclease fingerprinting of viral DNA. *J Infect Dis* 140:295–304, 1979.
2. Kit S, Trkula D, Qavi H, et al: Sequential genital infections by herpes simplex viruses types 1 and 2. Restriction nuclease analysis of viruses from recurrent infections. *Sex Transm Dis* 10:67–71, 1983.
3. Fife KH, Schmidt O, Remington M, et al: Primary and recurrent concomitant genital infection with herpes simplex virus types 1 and 2. *J Infect Dis* 147:163, 1983.
4. *Sexually Transmitted Disease Statistics. Calendar Year 1987.* U.S. DHHS, Public Health Service CDC, 1988, issue No. 136.
5. Anonymous: Sexually transmitted disease surveillance 1979. *Br Med J* 282:155–156, 1981.
6. MacDougall ML: Genital herpes simplex in the female 1968–1973. *NZ Med J* 82:333–335, 1975.
7. Mroczkowski TF: Genital herpes as a sexually transmitted disease. *Przegl Derm* 6:747–753, 1977.
8. Morton RS: Control of sexually transmitted diseases today and tomorrow. *Genitourin Med* 63:202–209, 1987.
9. *STD Fact Sheet.* (35th ed.) U.S. DHHS Public Health Service CDC, 1981, pp. 5–12, 1981.
10. Baker DA: Herpesvirus. *Clin Obstet Gynecol* 26:165–172, 1983.
11. Sumaya CV, Marx J, Ullis K: Genital infections with herpes simplex virus in university student populations. *Sex Transm Dis* 7:16–20, 1980.
12. Chuang T-Y, Su WPD, Perry HO, et al: Incidence and trend of herpes progenitalis. *Mayo Clin Proc* 58:436–441, 1983.
13. Corey L, Adams HG, Brown ZA, et al: Genital herpes simplex virus infections: Clinical manifestations, course, and complications. *Ann Intern Med* 98:958–972, 1983.
14. Nerurkar LS, West F, May M, et al: Survival of herpes simplex virus in water specimens collected from hot tubs in spa facilities and on plastic surfaces. *JAMA* 250:3081–3083, 1983.
15. Roizman B: An inquiry into the mechanism of recurrent herpes infections of man. *Perspect Virol* 4:283–301, 1965.

16. Klein RJ: The pathogenesis of acute, latent, and recurrent herpes simplex virus infection. *Arch Virol* 72:143–168, 1982.

17. Reeves WE, Corey L, Adams HG, et al: Risk of recurrence after first episodes of genital herpes: Relation to HSV types and antibody response. *N Engl J Med* 305:315–319, 1981.

18. Kaufman RH, Gardner HL, Rawls WE, et al: Clinical features of herpes genitalis. *Cancer Res* 33:1446–1451, 1973.

19. Stadler H: Herpes virus infection: Its spectrum in immunosuppressed patients, in Klatersky J (ed), *Infections in Cancer Patients.* New York, Raven Press, 1982, p. 189.

20. Callen JP: Epidemic herpes simplex virus infection. *Am J Dis Child* 137:182–184, 1983.

21. Cunningham AL, Merigan TC: Gamma-interferon production appears to predict time of recurrence of herpes labialis. *J Immunol* 130:2397–2400, 1983.

22. Schooley RT, Hirsch MS, Colvin RB, et al: Association of herpesvirus infections with T-lymphocyte-subset alterations, glomerulopathy and opportunistic infections after renal transplantation. *N Engl J Med* 308:307–313, 1983.

23. O'Reilly RJ, Chibbaro A, Anger E, et al: Cell-mediated immune responses in patients with recurrent herpes simplex infections. Infection-associated deficiency of lymphokine production in patients with recurrent herpes labialis or herpes progenitalis. *J Immunol* 118:1095–1102, 1977.

24. Spruance SL, Green JA, Chiu G, et al: Pathogenesis of herpes simplex labialis: Correlation of vesicle fluid interferon with lesion age and virus titer. *Infect Immun* 36:907–910, 1982.

25. Sheridan JF, Donnenberg AD, Aurelian L, et al: Immunity to herpes simplex virus type 2. IV. Impaired lymphokine production during recrudescence correlates with an imbalance of T-lymphocyte-subset. *J Immunol* 129:326–331, 1982.

26. Centifanto YM, Drylie DM, Deardourff SL, et al: Herpes virus type-2 in the male genitourinary tract. *Science* 178:318–319, 1972.

27. Goodell SE, Quinn TC, Mkrtichian E, et al: Herpes simplex proctitis in homosexual men. Clinical, sigmoidoscopic, and histopathological features. *N Engl J Med* 308:868–871, 1983.

28. Goldmeier D: Proctitis and herpes simplex virus in homosexual men. *Br J Vener Dis* 56:111–114, 1980.

29. Oates JK, Greenhouse PR: Retention of urine in anogenital herpetic infection. *Lancet* 1:691–692, 1978.

30. Corey L, Reeves WC, Holmes KK: Cellular immune response in genital herpes simplex virus infection. *N Engl J Med* 299:986–991, 1978.

31. Scher J, Bottone E, Desmond E, et al: The incidence and outcome of asymptomatic herpes genitalis in an obstetric population. *Am J Obstet Gynecol* 144:906–909, 1982.

32. Barton SE, Davis JM, Moss VW, et al: Asymptomatic shedding and subsequent transmission of genital herpes simplex virus. *Genitourin Med* 63:102–105, 1987.

33. Corey L: Genital herpes, in Holmes KK, Mardh P-A, Sparling PF, Wiesner PJ (eds), *Sexually Transmitted Disease.* New York, McGraw-Hill, 1984, pp. 449–474.

34. Blyth WA, Hill TJ, Field HJ, et al: Reactivation of herpes simplex virus infection by ultraviolet light and possible involvement of prostaglandins. *J Gen Virol* 33:547–550, 1976.

35. Hill TJ, Blyth WA, Harbour DA: Trauma to the skin causes recurrence of herpes simplex in the mouse. *J Gen Virol* 39:21–28, 1978.

36. Harbour DA, Blyth WA, Hill TJ: Prostaglandins enhance spread of herpes simplex virus in the cell culture. *J Gen Virol* 41:87–95, 1978.

37. Trofatter KF Jr, Daniels CA: Interaction of human cells with prostaglandins and cyclic AMP modulators. *J Immunol* 122:1363–1370, 1979.

38. Chang T-W, Fiumara NJ, Weinstein L: Genital herpes. Some clinical and laboratory observations. *JAMA* 229:544–545, 1974.

39. Adam E, Dreesman GE, Kaufman RH, et al: Asymptomatic virus shedding after herpes genitalis. *Am J Obstet Gynecol* 137:827–830, 1980.

40. Rattray MC, Corey L, Reeves WC, et al: Recurrent genital herpes among women: Symptomatic v. asymptomatic viral shedding. *Br J Vener Dis* 54:262–265, 1978.

41. Willmott FE, Mair HJ: Genital herpesvirus infection in women attending a venereal diseases clinic. *Br J Vener Dis* 54:341–343, 1978.

42. Guinan ME, MacCalman J, Kern ER, et al: The course of an untreated recurrent genital *herpes simplex* infection in 27 women. *N Engl J Med* 304:759–763, 1981.

43. Traub RG, Madden DL, Fuccillo DA, et al: The male as a reservoir of infection with Cytomegalovirus, herpes, and mycoplasma. *N Engl J Med* 289:697, 1973.

44. Deture FA, Drylie DM, Kaufman HE, et al: Herpes virus type 2: Study of semen in male subjects with recurrent infections. *J Urol* 120:449–451, 1978.

45. Adam E, Kaufman RH, Mirkovic RR, et al: Persistence of virus shedding in asymptomatic women after recovery from herpes genitalis. *Obstet Gynecol* 54:171–173, 1979.

46. August MJ, Nordlund JJ, Hsiung GD: Persistence of herpes simplex virus types 1 and 2 in infected individuals. *Arch Dermatol* 115:309–310, 1979.

47. Person DA, Kaufman RH, Gardner HL, et al: *Herpesvirus* type 2 in genitourinary tract infection. *Am J Obstet Gynecol* 116:993–995, 1973.

48. Stamm WE, Wagner KF, Amsel R, et al: Causes of the acute urethral syndrome in women. *N Engl J Med* 303:409–415, 1980.

49. Levine JB, Saeed M: Herpes virus hominis (type 1) proctitis. *J Clin Gastroenterol* 1:225–229, 1979.

50. Quinn TC, Corey L, Chaffee RG, et al: The etiology of anorectal infections in homosexual men. *Am J Med* 71:395–406, 1981.

51. Skoldenberg B, Jeansson S, Wolontis S: Herpes simplex virus type 2 and acute aseptic meningitis: Clinical feature of cases with isolation of herpes simplex virus from cerebrospinal fluids. *Scanl J Infect Dis* 7:227–232, 1975.

52. St. Geme JW, Prince JT, Burke BA: Impaired cellular resistance to Herpes simplex virus in Wiskott-Aldrich syndrome. *N Engl J Med* 273:229–234, 1965.

53. Sutton AL, Smithwick EM, Seligman SJ, et al: Fatal disseminated *Herpesvirus hominis* type 2 infection in an adult with associated thymic dysplasia. *Am J Med* 56:545–553, 1974.

54. Siegal FP, Lopez C, Hammer GS, et al: Severe acquired immunodeficiency in male homosexuals, manifested by chronic perianal ulcerative *herpes simplex* lesions. *N Engl J Med* 305:1439–1444, 1981.

55. Fauci AS, Macher AM, Longo DL, et al: Acquired immunodeficiency syndrome: Epidemiologic, clinical, immunologic, and therapeutic considerations. *Ann Intern Med* 100:92–106, 1984.

56. Goyette RE, Donowho EM, Hieger LR, et al: Fulminant *Herpesvirus hominis* hepatitis during pregnancy. *Obstet Gynecol* 43:191–196, 1974.

57. Kobberman T, Clark L, Griffin WT: Maternal death secondary to disseminated *Herpesvirus hominis*. *Am J Obstet Gynecol* 137:742–743, 1980.

58. Mailman CJ, Miranda JL, Spock A: Recurrent eczema herpeticum. *Arch Dermatol* 89:815–818, 1964.

59. Wheeler CE, Abele DC: Eczema herpeticum, primary and recurrent. *Arch Dermatol* 93:162–173, 1966.

60. Joseph TJ, Vogt PJ: Disseminated herpes with hepatoadrenal necrosis in adult. *Am J Med* 56:735–739, 1974.

61. Nahmias AJ: Disseminated herpes simplex virus infection. *N Engl J Med* 282:684–685, 1970.

62. Friedman HM, Pincus T, Gibilisco P, et al: Acute monoarticular arthritis caused by herpes simplex virus and cytomegalovirus. *Am J Med* 69:241–247, 1980.

63. Whittaker JA, Hardison MD: Severe thrombocytopenia after generalized herpes simplex virus-2 (HSV-2) infection. *South Med J* 71:864–865, 1978.

64. Riehle RA, Williams JJ: Transient neuropathic bladder following herpes simplex genitalis. *J Urol* 122:263–264, 1979.

65. Naseman T, Saurbrey W, Burgdorf WHC: *Fundamentals of Dermatology.* New York, Springer-Verlag, 1983, pp. 34–36.

66. Atherton, DJ, Marshall WC: Eczema herpeticum. Practitioner 226:971–973, 1982.

67. Hazen PG: Eczema herpeticum caused by herpes simplex virus type 2. *Arch Dermatol* 113:1085–1086, 1977.

68. Robinson GE, Underhill GS, Forster GE, et al: Treatment with acyclovir of genital herpes simplex virus infection complicated by eczema herpeticum. *Br J Vener Dis* 60:241–242, 1984.

69. Straus SE, Rooney JF, Sever JL, et al: Herpes simplex virus infection: Biology, treatment, prevention. *Ann Intern Med* 103:404–413, 1985.

70. Nahmias AJ, Alford CA, Korones SB: Infection of the newborn with herpes virus hominis. *Adv Pediatr* 17:185–226, 1970.

71. Hanshaw JB: *Herpesvirus hominis* infections in the fetus and the newborn. *Am J Dis Child* 126:546–555, 1973.

72. Quinn TC, Horn JE: Viral STDs: Herpes simplex and human papillomavirus. *Md Med J* 36:64–72, 1987.

73. Nahmias AJ, Josey WE, Naib ZM, et al: Perinatal risk associated with maternal genital herpes simplex virus infection. *Am J Obstet Gynecol* 110:825–834, 1971.

74. Amstey MS, Monif GR: Genital herpes virus infection in pregnancy. *Obstet Gynecol* 44:394–397, 1974.

75. Whitley RJ, Nahmias AJ, Visintine AM, et al: The natural history of herpes simplex virus infection of mother and newborn. *Pediatrics* 66:489–494, 1980.

76. Yeager AS, Arvin AM, Urbani LJ, et al: Relationship of antibody to outcome in neonatal herpes simplex virus infections. *Infect Immun* 29:232–238, 1980.

77. Parvey LS, Chien LT: Neonatal herpes simplex virus infection introduced by fetal-monitor scalp electrodes. *Pediatrics* 65:1150–1153, 1980.

78. Light IJ: Postnatal acquisition of herpes simplex virus by the newborn infant: A review of the literature. *Pediatrics* 63:480–482, 1979.

79. Sullivan-Bolyai J, Hull HF, Wilson C, et al: Neonatal herpes simplex virus infection in King County, Washington: Increasing incidence and epidemiologic correlates. *JAMA* 250:3059–3062, 1983.

80. Hanshaw JB, Dudgeon JA: Herpes simplex infection of the fetus and newborn, in *Viral Diseases of the Fetus and Newborn.* Philadelphia, W.B. Saunders, 1978, pp. 153–181.

81. Correy L, Spear PG: Infections with Herpes simplex virus. *N Engl J Med* 314:749–756, 1986.

82. Whitley RJ, Alford CA, Hirsch MS, et al: Vidarabine versus acyclovir therapy in herpes simplex encephalitis. *N Engl J Med* 314:144–149, 1986.

83. Schaffer AJ: *Diseases of the Newborn* (2nd ed). Philadelphia, W.B. Saunders, 1965, p. 733.

84. South MA, Tompkins WAF, Morris CR, et al: Congenital malformation of the central nervous system associated with genital type (type 2) herpesvirus. *J Pediatr* 75:13–18, 1969.

85. Montgomery JR, Flanders RW, Yow MD: Congenital herpesvirus infection with possibly related abnormalities. *Am J Dis Child* 125:364–366, 1973.

86. Nahmias AJ, Vistine AM: Herpes simplex, in Remington JS, Klein JO (eds), *Infectious Diseases of the Fetus and Newborn Infant.* Philadelphia, W.B. Saunders, 1976, pp. 156–190.

87. Amstey MS: Management of pregnancy complicated by genital herpes virus infection. *Obstet Gynecol* 37:515–520, 1971.

88. Light IJ, Linnemann CC: Neonatal herpes simplex infection following delivery by Caesarean section. *Obstet Gynecol* 44:496–499, 1974.

89. Kibrick S: Herpes simplex infection at term. What to do with mother, newborn, and nursery personnel. *JAMA* 243:157–160, 1980.

90. Meissner, HC: Herpes simplex virus infections in the newborn. *Clin Dermatol* 2:23–28, 1984.

91. Grossman JH, Wallen WC, Sever JL: Management of genital herpes simplex virus infection during pregnancy. *Obstet Gynecol* 58:1–4, 1981.

92. Rawls WE, Tompkins WAF, Melnick JL: The association of herpesvirus type 2 and carcinoma of the uterine cervix. *Am J Epidemiol* 89:547–554, 1969.

93. Aurelian L: Possible role of herpesvirus hominis type 2 in human cervical cancer. *Fed Proc* 31:1651–1659, 1972.

94. Ory HW, Jenkins R, Byrd J: The epidemiology and interrelationship of cervical dysplasia and type 2 herpes virus in a low-income housing project. *Am J Obstet Gynecol* 123:269–275, 1975.

95. Nahmias AJ, Naib ZM, Josey WE: Epidemiological studies relating genital herpetic infection to cervical carcinoma. *Cancer Res* 34:1111–1117, 1975.

96. Skinner GRB, Whitney JE, Hartley C: Prevalence of type-specific antibody against type 1 and type 2 herpes simplex virus in women with abnormal cervical cytology. Evidence towards pre-pubertal vaccination of seronegative female subjects. *Arch Virol* 54:211–221, 1977.

97. Freedman RS, Joosting AC, Ryan JT, et al: A study of associated factors including genital herpes in black women with cervical carcinoma in Johannesburg. *S Afr Med J* 48:1747–1752, 1974.

98. Catalano LW, Johnson LO: Herpesvirus antibody and carcinoma in situ of the cervix. *JAMA* 217:447–450, 1971.

99. Naib ZM, Nahmias AJ, Josey WE, et al: Relation of cytohistopathology of genital herpes virus infection to cervical anaplasia. *Cancer Res* 33:1452–1463, 1973.

100. Naib ZM, Nahmias AJ, Josey WE: Cytology and histopathology of cervical herpes simplex infection. *Cancer* 19:1026–1031, 1966.

101. Aurelian L: Herpes simplex virus type 2 and cervical cancer. *Clin Dermatol* 2:90–99, 1984.

102. Nahmias AJ, Norrild B: HSV-1 and 2—Basis and clinical aspects. *Disease a Month* 25:4–49, 1979.

103. Rapp F, Reed C: Experimental evidence for the oncogenic potential of herpes simplex virus. *Cancer Res* 36:800–806, 1976.

104. Wentz WB, Reagan JW, Fu JS, et al: Experimental studies of carcinogenesis of the uterine cervix in mice. *Gynecol Oncol* 12(Suppl):90–98, 1981.

105. Wentz WB, Haggie AD, Anthony DD, et al: Prevention of herpes simplex virus type 2 (HSV-2) induced cervical carcinoma in mice by pre-exposure immunization against HSV-2, in *Proceedings of the International Herpesvirus Workshop*, Oxford, 1983, p. 196.

106. Galloway DA, McDougall JK: The oncogenic potential of herpes simplex viruses: Evidence for a "hit and run" mechanism. *Nature* 302:21–24, 1983.

107. Iwasaka T, Smith CC, Aurelian L, et al: Proteins encoded by a fragment of HSV-2 DNA (Bg 1 IIC) that has neoplastic transformation potential, in *Proceedings of the International Herpesvirus Workshop*, Oxford, 1983, p. 75.

108. Aurelian L, Kessler II, Rosenshein NB, et al: Viruses and gynecologic cancers: herpes virus protein (ICP 10/AG-4), a cervical tumor antigen that fulfills the criteria for a marker of cancerogenicity. *Cancer* 48:455–471, 1981.

109. McDougall JK, Crum CP, Fenoglio CM, et al: *Herpesvirus* specific RNA and protein in carcinoma of the uterine cervix. *Proc Natl Acad Sci USA* 79:3853–3857, 1982.

110. Kaufman RH, Dreesman GR, Burek J, et al: Herpes virus-induced antigens in squamous-cell carcinoma in situ of the vulva. *N Engl J Med* 305:483–488, 1983.

111. Luleci G, Sakizli M, Gunlap A, et al: Herpes simplex type 2 neutralization antibodies in patients with cancers of urinary bladder, prostate, and cervix. *J Surg Oncol* 16:327–331, 1981.

112. Zur Hausen H: Human genital cancer: Synergism between two virus infections or synergism between a virus infection and initiating events. *Lancet* 2:1370–1372, 1982.

113. Tomita Y: Detection of Human papilloma virus DNA in genital warts, cervical dysplasia and neoplasms. *Intervirology* 25:151–157, 1986.

114. Rudolph J: Cancer of the female genital tract, in Rubin P (ed), *Clinical Oncology*. New York, American Cancer Society, 1974, pp. 216–257.

115. Hsiung GD, Landry ML, Mayo DR, et al: Laboratory diagnosis of herpes simplex virus type 1 and type 2 infections. *Clin Dermatol* 2:67–82, 1984.

116. Solomon AR, Rasmussen JE, Varani J, et al: The Tzanck smear in the diagnosis of cutaneous herpes simplex. *JAMA* 251:633–635, 1984.

117. Brown ST, Jaffe HW, Zaidi A, et al: Sensitivity and specificity of diagnostic tests for genital infection with herpes virus hominis. *Sex Transm Dis* 6:10–13, 1979.

118. Solomon AR: The Tzanck smear. Viable and valuable in the diagnosis of herpes simplex zoster and varicella. *Int J Dermatol* 25:169–170, 1986.

119. Lopez C, Roizman B: *Human Herpes Virus Infections*. New York, Raven Press, 1986.

120. Volpi A, Lakeman AD, Pereira L, et al: Monoclonal antibodies for rapid diagnosis and typing of genital herpes infections during pregnancy. *Am J Obstet Gynecol* 146:813–815, 1983.

121. Schmidt NJ, Gallo D, Devlin V, et al: Direct immunofluorescence staining for detection of herpes simplex and varicella-zoster virus antigens in vesicular lesions and certain tissue specimens. *J Clin Microbiol* 12:651–655, 1980.

122. Pearson NS, Fleagle G, Dorherty JJ: Detection of herpes simplex virus infection of female genitalia by the peroxidase-antiperoxidase method alone or in conjunction with the Papanicolaou stain. *J Clin Microbiol* 10:737–746, 1979.

123. Pereira L, Dondero DV, Gallo D, et al: Serological analysis of herpes simplex virus type 1 and 2 with monoclonal antibodies. *Infect Immun* 35:363–367, 1982.

124. Balachandran N, Frame B, Chernesky M, et al: Identification and typing of herpes simplex viruses with monoclonal antibodies. *J Clin Microbiol* 16:205–208, 1982.

125. Nilheden E, Jeansson S, Vahlne A: Typing of herpes simplex virus by an enzyme-linked immunosorbent assay with monoclonal antibodies. *J Clin Microbiol* 17:677–780, 1983.

126. Bernstein MT, Stewart JA: Method for typing antisera to herpesvirus hominis by indirect hemagglutination inhibition. *Appl Microbiol* 21:680–684, 1971.

127. Buchman TG, Roizman B, Adams G, et al: Restriction endonuclease fingerprinting of herpes simplex virus DNA: A novel epidemiological tool applied to a nosocomial outbreak. *J Infect Dis* 138:488–498, 1978.

128. Peterson E, Schmidt OW, Goldstein LC, et al: Typing of clinical herpes simplex isolates with mouse monoclonal antibodies to herpes simplex virus types 1 and 2. Comparison with type specific rabbit antisera and restriction endonuclease analysis of viral DNA. *J Clin Microbiol* 17:92–96, 1983.

129. Brautigam AR, Richman DD, Oxman MN: Rapid typing of herpes simplex virus isolates by deoxyribonucleic acid: Deoxyribonucleic acid hybridization. *J. Clin Microbiol* 12:226–234, 1983.

130. Cheng YC, Schinazi RP, Dutschman GE, et al: Virus-induced thymidine kinase as markers for typing herpes simplex virus and for drug sensitivity assays. *J Virol Methods* 5:209–217, 1982.

131. Elion GB: Mechanism of action and selectivity of acyclovir. *Am J Med* 73:7–13, 1982.

132. Corey L, Fife KH, Benedetti JK, et al: Intravenous acyclovir for the treatment of primary genital herpes. *Ann Intern Med* 98:914–921, 1983.

133. Bryson YJ, Dillon M, Lovett M, et al: Treatment of first episodes of genital herpes simplex virus infection with oral acyclovir: A randomized double-blind controlled trial in normal subjects. *N Engl J Med* 308:916–921, 1983.

134. Corey L, Nahmias AJ, Guinan ME, et al: A trial of topical acyclovir in genital herpes simplex virus infection. *N Engl J Med* 306:1313–1319, 1982.

135. Thin RN, Nabarro JM, Parker JD, et al: Topical acyclovir in the treatment of initial genital herpes. *Br J Vener Dis* 59:116–119, 1983.

136. Sacks SL, Fox R, Levendusky P, Stiver HG, et al: Chronic suppression for six months compared with intermittent lesional therapy of recurrent genital herpes using oral acyclovir: Effects on lesions and nonlesional prodromes. *Sex Transm Dis* 15:58–62, 1988.

137. Pazin GJ, Armstrong JA, Lam MT, et al: Prevention of reactivated herpes simplex infection by human leukocyte interferon after operation on the trigeminal root. *N Engl J Med* 301:225–230, 1979.

138. Grebeniuk VN, Kuznetsov VP, Rykova MP, et al: The effect of human leukocytic interferon in recurrent genital herpes. *Vestn Dermatol Venerol* 10:15–19, 1983.

6

GENITAL WARTS

Genital warts is a disease of the skin and/or mucous membranes caused by different types of human papillomavirus (HPV). The disease is mainly sexually transmitted; however, in certain cases autoinoculation cannot be ruled out. Clinical diseases include various types of macroscopically apparent anogenital warts while subclinical disease affects any part of the anogenital epithelium including the cervix, where it is most frequently encountered. Synonyms for genital warts are *condylomata acuminata, venereal warts, venereal vegetations,* and *figs.*

EPIDEMIOLOGY

Genital warts are one of the most common conditions seen in VD clinics in the United States and Europe. Their incidence has been rising steeply during the last two decades (Figure 6.1).[1-6] Approximately 500,000 cases are seen each year in the United States,[1] and the incidence of genital warts in England is over 60 cases per 100,000.[4] The disease is seen primarily in young sexually active persons, the majority of whom are from 16 to 25 years of age, with a frequency peak of 22 years for men and 19 years for women.[7,8]

There is sufficient evidence for the sexual transmission of genital warts, and a number of studies have shown that 50–70% of sexual partners of patients with genital warts also have the disease.[2,3,7-10] Not all infectious contacts must produce genital lesions. Resistance factors, although not completely understood, can be related to the presence or absence of skin abrasions, the quantity of infecting material, the age of the lesions (new warts are more infectious than old ones), and the immunological status of the host.[7,11]

Condylomata acuminata commonly affect genitalia but may also appear in the urethral or oral mucosa and in the anorectal region. Anal warts in women usually follow or accompany the development of genital warts,[7] but they may result from anal intercourse as well. Isolated warts in the anorectal region in men strongly suggest homosexual practices.[12] Among homosexual men, they are much more common than penile lesions.[12,13]

134

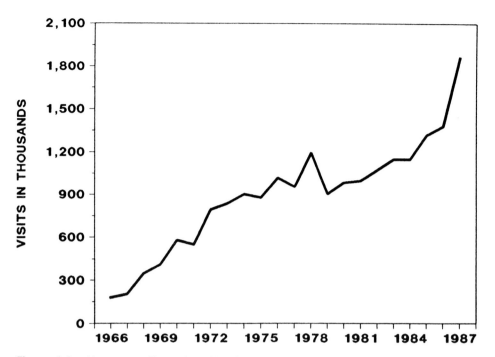

Figure 6.1. Human papillomavirus. Number of visits to private physicians' offices in the United States in 1966–1987.

Venereal warts in the mouth are very rare, and they may be associated with warts on the hands or with anogenital lesions.[14,15] Clinically they resemble verrucae vulgares or condylomata. Transmission probably occurs either through oral intercourse or self-inoculation.[2,15-17]

Although genital warts is a disease of young, sexually active adults, it has also been seen in children.[18-24] The origin of the disease in this group is not clear, but the mothers of some of these children may have been the source of infection.[19,20] In rare instances, the child may contract infection from the father, presumably through accidental inoculation.[21] In some cases, sexual child abuse has been incriminated.[18,22] The most common form of genital warts among children are vulval condylomata;[19,20] however, penile and anal warts also have been described.[18,21,23]

Transmission of the virus from mother to a child may occur during gestation, during labor, or after delivery promoted by close contact between mother and child. Maternal transmission of the disease may be confirmed by identification of HPV-6 and HPV-11 in juvenile laryngeal papillomas, very much as seen in vulval and cervical warts.[25] Of great importance is the information regarding two newborns who developed laryngeal papillomas during the first week of life after delivery by cesarean section. This suggests that the placenta should be considered as a possible route of infection.[26]

There has been much controversy about the relationship between genital and cutaneous warts. According to some studies, patients with genital warts do not have skin warts more often than the control population.[7,10] On the other hand, about 2% of genital warts clinically resemble common skin warts,[7] and it may be that in these cases the virus has been transferred to the genitals by the hands. Additional proof comes from viral studies showing the presence of HPV-1, HPV-2, and HPV-3 in anogenital lesions.[27,28]

CHARACTERISTICS OF HPV

The human papillomaviruses are host- and tissue-specific DNA viruses that are widespread in nature, causing characteristic proliferations on the skin and mucous membranes. The papillomaviruses are one of two members that make up the family of Papovaviridae and are further subdivided into specific types according to their nucleotide sequence homology. The HPVs comprise three clinicopathologic groups: cutaneotropic viruses found in immunologically normal individuals, cutaneotropic viruses found in epidermodysplasia verruciformis (EV), and mucosotropic viruses infecting the mucous membranes of the anogenital region, the mouth, and the respiratory tract.

Human papillomaviruses have a relatively simple structure. The viral particles are small, unenveloped spheres, about 55 nm in diameter, showing cubic symmetry in the arrangement of their subunits. All of them have a genome composed of a single molecule of a double-stranded supercoiled circular DNA complexed with histones, condensed into nucleosomes, and encapsulated in a isosahedral virion. The target cells for HPV infection seem to be the basal layer of the affected part of the epidermis or mucosa, where the virus remains undetectable, presumably latent, and progresses to active expression as progeny cells differentiate during their migrations toward the epithelial surface. This fact can be supported by the findings that productive viral DNA synthesis was detected only in the layer of differentiating epithelial cells but not in the basal layer or in the fibroblasts.[29,30]

Although the morphology of the virions of HPV species recovered from various clinical varieties of warts are identical, their types vary depending on the clinical features of the lesions. It seems likely that the different clinical types of lesions associated with an HPV are in fact distinct diseases caused by different types of human papillomaviruses (Table 6.1).[31-35] To date more than 50 types have been identified, and among them several subtypes have been characterized.

The HPV-associated lesions differ in their anatomic localization, their epidemiologic characters, their viral content, and their clinical evolution. Analysis of genital wart tissue has shown that the lesions may contain several different types of DNA. The most common HPV types found in condylomata acuminata were HPV-6 and HPV-11, whereas types 16, 18, and 31 were most often detected in high-grade premalignancies and invasive cancers.[9,36,37] Infrequently genital lesions contained a genome sequence related to HPV-1, HPV-2, and HPV-3, which are found in common skin warts.[28,38]

CLINICAL FEATURES

The incubation period of genital warts ranges from 6 weeks to 8 months, with an average of about 3 months.[7] The clinical features of genital warts depend on the type of virus and the location and duration of the lesions.

TABLE 6.1. Human Papillomavirus (HPV) Types and Their Clinical Manifestations

HPV Type	Clinical Manifestations
1a–c	Deep plantar warts (myrmecia warts)
2a–e	Mosaic plantar warts, common warts, palatal warts, filiform warts
3a,b	Flat warts, juvenile warts, mild forms of EV
4	Small hyperkeratotic palmar and plantar warts
5a,b, 8	Macular lesions of EV
6a–f	Condylomata acuminata, Buschke-Löwenstein tumors, CIN, GIN, laryngeal papillomas
7	Common hand warts in meat handlers and butchers
9,12,14, 15,17,19–29	Macular and flat wart lesions of EV
10a,b	Flat warts
11a,b	Condylomata acuminata, Buschke-Löwenstein tumors, laryngeal papillomas, conjunctival papillomas
13a,b, 32	Focal epithelial hyperplasia in mouth (Heck's disease)
16, 18	CIN, GIN, SSC of the uterine cervix, flat condylomata of the uterine cervix, vulvar and penile carcinoma, condylomata acuminata
30, 40	Laryngeal carcinoma
31, 35	CIN, SSC of the uterine cervix
33	CIN, GIN, carcinoma of the uterine cervix
34	GIN, Bowen's disease
36	Actinic keratosis, keratoacanthoma
37	Keratoacanthoma, malignant melanoma
38	Malignant melanoma
39	Carcinoma of the uterine cervix
41	Multiple flat wart lesions of the skin
42–45	Flat condylomas, genital papillomas, GIN

Key to abbreviations: EV = Epidermodysplasia verruciformis; CIN = Cervical intraepithelial neoplasia; GIN = Genital intraepithelial neoplasia; SSC = Squamous cell carcinoma
Compiled from the following: Syrjänen,[31,34] Silva et al.,[32] Mroczkowski and McEwen,[33] and Orth and Favre.[35] Holmes K.K.—personal communication.

Penile Warts

The most common clinical moiety of penile warts are condylomata acuminata (exophytic warts) caused by HPV-6 and HPV-11.[39] These kinds of lesions usually occur on surfaces subject to trauma, such as the margin of the corona of the glans, the frenulum, and the inner lining of the prepuce (Figure 6.2). Intraurethral condylomata can occur with the meatus commonly affected (Figure 6.3). Infrequently, condylomata acuminata may appear on the scrotum or in the groin (Figure 6.4).

The individual lesions are soft, white to grey or pink in color, elongated, filiform or pedunculated, and solitary or multiple. Initially small, they may grow and coalesce, taking on the so-called "cauliflower" appearance.

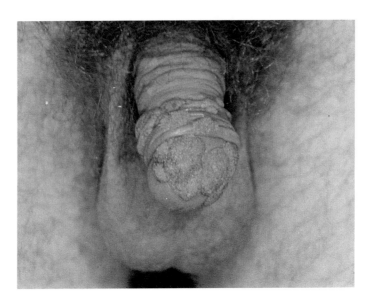

Figure 6.2. Warts on the glans of the penis, the inner surface of the prepuce, and the skin of the penis.

The second common type of warts found in the male genitalia are small, discrete, sessile warts commonly present on the shaft of the penis.[7] These kinds of warts can be the only warts present or are associated with typical condylomata on the glans. They resemble the flat warts on the nongenital skin. Subclinical infection of the penis with HPV is not uncommon. It can be revealed by application of 5% acetic acid and examination under magnification. The subclinical changes appear as irregular areas of white epithelium frequently found near macroscopically visible

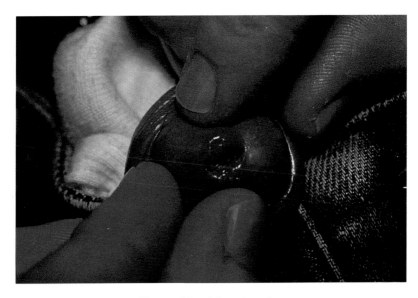

Figure 6.3. Meatal warts.

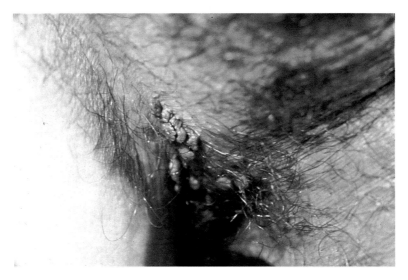

Figure 6.4. Condylomata acuminata in the groin.

warts but may also occur separately. Subclinical lesions are particularly important because of the possibility of unwitting infection of the sex partners.

Anal Warts

Anal warts are seen more frequently in men than in women and most commonly in homosexuals who engage in anal-receptive intercourse.[13] Since the anorectal area provides environmental conditions favorable for epithelial proliferation and microbial infection such as warmth, moisture, and mechanical friction, warts located in this area usually grow large and may be secondarily infected. Anorectal warts frequently assume the above-mentioned cauliflower-like appearance (Figure 6.5). In a high proportion of patients with anal warts, the lesions extend into the anal canal,[13] so examination by anoscopy is indicated for all patients so affected.

Vulval and Vaginal Warts

Condylomata acumata in females start as small, soft, verrucous papules at the fourchette, on the labia, the perineum, and the adjacent regions. They may involve vaginal, urethral, and anal mucosae as well as the cervix. At times the small lesions may coalesce to give an almost velvety appearance over large areas or form cock's comb-like excrescences along the labia (Figure 6.6). Between the labia majora and minora and around the introitus, the warts may form small warty or fleshy streaks. The lesions extending to the genitocrural folds are less soft and look more like common warts. In rare instances, the warts may develop into sessile, grapelike masses that completely mask the vulva. In pregnant women, genital warts may grow rapidly and become severe, with enlargement, maceration, and secondary infection.

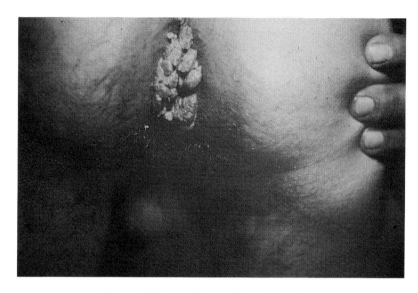

Figure 6.5.   Cauliflower-like anal warts.

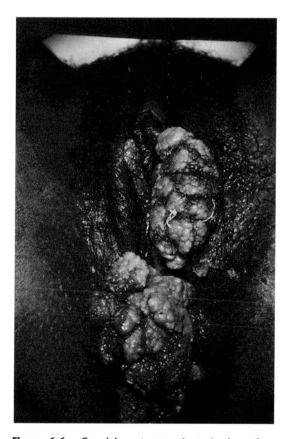

Figure 6.6.   Condylomata acuminata in the vulva.

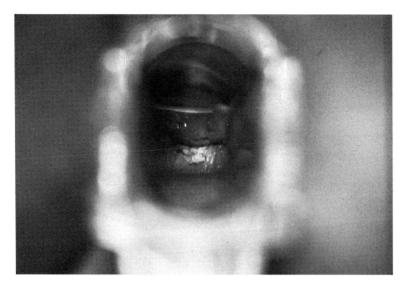

Figure 6.7. Exophytic warts on the cervix.

Similarly to microscopically invisible penile lesions, grossly inapparent warts may appear in the vulva or on the vaginal wall. They can be visualized by application of 5% acetic acid and are best visible by coloscope. They are usually symptomless but also have been incriminated as a possible cause of vulvodynia (long-standing burning and "rawness" in the vulva) or vulva vestibulitis syndrome (introital dyspareunia with tender red plaques in the vulva).[40]

Cervical Warts

Condylomatous lesions on the cervix present as classical exophytic (Figure 6.7) papillary condylomata acuminata or more frequently as flat lesions (condylomata plana).[41,42] The latter are macroscopically invisible and are recognized colposcopically as an acetowhite reaction. Both types of lesions show the same histological pattern. The flat condylomas are frequently indistinguishable from cervical intraepithelial neoplasia,[41,43] especially when they appear as a white epithelium in the transformation zone. Their surface is flat and mosaic pattern and/or punctuation can be seen. Their borders, however, are less sharply defined than those in cervical intraepithelial neoplasia.[41,43] These lesions should be viewed suspiciously if they are multiple, if they are outside the transformation zone, if the surrounding epithelium shows dilated capillaries, and if condylomata are present elsewhere in the genital tract.[41,43] Some cervical lesions may escape detection by colposcopy, thus necessitating the use of biopsy and cytology in the diagnosis.[42] The viral etiology of flat condylomata has been confirmed by electron microscopic observation of HPV particles,[41,44,45] by the peroxidase-antiperoxidase technique,[46] and by demonstrating the presence of an HPV DNA sequence using molecular cloning and hybridization techniques.[40,47,48] Many reports have emphasized their association with dysplastic and neoplastic lesions.[11,49-51]

Cervical warts are frequently associated with genital warts of other localization.[52] Therefore, identification of flat or exophytic warts on the cervix should prompt the physician to carefully inspect the vulva, vagina, and perianal regions and to use acetic acid to localize and treat all affected sites.

Buschke-Löwenstein Tumor

Buschke-Löwenstein (B-L) tumors are rare giant condylomata. Based on their clinical appearance and histologic features, they have been called "carcinoma-like condylomata" or "condylomata-like carcinomas." B-L tumors have a malignant fungating gross appearance and can be distinguished from typical condylomata by their deep penetration and compression of adjacent tissues. Despite these characteristics, they are histologically benign lesions and can be distinguished from true carcinomas by the absence of metastases.

A B-L tumor starts as a warty growth which gradually becomes nodular and penetrates underlying tissues. Fistulas may develop that exude putrid-smelling purulent fluid. Subsequently, the whole genitalia may be overgrown with luxuriant condylomatous masses. Secondary infection may cause maceration and erosions, with regional lymph node enlargement. B-L tumors appear mainly on the penis[53] but may also occur in the vulva, scrotum, perianum, groin, and oral mucosa.[54] The lesions contain HPV-6 and the closely related HPV-11 (Figures 6.8 and 6.9).[55]

Genital Intraepithelial Neoplasia

Genital intraepithelial neoplasia (GIN) is a relatively new clinical entity presumably caused by HPV types 16 and 18. The lesions usually appear on the external genitalia and have been previously described under different names such as multicentric pigmented Bowen's disease, multicentric Bowen's disease of the genitalia, bowenoid papulosis, erythroplasia of Queyrat, vulval intraepithelial neoplasia, penile intraepithelial neoplasia, and carcinoma in situ of the vulvae, just to name the most frequently used. GIN has the histologic feature of Bowen's disease but is clinically different.

The lesions of GIN may appear as small, flat, multicentric papules that are often irregular in outline and coalescent. They may be translucent or reddish to brown in color. In men GIN occur most commonly on the penile shaft but also have been found on the foreskin and the glans of penis (Figure 6.10). The surface of the lesions is mostly smooth and velvety, but in some instances small translucent papules may be difficult to distinguish from genital herpes.[56] The number of lesions may vary from a single papule to numerous and confluent papules throughout the whole glans of the penis in men and extending to the anal canal in women.[56,57]

In women the lesions may be multicentric or confluent, light or dark brown, and sometimes slightly elevated and papillomatous (Figure 6.11). They are usually located on labia majora and minora and may coalesce to form velvety plaques over a wide area of the anogenital skin.

The disease has been found mainly in relatively young sexually active adults but has been also described in a patient over 60 years old.[58]

The natural course of GIN is not well known since it has been recognized

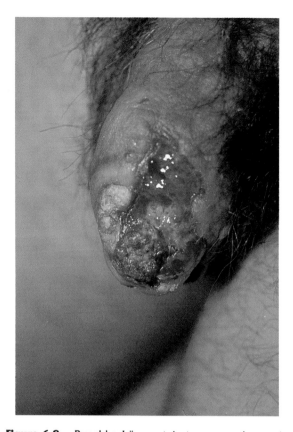

Figure 6.8. Buschke-Löwenstein tumor on the penis.

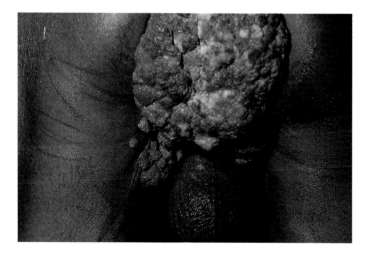

Figure 6.9. Buschke-Löwenstein tumor around the anus forming a huge cauliflower-like mass with superficial erosions.

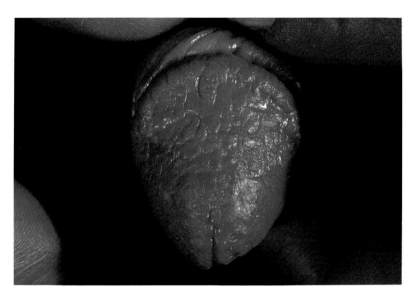

Figure 6.10. Genital intraepithelial neoplasia (GIN) on the glans of the penis (Bowenoid papulosis). Courtesy of Prof. S. Jabłońska.

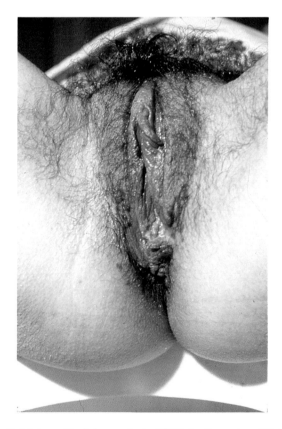

Figure 6.11. Genital intraepithelial neoplasia (GIN) in the vulva. (Multicentric Bowen's disease) Courtesy of Prof. S. Jabłońska.

recently and the number of cases followed is small. Genital intraepithelial neoplasia usually behave in a benign fashion, and in many instances spontaneous regression has been reported, especially in young women after delivery,[59] after repeated removal of single papules, or after destruction or removal of all lesions.[56,60] Some authors, however, reported single cases that progressed to squamous cell carcinoma[61] and to classic Bowen's disease.[62] An association of GIN with carcinoma in situ and invasive carcinoma has been also reported.[63,64]

COMPLICATIONS

In both sexes genital warts may cause the patients much trouble because of their size, common secondary bacterial infections, and occasional bleeding usually due to mechanical trauma.

In pregnant women in whom the genital warts tend to grow rapidly, they may cause problems in the management of pregnancy and labor. At times even small warts can be the cause of dyspareunia both in males and females.

Giant warts, for example, Buschke-Löwenstein tumors, may cause extensive tissue destruction[54,65] and/or formation of multiple fistulas and bleeding.[54,66] Warts located in the urethral meatus may interfere with urination, and the warts around anus may cause problems with defecation.

However, the most dangerous complication associated with HPV infection is its influence on cell-mediated immunity[67-69] and the relationship with genital cancer.[31,34,50,70,71]

HPV Infection and Malignancy

An increasing body of evidence supports the concept of a close relationship between HPV infection and malignant and premalignant lesions of genitalia and elsewhere. Certain papillomas that occur in rabbits and caused by Shope papillomavirus have been known for years to carry a high risk of conversion to squamous cell carcinoma. This transformation seems to be catalyzed by environmental carcinogens as well as by genetic constitution. In a similar way esophageal carcinoma in cattle living in areas where bracken ferns grow seems to be induced by the synergistic effect of bovine papillomavirus and carcinogens or immunodepressants, or both, present in the bracken.

There is no doubt that there is a close relationship between genital warts caused by different types of HPV and genital malignancy, and at least three types of associations can be pointed out: epidemiologic, virologic, and anatomic.

Numerous epidemiologic studies have suggested that genital carcinoma and its precursors are a venereally linked disease.[72-77] For example, cervical cancer occurs more often in countries with poor hygienic conditions[72,73] or in women living at a low socioeconomic level.[72,74] It has been found more often in persons with an early age of first intercourse and a higher number of different sexual partners[75,76] and almost nonexistent among virgins and nuns. Moreover, genital carcinomas develop 10–15 years earlier in patients who have condylomata acuminata than in those who do not.[77]

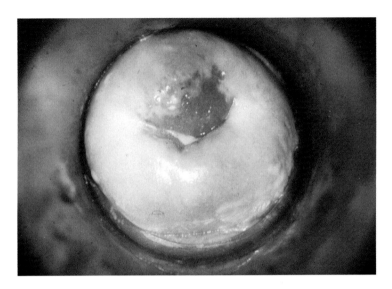

Figure 6.12. Cervical neoplasia has been frequently associated with HPV types 16, 18, 31, 33 and 35.

The second indication for a relationship between HPV and genital carcinomas is provided by the demonstration of HPV genomes within cancer tissues.[52,55,78] Five of the HPV types identified so far, 16, 18, 31, 33, and 35, have been related to cervical neoplasia (Figure 6.12).[9,78-80] Moreover, HPV-16 and HPV-18 sequences were found in vulvar and penile cancers (Figure 6.13) as well as in GIN and Bowen's disease of the genitalia.[56,81,82]

There is good evidence that premalignant genital lesions contain the same

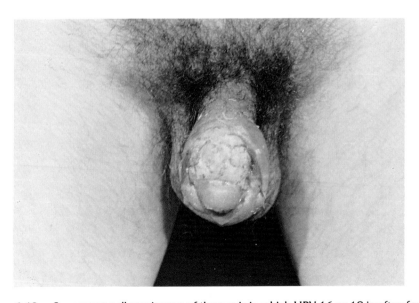

Figure 6.13. Squamous cell carcinoma of the penis in which HPV 16 or 18 is often found.

papillomavirus types that have been found in malignant tumors.[52,55,56,78-82] Studies by electron microscopy have revealed the presence of human papillomavirus particles in sections immediately adjacent to that of the carcinoma.[83,84] Isolated foci of squamous cell carcinomas (usually in situ) were found in sections of lesions which appear to be typical condylomata acuminata.[77] Moreover, an unexpectedly high proportion of patients with genital neoplasia have genital warts in the skin surrounding the cancerous lesions.[50,85]

Although the current opinion is that the association between HPV and genital neoplasia cannot be casual, the mere presence of these types of HPV in lesions does not seem to be sufficient to ensure their transformation into the carcinomas. Other cofactors seem to be necessary for this process to occur;[34] those seriously considered are

- The presence of other viral (herpes simplex virus or cytomegalovirus) or microbial (*Chlamydia trachomatis, Trichomonas vaginalis*) infections which may result in alterations of host and papillomavirus gene expression
- Local inflammatory responses to antigens and metabolites
- Genetic predisposition and host immune status
- Growth factor and oncogenic activation
- Radiation and other physical and/or chemical carcinogens (including tobacco products)
- Natural and contraceptive hormones
- Mechanical irritation resulting in the recurrent presence of wound epithelium

DIAGNOSIS

Histopathology

The diagnosis of genital warts is made predominantly on clinical grounds; however, histopathology may be necessary in some circumstances. In the case of cervical lesions, cytologic examination in addition to biopsy is recommended.

The histopathology of typical condyloma acuminatum in early lesions shows disk-like thickening of the epithelium above a flattened area of papillar dermis with dilated capillaries. The fully developed condyloma acuminatum shows extreme acanthosis and papillomatosis. The stratum corneum is thickened and shows focal parakeratosis. The prickle cells are larger than those of the adjacent normal epithelium. The most characteristic feature, however, is the presence of epithelial cells with perinuclear vacuolization.

The histology of the Buschke-Löwenstein tumor is similar to that of typical condyloma acuminata: acanthosis, papillomatosis with hyperplasia of the prickle cell layer, variable hyperkeratosis and parakeratosis with frequent underlying inflammation. The difference between typical condyloma acuminata and B-L tumors lies in the fact that ordinary conylomata are always superficial and spare underlying tissue, whereas the B-L tumors have a pronounced tendency to downward growth, simulating malignant invasion.

The histology of genital intraepithelial neoplasia has the feature of Bowen's atypia. The characteristic findings are epidermal hyperplasia with numerous, often abnormal mitotic figures, atypical cells with large hyperchromatic pleomorphic nuclei, multinucleated cells containing clusters of nuclei, and large dyskeratotic cells. The epidermal-dermal border is preserved. There may be slight inflammatory infiltrates and dilated papillary capillaries. Histologic differentiation between GIN and Bowen's disease is not possible in most instances. Histologically GIN is graded from I to IV according to the amount of change within the epithelium.

Colposcopy

Identification of cervical lesions and lesions of GIN may require colposcopic examination. Typical condyloma acuminatum on the cervix looks like exophytic papilloma. Condylomata plana which are macroscopically invisible can be recognized colposcopically with the use of 5% acetic acid. Even though the application of acetic acid should reveal the invisible lesions of GIN, the use of a colposcope can be very helpful in identifying lesions located on the vaginal wall and the small foci of GIN in the vulva. Colposcopy was also found to be very useful in evaluating male patients infected with HPV in whom penile lesions would not be visualized otherwise.[86] Despite the fact that in experienced hands colposcopy is a reliable method of detection of HPV-induced lesions, some of them may escape detection by this method.[87]

Cytology

The presence of koilocytes in the Papanicolaou-stained smear is regarded as a pathognomonic sign of HPV infection[48] and is considered to be a cytopathic effect caused by HPV.[88] Koilocytes are the cells characterized by a perinuclear cavity (perinuclear clearing) surrounded by dense peripheral cytoplasm. The nuclei of the cells may be single, but binucleation or multinucleation is frequent. The nuclei of koilocytes often exhibit hyperchromasia and a loss of chromatin pattern.

Other characteristic cytologic features of HPV infection of the cervix is the almost constant shedding of dyskeratotic cells.[89] Dyskeratocytes, which are small, keratinized squamous cells, exhibit on Pap smear an intensely orangeophilic cytoplasm and an enlarged, usually pyknotic, nucleus. Sometimes the nuclei may display dyskeratotic changes depending on whether intraepithelial neoplasia are present.[70,89]

Evaluation of the nuclear/cytoplasmic ratio in both koilocytes and dyskeratotic cells may enable one to assess whether the examined lesion is accompanied by intraepithelial neoplasia, which is very important from a prognostic viewpoint.[90,91]

HPV Identification

- Electron microscopy reveals viral particles in tissues from biopsies or in cells from smears. However, the method is laborious and time consuming because the genital lesions contain scanty HPV particles.
- DNA hybridization is so far the most precise technique for identifying the presence of viral DNA in tissue. Techniques available for typing HPV DNA include Southern blot, dot blot, filter in situ, sandwich, and in situ hybridization.

- Immunoperoxidase reaction enables the visualization of the papillomavirus antigen by light microscopy using an antiserum prepared with HPV.[92] A positive reaction results in a dark, gold-brown staining of nuclei. The positive reaction is preferentially localized in the nuclei of koilocytes and dyskeratocytes.

Differential Diagnosis

- *Condylomata lata in secondary syphilis:* flat papules in genital and intertriginous areas; positive dark-field examination; positive serology (usually high titer).
- *Pearly penile papules:* parallel rows of tiny filiform papules around the corona; histology demonstrates hypertrophic papillae with normal epidermis.
- *Molluscum contagiosum:* small lesions may resemble genital warts; however, round opening at the summit of the lesion and the presence of an expressible white caseous material will help to establish diagnosis.
- *Genital carcinoma:* may cause great difficulty in differential diagnosis; biopsy is essential; penile carcinomas are usually hard and nonmovable, frequently with inguinal node involvement. Vulvar carcinoma may be indistinguishable from condylomata acuminata which in fact may precede it; early biopsy is the only method of diagnosis.
- *Benign neoplasms:* fibromas, lipomas, hidradenomas, and adenomas can all be ruled out by biopsy.
- *Lichen planus:* small, flat-topped, shiny whitish to violaceous papules, grouped or linearly arranged; histology is decisive.
- *Genital herpes:* painful grouped blisters; frequent recurrences; Tzanck smear positive; positive viral culture.
- *Multiple pigmented papillomas:* biopsy, histologic pattern of papillomas without Bowenoid atypia.
- *Bowen's disease:* usually solitary, nonpigmented lesion; slowly progressive course without tendency to spontaneous regression, older age of patients; histology may be indistinguishable from GIN.
- *Anal warts:* should be distinguished from *rectal cancer* and *hemorrhoids.*
- *Cervical lesions:* should be distinguished from *intraepithelial dysplasia;* cytology is necessary; histology.

TREATMENT

Condylomata Acuminata:

Cryotherapy with liquid nitrogen or dry ice is currently the most frequently used of all the destructive methods of the treatment of warts. It is easy because no anesthetic is required and it is relatively very precise.[93] Liquid nitrogen is applied to the wart either with the use of cotton-tipped swabs or with a specially constructed apparatus with changeable nozzles adapted to the shape and diameter of lesions. The diameter of the metal or cotton tip cryoapplicator should be, more or less, the same as the diameter of the lesion, and the entire lesion plus a surrounding area should be frozen.[94] Genital warts are very responsive to cryotherapy (more than skin warts), and the best results were observed in anal warts.[94] The genital warts treated with liquid nitrogen disappeared more rapidly than after treatment with podophyllin, and complications were less frequent.[95] Cryotherapy has been successfully used to treat cervical lesions with no consequences for future pregnancies and labor.[96]

Podophyllin, 10–25 percent in compound tincture of benzoin, should be applied carefully to each wart, avoiding normal tissue, and left in contact with the wart for 2–4 hours and thoroughly washed out. Some specialists use a longer period, but this should be individualized after the patient's tolerance and compliance have been established. This procedure can be repeated once or twice weekly. Podophyllin should not be used during pregnancy and with oral and meatal warts. It should be used with extreme caution for vaginal or cervical warts and abandoned if other methods of treatment are available. Podophyllin is ineffective in Buschke-Löwenstein tumors and GIN.

Use of a carbon dioxide laser is the newest of the destructive methods available. It seems that this method affords more precise tissue ablation, leaves less necrotic tissue, and heals slightly faster than any other method. Also, patients treated with a laser for cervical intraepithelial neoplasia found the laser less objectionable when cost was not considered. However, compared with cryotherapy, laser therapy is much more expensive.[97] The carbon dioxide laser was highly successful for the treatment of persistent or extensive urogenital and anal condyloma.[98] It was also successfully used in the treatment of genital warts in pregnant women.[99]

Electrosurgical removal is highly effective and should be applied in meatal warts or when the lesions are extensive. Surgical removal should be considered in cases where podophyllin is contraindicated or cryotherapy or laser therapy is not available.

5-Fluorouracil (5% fluorinated pyrimidine) has been successfully used, including in the treatment of intraurethral condylomata.[100]

Immunotherapies using different interferons[101,102] or inosine pranobex (Immunovir®),[103] have been tested in the treatment of genital warts. These relatively new methods, which seem to be effective and fairly well tolerated, hold great promise for the therapy of genital warts in the future, although further trials are desirable and reduction of cost necessary.

Buschke-Löwenstein Tumors

Surgical removal or Moh's fresh-tissue histographic surgery is recommended for this giant condyloma.[104]

Genital Intraepithelial Neoplasia

Cryotherapy,[105] carbon dioxide laser,[106] electrocautery,[107,108] surgical excisions,[56,109] and excision with skin graft[110] have all been recommended for the treatment of genital intraepithelial neoplasia. Because of possible spontaneous regression, any radical approach in young patients, for example, total vulvectomy or amputation of the penis, should be avoided.

MANAGEMENT OF SEX PARTNERS AND PREVENTION

All patients with genital warts should be urged to encourage their sex partners to seek examination as soon as possible so that treatment can be provided if necessary. To reduce recurrence rates due to reinfection, the patients should use condoms until their partner has been examined and shown to be free of disease. However, bearing in mind the fact that the incubation period may be as long as 8 months, a single examination may not be enough, and the sex partners of patients with genital warts should be evaluated on several occasions. Of special consideration should be reports that 53% of male sex partners of women with cervical intraepithelial neoplasia have HPV-induced genital lesions,[111] that the male consorts of cervical cancer patients are at risk for penile carcinoma,[112] and that second wives of men whose first wives died of cervical cancer are at increased risk of developing cervical cancer.[113]

If the association between HPV infection and genital cancer is not casual and the human papillomavirus can be sexually transmitted, the conclusion that genital cancer can be a sexually transmitted disease sounds logical. If this is true, appropriate patient education and more rigorous epidemiologic measures seem to be necessary to prevent the spread of HPV-induced disease.

REFERENCES

1. Condyloma acuminatum, United States, 1966–1981, *MMWR* 23:306–308, 1983.
2. Oriel JD: Genital warts. *Sex Transm Dis* 4:153–159, 1977.
3. Wallin J: Sexually transmitted diseases: The present situation in Sweden. *Br J Vener Dis* 54:24–27, 1978.
4. Annual Report of the Chief Medical Officer 1981: Sexually transmitted diseases. *Br J Vener Dis* 59:206–210, 1983.
5. Felman YM: Condylomata acuminata. *Cutis* 33:118–120, 1984.
6. Annual report of the Chief Medical Office DHSS for the year 1982: Sexually transmitted disease. *Br J Vener Dis* 60:199–203, 1984.
7. Oriel JD: Natural history of genital warts. *Br J Vener Dis* 47:1–13, 1971.
8. Eftaiha MS, Amshel AL, Shonberg IL, et al: Giant and recurrent condyloma acuminatum: Appraisal of immunotherapy. *Dis Colon Rectum* 25:136–138, 1982.
9. Sand PK, Bowen L, Blischke SO, et al: Evaluation of male consorts of women with genital human papilloma virus infection. *Obstet Gynecol* 68:679–681, 1986.
10. Teokharov BA: Nongonococcal infections of the female genitalia. *Br J Vener Dis* 45:334–339, 1969.
11. Powell LC: Condyloma acuminatum: Recent advances in development, carcinogenesis and treatment. *Clin Obstet Gynecol* 21:1061–1079, 1978.

12. Oriel JD: Anal warts and anal coitus. *Br J Vener Dis* 47:373–376, 1971.

13. Carr G, William DC: Anal warts in a population of gay men in New York City. *Sex Transm Dis* 4:56–57, 1977.

14. Lutzner M, Kuffer R, Blanchet-Bardon C, et al: Different papillomaviruses as the cause of oral warts. *Arch Dermatol* 118:393–399, 1982.

15. Anneroth G, Anniko M, Romander H: Oral condyloma acuminatum: A light and electronmicroscopic study. *Int J Oral Surg* 11:260–264, 1982.

16. Judson FN: Condyloma acuminatum of the oral cavity: A case report. *Sex Transm Dis* 8:218–219, 1981.

17. Fiumara NJ: The management of warts of the oral cavity. *Sex Transm Dis* 11:267–270, 1984.

18. Sait MA, Garg BR: Condylomata acuminata in children: Report of four cases. *Genitourin Med* 61:338–342, 1985.

19. Patel R, Groff DB: Condylomata acuminata in childhood. *Pediatrics* 50:152–153, 1972.

20. Grace DA, Ochsner JA, McClain CR, et al: Vulvar condylomata acuminata in prepubertal females. *JAMA* 201:137–138, 1967.

21. Baruah MC, Sardari L, Selvaraju M, et al: Perianal condylomata acuminata in a male child. *Br J Vener Dis* 60:60–61, 1984.

22. Storrs FJ: Spread of condylomata acuminata to infants and children. *Arch Dermatol* 113:1294, 1977.

23. Eftaiha MS, Amshel AL, Shonberg IL: Condylomata acuminata in an infant and mother: Report of a case. *Dis Colon Rectum* 21:369–371, 1978.

24. Bender ME: New concept of condyloma acuminata in children. *Arch Dermatol* 122:1121–1123, 1986.

25. Gissmann L, Diehl V, Schultz-Coulon H-J, et al: Molecular cloning and characterization of human papilloma virus DNA derived from a laryngeal papilloma. *J Virol* 44:393–400, 1982.

26. Steinberg BM, Abramson AL: Laryngeal papillomas. *Clin Dermatol* 3:130–137, 1985.

27. Orth G, Jablonska S, Breitburd F, et al: The human papillomaviruses. *Bull Cancer* 65:151–164, 1978.

28. Krzyzek RA, Watts SL, Anderson DL, et al: Anogenital warts contain several distinct species of human papillomavirus. *J Virol* 36:236–244, 1980.

29. Gupta J, Gendelman HE, Naghashfar Z, et al: Specific identification of human papillomavirus type in cervical smears and paraffin sections by in situ hybridization with radioactive probes: A preliminary communication. *Int J Gynecol Pathol* 4:211–218, 1985.

30. Syrjänen S, Von Krogh G, Syrjänen K: Detection of human papillomavirus (HPV) DNA in anogenital condylomata using in situ DNA-hybridization applied to paraffin-sections. *Genitourin Med* 63:32–39, 1987.

31. Syrjänen KJ: Current concepts of human papillomavirus infections in the genital tract and their relationship to intraepithelial neoplasia and squamous cell carcinoma. *Obstet Gynecol Surv* 39:252–256, 1984.

32. Silva PD, Micha JP, Silva DG: Management of condyloma acuminatum. *J Am Acad Dermatol* 13:457–463, 1985.

33. Mroczkowski TF, McEwen C: Warts and other human papillomavirus infections. *Postgrad Med* 78:91–98, 1985.

34. Syrjänen KJ: Genital papillomavirus infections and their sequelae. 1. Virology and pathogensis, in *Proceedings of an International Symposium Held During the 17th World*

Congress of Dermatology, Berlin, May, 1987, pp. 5–15. Update—Siebert Publications Ltd. Guilford, UK.

35. Orth G, Favre M: Human papillomavirus. Biochemical and biologic properties. *Clin Dermatol* 3:27–42, 1985.

36. Zachow KR, Ostrow RS, Bender M: Detection of human papillomavirus DNA in anogenital neoplasia. *Nature* 300:771–773, 1982.

37. Durst M, Gissmann L, Ikenberg H, et al: A papillomavirus DNA from a cervical carcinoma and its prevalence in cancer biopsy samples from different geographic regions. *Proc Natl Acad Sci USA* 80:3812–3815, 1983.

38. Jabłońska S, Orth G: Human papovaviruses, in Rook A, Maibach HJ (eds), *Recent Advances in Dermatology*. Churchill Livingstone, 1983, p. 1.

39. Gissmann L, Wolnik L, Ikenberg H, et al: Human papillomavirus type 6 and 11 DNA sequences in genital and laryngeal papillomas and in some cervical cancers. *Proc Natl Acad Sci USA* 80:560–563, 1983.

40. Turner MC, Marinoff S, Lancaster W, et al: The association of human papillomavirus with vulvodynia and vulva vestibulitis syndrome. Poster presented at the American Academy of Dermatology, Washington, DC, December, 1988.

41. Meisels A, Fortin R, Roy M: Condylomatous lesions of the cervix. II. Cytologic, colposcopic and histopathologic study. *Acta Cytol* 21:379–390, 1977.

42. Purola E, Savia E: Cytology of gynecologic condyloma acuminatum. *Acta Cytol* 21:26–31, 1977.

43. Meisels A, Roy M, Fortier M: Condylomatous lesions of the cervix: Morphologic and colposcopic diagnosis. *Am J Diag Gynecol Obstet* 1:109–116, 1979.

44. Hills E, Laverty CR: Electron microscopic detection of papillomavirus particles in selected koilocytotic cells in a routine cervical smear. *Acta Cytol* 23:53–56, 1979.

45. Morin C, Meisels A: Papillomavirus infection of the uterine cervix. *Acta Cytol* 24:82–84, 1980.

46. Ferenczy A, Braun L, Shah KV: Human papillomavirus (HPV) in condylomatous lesions of cervix. *Am J Surg Pathol* 5:661–670, 1981.

47. DeVilliers M, Gissmann L, zur Hausen H: Molecular cloning of viral DNA from human genital wart. *J Virol* 40:932–935, 1981.

48. Meisels A, Casas-Cordero M, Morin C: Cervical condyloma planum. *Clin Dermatol* 3:114–123, 1985.

49. Meisels A, Morin C: Human papillomavirus and cancer of the uterine cervix. *Gynecol Oncol* 2:S111–S123, 1981.

50. zur Hausen H: Human papillomaviruses and their possible role in squamous cell carcinomas. *Curr Top Microbiol Immunol* 78:1–31, 1977.

51. Ludwig ME, Lowell DM, Livolsi VA: Cervical condylomatous atypia and its relationship to cervical neoplasia. *Am J Clin Pathol* 76:255–262, 1981.

52. Schneider A, Sawada E, Gissmann L, et al: Human papillomavirus in women with a history of abnormal Papanicolau smears and their male partners. *Obstet Gynecol* 69:554–559, 1987.

53. Ananthakrishan N, Ravidran R, Veliath AJ, et al: Löwenstein-Buschke tumor of the penis—a carcinomimic. Report of 24 cases with a review of the literature. *Br J Urol* 53:460–465, 1981.

54. Grussendorf-Conen E-I: Condylomata acuminata. *Clin Dermatol* 3:97–103, 1985.

55. Gissmann L: Papillomaviruses and their association with cancer in animals and in man. *Cancer Surv* 3:162–181, 1984.

56. Obałek S, Jabłońska S, Orth G: HPV-associated intraepithelial neoplasia of external genitalia. *Clin Dermatol* 3:104–113, 1985.

57. Kaplan AL, Kaufman RH, Birken RA, et al: Intraepithelial carcinoma of the vulva with extension to the anal canal. *Obstet Gynecol* 58:368–371, 1981.

58. Kimura S: Bowenoid papulosis of the genitalia. *Int J Dermatol* 21:432–436, 1982.

59. Friedrich EG: Reversible vulvar atypia: A case report. *Obstet Gynecol* 39:173–181, 1972.

60. Zelickson AS, Prawer SE: Bowenoid papulosis of the penis: Demonstration of intranuclear viral-like particles. *Am J Dermatopathol* 2:305–308, 1980.

61. Hirai A, Inamoto N, Harada R, et al: So-called multicentric pigmented Bowen's disease progressing to squamous cell carcinoma. *J Dermatol* (Tokyo) 89:380–383, 1979.

62. De Villez RL, Stevens Ch S: Bowenoid papules of the genitalia: A case progressing to Bowen's disease. *J Am Acad Dermatol* 3:149–152, 1980.

63. King CM, Yates VM, Dave VK: Multicentric pigmented Bowen's disease of the genitalia associated with carcinoma in situ of the cervix. *Br J Vener Dis* 60:406–408, 1984.

64. Friedrick EG, Wilkinson EJ, Fu YS: Carcinoma in situ of the vulva: A continuing challenge. *Am J Obstet Gynecol* 136:830–838, 1980.

65. Harvey JM, Glen E, Watson GS: Buschke-Löwenstein tumor of the penis: A case report. *Br J Vener Dis* 59:273–276, 1983.

66. Saeks EH, Goldman L, Schwarz J: Giant condyloma acuminatum of Buschke and Löwenstein. *Cutis* 26:386–388, 1980.

67. Avgerinou G, Georgala S, Theodoridis A, et al: Reduction of cell mediated immunity in patients with genital warts of long duration. *Genitourin Med* 62:396–398, 1986.

68. Mohanty KC, Roy RB: Thymus derived lymphocytes (T-cells) in patients with genital warts. *Br J Vener Dis* 60:186–188, 1984.

69. Chardonnet Y, Viac J, Staquet MJ, et al: Cell-mediated immunity to human papillomavirus. *Clin Dermatol* 3:156–164, 1985.

70. Syrjänen KJ: Human papillomavirus (HPV) infections of the female genital tract and their association with intraepithelial neoplasia and squamous cell carcinoma. *Pathol Ann* 21:53–89, 1986.

71. zur Hausen H: Intracellular surveillance of persisting viral infections. Human genital cancer results from deficient cellular control of papillomavirus gene expression. *Lancet* 2:489–491, 1986.

72. Lunt R: Worldwide early detection of cervical cancer. *Obstet Gynecol* 63:708–713, 1984.

73. *Report of the Surgeon General: Cancer Incidence in Five Continents.* Washington, DC, 1982, Vol. 4.

74. Jones EG, MacDonald I, Breslow L: Study of epidemiologic factors in carcinoma of uteri cervix. *Am J Obstet Gynecol* 76:1–10, 1958.

75. Rotkin ID: A comparison review of key epidemiological studies in cervical cancer related to current searches for transmissible agents. *Cancer Res* 33:1353–1367, 1973.

76. Beral V: Cancer of the cervix: A sexually transmitted infection? *Lancet* 1:1037–1040, 1974.

77. Josey WE, Nahmias AJ, Naib ZM: Viruses and cancer of the lower genital tract. *Cancer* 38(Suppl):526–533, 1976.

78. Boshart M, Gissmann L, Ikenberg H, et al: A new type of papillomavirus DNA: Its presence in genital cancer biopsies and in cell lines derived from cervical cancer. *EMBO J* 3:1151–1157, 1984.

79. Reid R, Greenberg M, Jenson AB, et al: Sexually transmitted papilloma infections. I: The anatomic distribution and pathologic grade neoplastic lesions associated with different viral types. *Am J Obstet Gynecol* 156:212–222, 1987.

80. McCanse DJ, Campion MJ, Clarkson PK, et al: Prevalence of human papillomavirus type 16 DNA sequence in cervical intraepithelial neoplasia and invasive carcinoma of the cervix. *Br J Obstet Gynaecol* 92:1101–1105, 1985.

81. Ikenberg H, Gissmann L, Gross G, et al: Human papillomavirus type 16 related DNA in genital Bowen's disease and in bowenoid papulosis. *Int J Cancer* 32:563–565, 1983.

82. Gissmann L, Gross G: Association of HPV with human genital tumors. *Clin Dermatol* 3:124–129, 1985.

83. Grussendorf E-I, Bar T: Condylomata acuminata with M. Bowen: Carcinoma in situ: A light and electron microscopic study. *Dermatologica* 155:50–58, 1977.

84. Kovi J, Tillman RL, Lee SM: Malignant transformation of condyloma acuminatum: A light microscopic and ultrastructural study. *Am J Clin Pathol* 61:702–710, 1974.

85. Bender ME, Pass F: Papillomavirus and cutaneous malignancy. *Int J Dermatol* 20:468–474, 1981.

86. Comite SL, Castadot M-J: Colposcopic evaluation of men with genital warts. *J Am Acad Dermatol* 18:1274–1278, 1988.

87. Purola E, Halila H, Vesterinen E: Condyloma and cervical epithelial atypias in young women. *Gynecol Oncol* 16:34–40, 1983.

88. Meisels A, Fortin R, Roy M: Condylomatous lesions of cervix and vagina 1. Cytologic patterns. *Acta Cytol* 20:505–509, 1976.

89. Syrjänen KJ, Heinonen UM, Kauraniemi T: Cytological evidence of the association of condylomatous lesions with the displastic and neoplastic changes in the uterine cervix. *Acta Cytol* 25:17–22, 1981.

90. Syrjänen K, Väyrynen M, Saarikoski S, et al: Natural history of cervical human papillomavirus (HPV) infections based on prospective follow-up. *Br J Obstet Gynecol* 92:1086–1092, 1985.

91. Syrjänen KJ, Mantyjärvi R, Väyrynen M, et al: Cervical smears in assessment of natural history of human papillomavirus infections in prospective followed women. *Acta Cytol* 31:855–865, 1987.

92. Jenson AB, Rosenthal JR, Olson C, et al: Immunologic relatedness of papillomaviruses from different species. *J Natl Cancer Inst* 64:495–500, 1980.

93. Ghosh AK: Cryosurgery of genital warts in cases in which podohyllin treatment failed or was contraindicated. *Br J Vener Dis* 53:49–53, 1977.

94. Dachow-Siwiec E: Technique of cryotherapy. *Clin Dermatol* 3:185–188, 1985.

95. Mroczkowski TF, Dachow-Siwiec E: Cryotherapy in the treatment of genital warts. Paper presented at 4th meeting of ISSTDR, Heidelberg, Federal Republic of Germany, October, 1981.

96. Benrubi GI, Young M, Nuss RC: Intrapartum outcome of term pregnancy after cervical cryotherapy. *J Reprod Med* 29:251–254, 1984.

97. Wetchler SJ: Treatment of cervical intraepithelial neoplasia with the CO_2 laser: Laser versus cryotherapy. A review of effectiveness and cost. *Obstet Gynecol Surv* 39:469–473, 1984.

98. Ferenczy A: Laser therapy of genital condylomata acuminata. *Obstet Gynecol* 63:703–707, 1984.

99. Ferenczy A: Treating genital condyloma during pregnancy with the carbon dioxide laser. *Am J Obstet Gynecol* 184:9–12, 1984.

100. Dretler SP, Klein LA: The eradication of urethral condylomata acuminata with 5 percent 5-fluorouracil cream. *J Urol* 113:195–198, 1975.

101. Schoenfeld A, Nitke S, Schattner A, et al: Intramuscular interferon injections in the treatment of condylomata acuminata. *Lancet* 1:1038–1042, 1984.

102. Eron LJ, Judson F, Tucker S, et al: Interferon therapy for condylomata acuminata. *N Engl J Med* 315:1059–1064, 1986.

103. Mohanty KC, Scott CS: Immunotherapy of genital warts with inosine pranobex (Immunovir): Preliminary study. *Genitourin Med* 62:352–355, 1986.

104. Rees RB: The treatment of warts. *Clin Dermatol* 3:179–184, 1985.

105. Bergman A, Bhatia NM, Broen EM: Cryotherapy for treatment of genital condyloma during pregnancy. *J Reprod Med* 29:432–435, 1984.

106. Jobson VW, Homesley HD: Treatment of vaginal intraepithelial neoplasia with the carbon dioxide laser. *Obstet Gynecol* 62:90–93, 1983.

107. Wade TR, Kopf AW, Ackerman AB: Bowenoid papulosis of the genitalia. *Arch Dermatol* 115:306–308, 1979.

108. Hilliard GD, Massey FM, O'Toole RV: Vulvar neoplasia in the young. *Am J Obstet Gynecol* 135:185–188, 1979.

109. Ulbright TM, Stehman FB, Roth LM, et al: Bowenoid dysplasia of the vulva. *Cancer* 50:2910–2919, 1982.

110. Rutledge F, Sinclair M: Treatment of intraepithelial carcinoma of the vulvae by skin excision and graft. *Am J Obstet Gynecol* 102:806–818, 1968.

111. Levine RU, Crum CP, Herman E, et al: Cervical papillomavirus infection and intraepithelial neoplasia: A study of male sexual partners. *Obstet Gynecol* 64:16–20, 1984.

112. Boxer RJ, Skinner DG: Condylomata acuminata and squamous cell carcinoma. *Urology* 9:72–78, 1977.

113. Kessler II: Venereal factors in human cervical cancer: Evidence from marital clusters. *Cancer* 39:1912–1939, 1977.

7

MOLLUSCUM CONTAGIOSUM

Molluscum contagiosum is a superficial cutaneous infection of children and young adults caused by a member of the pox virus group. The disease is characterized by the presence of small umbilicated papules located on exposed skin in children or lower abdomen, thighs and the skin of genitals in adults. The disease in children seems to be transmitted by direct contact, while in adults it is often sexually transmitted.

Synonyms for molluscum contagiosum are *condyloma porcelaneum* and *epithelioma contagiosum.*

EPIDEMIOLOGY

Molluscum contagiosum is found worldwide and most commonly affects children and sexually active adults. In the South Pacific, where molluscum contagiosum is considered a childhood disease, an estimated incidence at one time was 10,000 cases per 100,000[1,2] with a peak incidence of 25 percent found among children under 5 years of age. Among children the disease is transmitted primarily by nonsexual means, and lesions presumably result from skin-to-skin or fomite-to-skin transmission of the virus. Usually boys are more frequently affected than girls.[3]

As with other viral STDs, the prevalence of molluscum contagiosum infections increased in recent years. In STD clinics in Great Britain, one case of molluscum contagiosum for every 60 cases of gonorrhoea was reported in 1978,[4] whereas selected STD clinics in the United States identified molluscum contagiosum once for every 42 cases of gonorrhoea during 1976–1980, or 1 for every 190 persons attending these clinics.[5] Data collected from the National Disease and Therapeutic Index Survey of private patients at selected STD clinics indicates that the greatest incidence of molluscum contagiosum is in the 15–29-year age group,[6] presumably the most sexually active segment of the population.

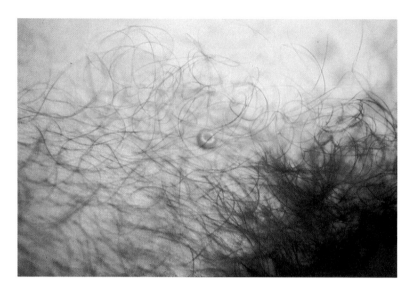

Figure 7.1. Molluscum contagiosum: typical hemispherical papule with umbilicated center.

There is little doubt that molluscum contagiosum is sexually transmitted among adults. The distribution of lesions,[7,8] the sexual promiscuity of the patients,[7-9] the same disease identified in sex partners,[8,9] and the common occurrence of other STDs in these patients[7,9,10] confirm this. However, nonsexual transmission has been reported among wrestlers,[11] patients of a surgeon with a hand lesion,[12] and masseurs and patrons of public baths and swimming pools.[3]

CLINICAL FEATURES

The incubation period of molluscum contagiosum ranges from 7 days to 6 months (average 2–3 months).[5] The typical lesion is a pinhead to pea-sized, firm, smooth-surfaced, shiny, hemispherical papule with an umbilicated center (Figure 7.1). Its color can be flesh, pearly white, translucent, or even yellow. When squeezed, caseous or curd-like material may be expressed from the lesion.

The number of lesions generally varies from 1 to 20, but hundreds of lesions may occur.[13,14] Multiple, widespread lesions often have been associated with atopy,[15-17] administration of corticosteroids,[18] or impaired immunity, either congenital or acquired, including AIDS.[19-21]

The lesions of molluscum contagiosum tend to occur in groups but may be solitary. The size of the lesions varies with their duration. The average lesions is 2–5 mm in diameter, but single lesions of more than 15 mm have been described.

In adults, in whom the disease is often sexually transmitted, the lesions are located in the lower abdomen; around the pubic hairs on the genitalia; on the upper, inner aspects of the thighs; in the perianal region; and on the buttocks (Figures 7.2 and 7.3). Lesions in children may appear on any part of the body but are most commonly seen on the face, chest, arms, and legs.

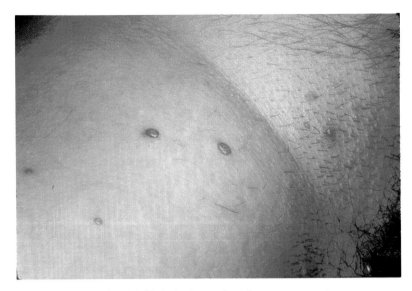

Figure 7.2. Multiple lesions of molluscum contagiosum.

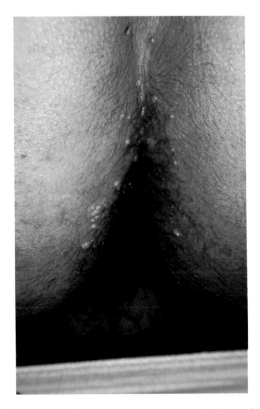

Figure 7.3. Mollusca contagiosa on the buttocks.

Molluscum contagiosum lesions may occur rarely on palms,[22] soles,[23] and eyelids and may infect conjunctiva.[24] At times the lesions may be linearly oriented, which would suggest that the disease may be autoinoculated by scratching (Koebner's phenomenon).[3]

Most patients with molluscum contagiosum are asymptomatical though a few may complain of pruritus, tenderness, or even mild pain at the site of the lesion. Some (about 10 percent) develop an eczematous reaction around the lesion, the so-called "molluscum dermatitis,"[25] often with secondary bacterial infection.[26]

Untreated lesions usually last 2–4 months, but single lesions may persist for years. However, most of them resolve spontaneously in 6–12 months as a result of the inflammatory response to secondary bacterial infection, trauma, or spontaneous rupture. It has been suggested that each of these releases viral antigen into the dermis eliciting an immune response.[27] Recurrences of lesions have also been observed in these same locations. It is not clear whether they were exacerbations of latent infection or simply reinfections.

Special consideration should be given to patients with AIDS who frequently develop molluscum contagiosum.[19-21] In these patients the lesions frequently appear on the skin of the face where, over a short period of time, they may increase in number and size, spreading to the forehead, scalp, and neck. In patients with AIDS, treatment of molluscum contagiosum is difficult because of poor local inflammatory response.

DIAGNOSIS

Diagnosis is largely clinical, based on the presence of small, pearly, umbilicated papules on exposed areas in children and in the lower abdomen or genital area of young sexually active adults. Occasionally the central umbilication may be inconspicuous, and gentle freezing with ethyl chloride may help accentuate this depression.

Laboratory Diagnosis

Although clinical diagnosis is usually quite reliable, it can be confirmed by identification of characteristic intracytoplasmic inclusion in histologic preparations or in smears. Molluscum contagiosum virions may be also identified by light microscope or by electron microscopy. Antigens of molluscum contagiosum may be detected using fluorescent antibody techniques.

Histology: Hematoxylin and eosin–stained tissue sections reveal a mass of hypertrophied, hyperplastic epidermis projecting down to, but not below, the basal membrane. It also extends above the surface, producing the skin papule. Characteristic intracytoplasmic inclusion bodies can be identified in cells of the stratum spinosum. As the virus develops in the cytoplasm, the nucleus is pushed to the cell periphery.[28] The dermis is essentially normal unless the lesion is inflamed.

Microscopy

After minimal incision of the papule, the core of the papule can be expressed. This caseous tissue should be squashed at once between the glass microscope slide. Very firm compression of the glass with a twisting motion is necessary to release the virus. The smear can be stained with a drop of Sedi-Stain* which is used for staining of urinary sediment and covered with a coverslip. The slide examined under "high dry" magnification will reveal myriad very small dark particles "streaming out of islands of amorphous compressed lesions."[29] They are the molluscum contagiosum virions, which are the largest of all known viruses, with a maximum diameter of more than 0.3 μm. Smears can be also stained with Wright's, Giemsa, Papanicolaou and Gram methods. They will reveal large, homogenous intracytoplasmic inclusions ("molluscum bodies") characteristic for the disease.

Electron Microscopy

The molluscum contagiosum virus can be also demonstrated in an electron micrograph of fixed material from the lesions.[30]

Differential Diagnosis

- *Plain warts:* especially in children may resemble molluscum contagiosum, but are usually smaller and more numerous; no umbilication at the top of single lesion.
- *Genital warts:* no umbilication at the summit; absence of expressible material; biopsy.
- *Common warts:* rough with hyperkeratotic surface and flesh-colored papules or nodules studded with black puncto.
- *Secondary syphilis (condylomata lata):* soft moist flat papules or nodules in the perineum or in groins; positive serology; positive dark-field test.
- *Nodular basal cell epithelioma:* pearly nodule (usually single) with telangiectasia often with a central depression or ulceration; occur in older people on sun-exposed skin; biopsy.
- *Syringomas:* small papules usually about the eyes and cheeks and sometimes on the trunk; no central umbilication; more frequent in females; biopsy.

Occasionally molluscum contagiosum has to be distinguished from varicella, fibroma, milium, pyogenic granuloma, lichen planus, histiocytoma, nevoxanthoendothelioma, granulomas, or small keloids. Freezing with ethyl chloride may help to discriminate, but biopsy may at times be necessary.

---

*Sedi-Stain (Clay Adams, Parsippany, NJ) has the following composition: crystal violet 0.10%, safranin 0.25%, ammonium oxalate 0.03%, ethyl alcohol (SD–3A) 10%, water and stabilizers 89.62%.[29]

TREATMENT

The natural history of molluscum contagiosum is that the majority of lesions resolve spontaneously over a period of a few months. However, since treatment may shorten the duration and prevent autoinoculation as well as transmission of the disease, the following may be advisable:[3]

- Curettage, with or without local anesthesia
- Cryotherapy with liquid nitrogen or dry ice
- Laser surgery, surgical excision, or electrocoagulation
- Expression of the content of the lesion followed by application of iodine tincture, silver nitrate, or phenol
- Topical application of cauterants or irritants: trichloracetic acid, podophyllin, carbolic acid, tretinoin

Since developing lesions may not be clinically evident at the time of initial treatment, the patient should be informed of such a possibility and a control visit may be scheduled. However, caution is advisable in all treatment as the natural history of the lesions is benign and they do not result in scarring unless there is secondary infection.

MANAGEMENT OF SEX PARTNERS AND CONTROL

Infected sex partners should be examined and treated simulatneously to prevent reinfection. One should keep in mind the long incubation period of the disease and the possibility of the development of skin lesions over the period of a few months. Siblings of children with molluscum contagiosum may have lesions as well, so examination of these persons should be arranged whenever possible.[32]

REFERENCES

1. Porteous IB: Molluscum contagiosum. *Br Med J* 1:898, 1979.
2. Sturt RJ, Mueller HK, Francis GD: Molluscum contagiosum in villages of the West Sepik District of New Guinea. *Med J Aust* 2:751–754, 1971.
3. Felman YM, Nikitas JA: Genital molluscum contagiosum. *Cutis* 26:28–32, 1980.
4. Chief Medical Officer of the Department of Health and Social Security: Extract from the Annual Report for the year 1978: Sexually transmitted diseases. *Br J Vener Dis* 56:178–181, 1980.
5. Brown ST, Nalley JF, Kraus SJ: Molluscum contagiosum. *Sex Transm Dis* 8:227–234, 1981.
6. Becker TM, Blount JH, Douglas J, et al: Trends in molluscum contagiosum in the United States, 1966–1983. *Sex Transm Dis* 13:88–92, 1986.
7. Brown ST, Weinberger J: Molluscum contagiosum: Sexually transmitted disease in 17 cases. *J Am Vener Dis Assoc* 1:35–36, 1974.
8. Jackobs PH: Molluscum contagiosum. *Aerospace Med* 41:1196–1197, 1970.

9. Wilkin JK: Molluscum contagiosum venereum in a women's outpatient clinic: A venerally transmitted disease. *Am J Obstet Gynecol* 128:531–535, 1977.

10. Cobbold RJC, Macdonald A: Molluscum contagiosum as a sexually transmitted disease. *Practitioner* 204:416–419, 1970.

11. Low RC: Molluscum contagiosum. *Edinburgh Med J* 53:657–670, 1946.

12. Paton EP: Seven cases in which operation wounds were infected with molluscum contagiosum. *Westminster Hosp Gaz* 16:11–15, 1909.

13. Lynch PJ, Minkin W: Molluscum contagiosum of the adult: Probable venereal transmission. *Arch Dermatol* 98:141–143, 1968.

14. Kaye JW: Problems in therapy of molluscum contagiosum. *Arch Dermatol* 94:454–455, 1966.

15. Solomon LM, Telner P: Eruptive molluscum contagiosum in atopic dermatitis. *Can Med Assoc J* 95:978–979, 1966.

16. Blattner RJ: Molluscum contagiosum: Eruptive infection in atopic dermatitis. *J Pedatr* 70:997–999, 1967.

17. Pauly ChR, Artis WM, Jones HE: Atopic dermatitis, impaired cellular immunity and molluscum contagiosum. *Arch Dermatol* 114:391–393, 1978.

18. Hellier FF: Profuse mollusca contagiosa of the face induced by corticosteroids. *Br J Dermatol* 85:398, 1971.

19. Lombardo PC: Molluscum contagiosum in the acquired immunodeficiency syndrome. *Arch Dermatol* 121:824–825, 1985.

20. Katzman M, Elmats CA, Lederman MM: Molluscum contagiosum in the acquired immunodeficiency syndrome. *Ann Intern Med* 102:413–414, 1985.

21. Warner LC, Fisher BK: Cutaneous manifestations of acquired immunodeficiency syndrome. *Int J Dermatol* 25:337–350, 1986.

22. Postlethwaite R, Watt JA, Hawley TG, et al: Features of molluscum contagiosum in the north-east of Scotland and in Fijian village settlements: *J Hyg* (Lond) 65:281–291, 1967.

23. Dickinson T, Tschen JA, Wolf JE: Giant molluscum contagiosum of the sole. *Cutis* 32:239–243, 1983.

24. Vannas S, Lapinleimu K: Molluscum contagiosum in the skin, caructe and conjunctiva: Detection of a cytopathic agent in tissue cultures. *Acta Ophthalmol* 45:314–321, 1967.

25. Kipping HF: Molluscum dermatitis. *Arch Dermatol* 103:106–107, 1971.

26. Johnson M-L: Molluscum contagiosum reactivation. *JAMA* 243:2526, 1980.

27. Postlethwaite R: Molluscum contagiosum: A review. *Arch Environ Health* 21:432–452, 1970.

28. Dourmashkin R, Bernhard W: A study with the electron microscope of the skin tumor of molluscum contagiosum. *J Ultrastruct Res* 3:11–38, 1959.

29. Shelley WB, Burmeister W: Office diagnosis of molluscum contagiosum by light microscopic demonstration of virions. *Cutis* 36:465–466, 1985.

30. Blank H, Davis C, Collins C: Electron microscopy for the diagnosis of cutaneous viral infections. *Br J Dermatol* 83:69–80, 1970.

31. Felman YM: Molluscum contagiosum. *Cutis* 33:113–117, 1984.

32. Brown ST: Molluscum contagiosum in Holmes KK, Mardh P-A, Sparling PF, Wiesner PJ (eds), *Sexually Transmitted Diseases.* New York, McGraw-Hill, 1984, p. 507.

8

SYPHILIS

Syphilis is a chronic sexually transmitted disease caused by the spirochete *Treponema pallidum*. Shortly after its inception, the disease is capable of involving any organ of the body. If left untreated, it may be self-limited or may progress through several stages, eventually causing serious complications several years after acquisition. Syphilis is characterized by a wide variety of manifestations as well as periods of completely asymptomatic latency. Untreated mothers may infect their offsprings transplacentally. A synonym for syphilis is *lues*.

ETIOLOGY

Treponema pallidum is a spirochete of the family Treponemataceae. Other pathogenic treponemas include *T. pertenue* which causes yaws, and *T. carateum*, which causes pinta. The latter diseases are endemic in certain subtropical and tropical regions. *Treponema pallidum* is a spiral or corkscrew-shaped microorganism approximately 6–15 μm in length and about 0.2 μm in width. It can be recognized under dark-field illumination as a bluish white, thin, delicate spirochete which has from 8 to about 24 regular coils (Figure 8.1). It has characteristic movements which include rotation, forward and backward movements, bending, compression, expansion, and looping. However, the angulation in which *T. pallidum* bends back on itself appears to be the most typical.

Treponema pallidum cannot be grown on artificial culture media (except for a short time), but the organism can be inoculated into certain experimental animals such as the rabbit or the monkey. Intratesticular inoculation of rabbits is used to maintain strains for the *Treponema pallidum* immobilization test. *Treponema pallidum* multiplies by transverse fission, and the replication time is about 30 hours.[1] It requires moisture for survival and will remain alive for only a few hours outside the human body except in blood, where it can survive for up to 72 hours. It is very sensitive to drying and temperature and is susceptible to common antiseptics, including ordinary soap.

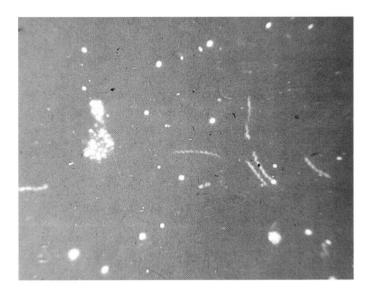

Figure 8.1. *Treponema pallidum* shown under dark-field illumination.

EPIDEMIOLOGY

Although the introduction of penicillin about 40 years ago raised hopes for the eradication of syphilis, the disease still exists and continues to be a serious problem in many countries.[2,3] However, in the developed countries syphilis has been successfully controlled primarily through routine blood testing of patients with other sexually transmitted diseases (STDs), blood donors, and pregnant women; proper health education; and adequate treatment of the disease, including administration of penicillin to individuals who have been exposed to the disease (epidemiologic treatment).[4,5] The total number of cases of syphilis in the United Kingdom in 1984 was 3,307 and the total number of cases of syphilis in the United States in 1987 was 86,542, where the rate per 100,000 was 35.8. Even though the incidence of this infection has declined since the Second World War, the resurgence of primary and secondary syphilis in recent years[6] might make the 1990 projections of the Centers for Disease Control (CDC) difficult to achieve.[7] Transmission of syphilis occurs primarily during sexual contact, and exposure to moist skin or mucous lesions is required for the infection to occur. It is still not clear whether *T. pallida* can penetrate an intact skin or mucous membranes and whether microscopic abrasions are necessary for them to produce infection. The disease is most contagious (mainly because of the presence of moist lesions) during the first 2 years of infection, gradually decreasing thereafter; it is rather rare for syphilis to be transmitted by intercourse after 5 years duration of illness.

Transmission by extragenital contact such as kissing or accidental infection of medical personnel (dentists and surgeons) is very rare. Similarly, transfusion of infected blood may cause syphilis, but this is extremely rare in developed countries where blood donors are tested for syphilis and where mostly refrigerated blood is being used for transfusion. Transmission to the fetus in utero by an untreated mother is well documented and can occur as early as in the ninth week of gesta-

TABLE 8.1. Characteristic Features of Primary Chancre

Usually single (multiple lesions are less common)
Located on genitals (most often)
Round or oval
Painless, unless secondarily infected
Indolent, persisting for several weeks before healing
Slightly raised, smooth, with sharply defined borders
Hard, finely granular, flesh-colored, indurated base
When squeezed does not change its shape and produces scanty serous discharge loaded with spirochetes
Heals without trace or leaves barely visible atrophic scar
Neighboring lymph nodes enlarged, hard and painless and nonsuppurating

tion.[8] Most infections of fetuses however take place in the second half of pregnancy when the placenta is fully developed.

PRIMARY SYPHILIS

Clinical Features

Primary Chancre

The incubation period of syphilis varies from 9 to 90 days following the day of exposure, with an average of 2–4 weeks. The primary lesion appears at the point of inoculation, which is most commonly on the genitals. It begins as a small papule which quickly erodes and become ulcerative. This ulcer is called the ''primary chancre'' and has very characteristic features (Table 8.1). The classical primary chancre* is usually a solitary, painless ulcer with an indurated base. It is regular in shape, usually round or oval with clearly defined, raised, smooth borders surrounded by a dull red areola or sometimes by normal skin. The base of it is finely granular, glistening, and clean unless secondarily infected. Some swelling of the surrounding tissues is not uncommon. On palpation the base of the ulcer has hard, buttonlike, or cartilaginous induration. Squeezing or abrading the ulcer produces serous or yellowish exudate containing spirochetes which can be visualized on dark-field examination. Unilaternal or bilateral inguinal lymphadenopathy follows the primary chancre located on genitalia in a few days (Figure 8.2). The enlarged nodes are firm on palpation, movable, and separate from one another, and the skin over them does not become reddened. They are usually painless and do not suppurate. If not treated, the chancre of primary syphilis will heal in 2–6 weeks, leaving a thin atrophic scar which in many instances becomes bearly visible. In some cases, however, the primary chancre may be so small and heals so rapidly that the patient does not notice it and does not seek medical advice.

Although the primary chancre may appear anywhere on the body, more than

---

*About 50 percent of primary chancres are atypical in some manner (Chapel[9]).

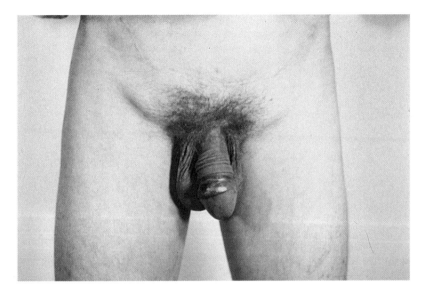

Figure 8.2. Primary chancre accompanied by bilateral lymphadenopathy.

90 percent of primary chancres occur on the genitalia or in the anorectal area. In men most chancres occur on the coronal sulcus, glans penis, inner surface of the prepuce, or near the frenulum. Some may be located in the urethral meatus, on the shaft of the penis, or on the scrotum. In homosexual men the most common sites are around the anal margin or on the skin around the perineum (Figure 8.3). Anal chancres may appear alone, mimicking fissures.[10] Chancres of the rectum are less commonly seen and may appear as indurated ulcerations resembling anal carcinoma.

In women, the most common sites are the labia (Figure 8.4), but primary chancres may also appear at the fourchette, the cervix, the urethra, the clitoris, and in the perineum. Some chancres in women may be inconspicuous and if located on the cervix may escape notice.

Extragenital primary chancres range in incidence from 2 to 10 percent[11,12] and usually result from contact with genital or extragenital lesions during sexual foreplay. They most commonly appear in the oral cavity (Figure 8.5) (the lips and tongue are most frequently affected), but they have been also found in the pubic area (Figure 8.6) and on the tonsils, the skin of the chin, the fingers (Figure 8.7), the eyelids, the nipple, the umbilicus, and even the skin of the arm.[13] Extragenital chancres are often atypical, and as early syphilis becomes more uncommon in the community, a high index of suspicion is essential for their diagnosis.[14]

Nontypical Primary Chancres. About half of primary chancres can be atypical.[9] They can be multiple, very small, and superficial, resembling genital herpes, or large and deep "primary ulcer phagoideum" (Figure 8.8). The latter frequently has been observed in alcoholics and patients with an impaired immune system. Although primary chancres are usually painless, secondarily infected lesions may be painful and may have undermined borders and necrotic bases covered with pus.

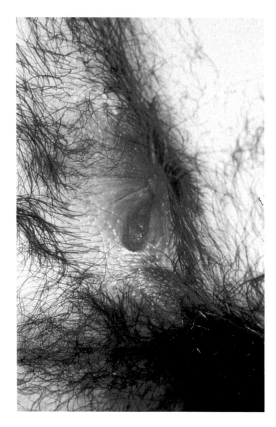

Figure 8.3.   Primary chancre in the anal margin mimicking a fissure.

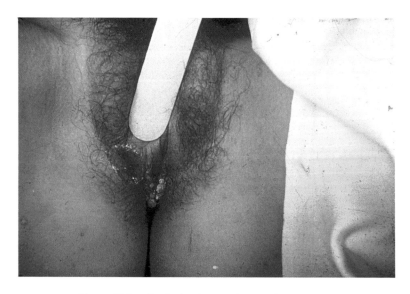

Figure 8.4.   Typical primary chancre in women.

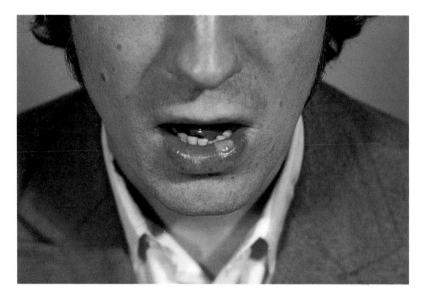

Figure 8.5. Primary chancre on the lower lip.

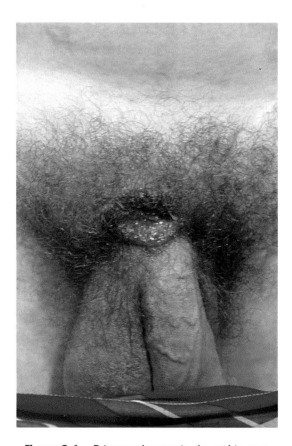

Figure 8.6. Primary chancre in the pubic area.

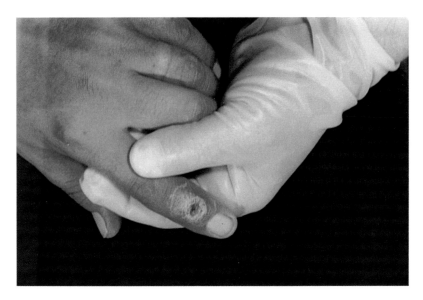

Figure 8.7. Primary chancre on the finger.

When this occurs lymphatic nodes may become painful and in very rare instances may suppurate. Also lesions around the nails are usually painful and may be mistaken for a herpetic withlow. Intraurethral chancre which occurs inside the urethra (usually in the meatus) may produce very few symptoms such as scanty serous discharge and induration felt on palpation. It is difficult to diagnose, and in some instances urethroscopy may be necessary to reveal the lesion. "Kissing chancre" is an example of a multiple primary lesion which occurs on contiguous opposite surfaces, usually the glans of the penis and reflect prepuce (Figure 8.9).

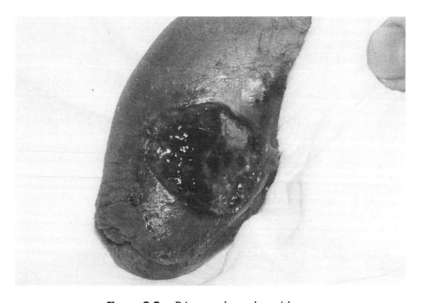

Figure 8.8. Primary ulcer phagoideum.

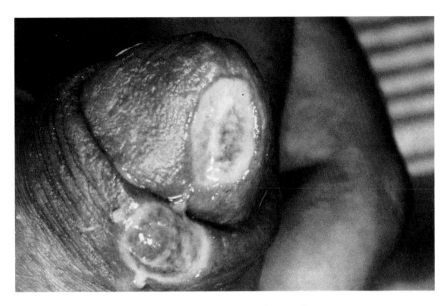

Figure 8.9. "Kissing chancre."

Complications

In uncircumcised men the most common complication of the primary lesion is *phimosis*, in which, as a result of edema, the foreskin cannot be retracted behind the coronal sulcus (Figure 8.10). *Paraphimosis* occurs when the retracted foreskin cannot be returned to its normal position (Figure 8.11). In circumcised men the most frequent complication is secondary infection causing pain, edema of the penis, and

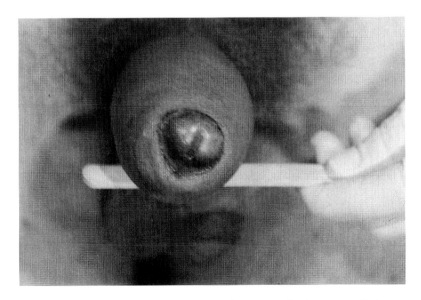

Figure 8.10. Phimosis caused by a primary chancre on the inner site of the prepuce.

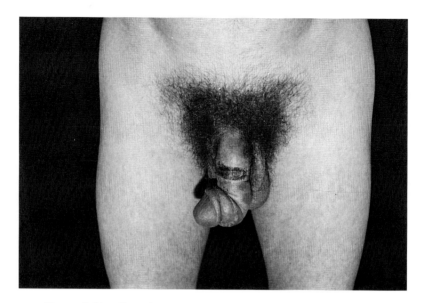

Figure 8.11. Paraphimosis as a complication of primary syphilis.

tender lymphadenopathy. Follmann's balanitis is a superficial infection of the glans of the penis caused by *T. pallidum*. It may involve the whole glans or only part of it and may accompany the primary chancre or follow it.[15] In women the most common complication is the edema of the labium on which the primary chancre occurs.

Diagnosis

The diagnosis of primary syphilis is based on clinical features (painless ulceration with accompanying regional lymphadenopathy) supported by the finding of *T. pallidum* on dark-field examination or a positive direct fluorescent antibody *T. pallidum* test.[16] Serologic tests are reactive in primary syphilis from 59–87 percent of the time (Venereal Disease Research Laboratory [VDRL] test) to 86–100 percent of the time (fluorescent treponemal antibody absorbtion [FTA-ABS] test).[17] Serologic tests are more likely to be negative if the chancre has been present for less than a week.

Dark-Field Examination

A specimen for dark-field (DF) examination should be obtained from the surface of the lesion. The lesion can be cleaned with a gauze or cotton swab soaked in sterile physiologic saline or water. All tissue debris, blood cells, and other contaminations should be carefully removed. In the case of secondary infection, administration of sulfonamides for 2–3 days (which do not affect *T. pallidum*) will help to clean the lesion and enable one to obtain a specimen. (All antibiotics should be withheld until a definite diagnosis is made.) The examined lesion should be firmly squeezed between the fingers and thumb (rubber globes should be worn) for a few minutes until serum emerges from its base. If the obtained specimen is contaminated with blood, other attempts should be undertaken to obtain clean serum. The serum should be collected on a cover slip, placed on microscope slide, and examined as soon as possible to avoid specimen drying. From hidden sites such as the cervix or oral cavity, material may be collected with a bacteriology loop. It is advisable to prepare more than one slide and examine them one after another. This procedure enhances the chance of finding motile *T. pallidum*. A microscope with a substage lamp and dark-field condensor should be used. *Treponema pallidum* appear under dark-field examination as bluish white spiral-shaped organisms with regular coils and a distinctive type of mobility (see p. 164). In syphilis, the majority of spirochetes will have the same size, shape, and motility pattern. Other, non-syphilitic spirochetes are usually mixed and appear under dark-field examination as organisms of various size, shape, and motility. When specimens from the mouth are examined, mistakes can be made with two common spirochetes residing in the oral cavity: *T. microdentium* and *T. macrodentium*. Even though these organisms possess certain distinctive features which allow the examiner to distinguish them from *T. pallidum*, dark-field examination of the mouth lesion is less reliable, and the diagnosis should be supported by syphilis serology tests. Failure to demonstrate *T. pallidum* in a suspect ulcer does not necessarily rule out the diagnosis of syphilis. Drying of the lesion, improperly obtained specimens, and use of topical antiseptics or creams containing antibiotics, not to mention the use of systemic antibiotics, may result in a failure to demonstrate *T. pallidum*. If serologic tests are negative in the early period of the disease, they should be repeated in 7–10 days, and more than one attempt should be made to identify the microorganism in the dark field.

Direct Fluorescent Antibody T. pallidum Test

The direct fluorescent antibody *T. pallidum* test (DFATP) can be used for wet mounts or fixed dried smears. The specimen is collected on a glass slide in the same manner as in dark-field examination. Fluorescin-labeled anti–*T. pallidum* globulin is used to visualize the spirochetes, and the smears are examined by fluorescent microscope. Even though the method seems to be more specific, it has not achieved widespread use.

Differential Diagnosis

The differential diagnosis of primary syphilis depends on the site of the primary chancre.

A primary chancre on the genitalia should be distinguished from (see Table 8.2)

- *Genital herpes:* multiple, grouped, superficial small ulcers on a slightly infiltrated base; frequently unbroken vesicles are also present; the lesions are nonindurated and painful; tender lymphadenopathy; history of recurrences at the same site; negative results from dark-field examination; a positive Tzanck test and/or culture. Caution: mixed infections are possible.
- *Chancroid:* shorter incubation period (3–7 days); single or multiple soft and tender ulceration; easily bleeds on palpation; painful lymphadenopathy with the nodes mated together; negative dark-field examination; positive culture for

TABLE 8.2. Short Characteristics of Sexually Transmitted Genital Ulcers

	Primary Syphilis	Genital Herpes	Chancroid	Lymphogranuloma Venereum	Donovanosis
Incubation period	9–90 days, Avg. 2–4 weeks	2–7 days	Range 1–35 days, Avg. 3–7 days	3 days to 3 weeks, Avg. 10–14 days	Precise data unavailable; probably from a few days to several months
Number of lesions	Usually one, may be multiple	Multiple; may coalesce, more with primary episodes than with recurrences	Usually 1–3, may be multiple	Usually single	Single or multiple
Description of genital ulcers	Sharply demarcated round or oval ulcer with slightly elevated edges; may be irregular, symmetrical ("kissing chancre")	Small, superficial, grouped vesicles and/or erosions; lesion may coalesce, forming bullae or large areas of ulcerations; lesions have irregular borders	Superficial, shallow, sharply demarketed ulcer; irregular, ragged undermined edge; size from a few millimeters to 2 cm in diameter	Papule, pustule, vesicle, or ulcer discrete, and transient; frequently overlooked	Sharply defined, irregular ulcerations or hypertrophic, verrucous, necrotic or cicatrical granulomas
Base	Red, smooth, and shiny or crust; oozing serous exudate when squeezed	Bright, red, and smooth	Rough, uneven, yellow to gray color	Variable	Usually friable, rough, beefy granulations; can be necrotic, verrucous, or cicatrical
Induration	Firm; does not change shape with pressure	None	Soft; changes shape with pressure	None	Firm granulation tissue

Pain	Painless; may become tender if secondarily infected	Common; more prominent with initial infection than with recurrences	Common	Variable	Rare
Inguinal lymphadenopathy	Unilateral or bilateral, firm, movable, and nontender; does not suppurate	Usually bilateral, firm, and tender; more common in primary episodes than in recurrences	Unilateral, bilateral rarely occurs; overlying erythema; matted, fixed, and tender; suppuration may occur	Unilateral or bilateral; initially movable, firm, and tender; later indolent; fixed and matted; "sign of groove" may suppurate; fistules	Pseudobuboes; subcutaneous perilymphatic granulomatous lesions that produce inguinal swellings
Constitutional symptoms	Rare	Common in primary episode; less likely in recurrences	Rare	Frequent	Rare
Course of untreated disease	Slowly (2–6 weeks) resolves to latency	Recurrence is the rule	May progress to erosive lesions	Local lesions heal; systemic disease may progress; disfiguring; late complications	Worsens slowly
Diagnostic tests	Dark-field exam, direct immunofluorescence, FTA-ABS, VDRL	Tzanck smear, culture, Pap smear, direct immunofluorescence, electromicroscopy, direct immunoperoxidase staining, serology and others	Culture, biopsy (rarely used), Gram-stained smears—low specificity	LGV complement fixation test, isolation of the microorganism by culture	"Donovan bodies" in tissue smears; biopsy

Hemophilus ducreyi; negative serologic test. Caution: in certain geographic regions, a mixed infection may occur.

- *Behçet's syndrome:* multiple, superficial genital ulcerations, aphthous stomatitis, and irydocyclitis; negative dark-field examination and syphilis serology. Other symptoms or signs are discussed on p. 381.
- *Balanitis or balanoposthitis:* superficial erosions mixed with rash on the glans or inner site of the prepuce usually on an inflamed background; negative dark-field examination; negative serology; positive culture for yeasts, other fungi, or bacteria. There is frequently a history of diabetes.
- *Lymphogranuloma venereum (LGV):* rarely seen; small, herpetiform, and transient initial lesion; enlarged inguinal lymph nodes which tend to suppurate; positive complement fixation test (CFT) or other tests for LGV; negative syphilis serology; history of recent travel to LGV endemic areas.
- *Genital cancer:* usually long lasting, easily bleeding, indurated lesion; lymph nodes can be enlarged in later stages of the disease and are very hard on palpation; negative dark-field examination and syphilis serology; biopsy is decisive. The disease is more likely to occur in older, uncircumcised men.
- *Scabies:* rarely, scabietic lesions on the genitalia may become ulcerated, usually due to secondary infection; history of itching which is worse at night and the presence of pruritic lesion (burrows) on other parts of the body; negative dark-field examination and syphilis serology; Scrapings of the lesion may demonstrate the causative mite.
- *Donovanosis:* Rare in temperate zones; may be considered in recent travelers to the endemic areas; bright red, raised chronic granulations; biopsy may reveal "Donovan bodies."
- *Traumatic lesions:* history of recent trauma; lack of induration and lymph node involvement; negative dark-field examination and syphilis serology.

Extragenital primary chancre is rare, but if it occurs it may be mistaken

- On the lips: for herpes labialis, squamous cell carcinoma, aphthous ulcers, angular cheilitis (perlèche);
- On the tongue: for aphthous ulcers, squamous cell carcinoma, tuberculosis;
- On the finger: for herpetic whitlow, paronychia, traumatic ulcer, and anthrax pustule.

A primary chancre in the anorectal region may be misdiagnosed as an anal fissure, an anal wart, carcinoma, hemorrhoids, or Bowen's disease.

SECONDARY SYPHILIS

Clinical Features

Symptoms and signs of secondary syphilis usually appear within 9–10 weeks of infection. The average interval between the appearance of the primary chancre and of the secondary lesions is 5–8 weeks. However, the rashes of secondary syphilis may follow the primary lesion by as early as several days or may be delayed for several months. Secondary syphilis represents a stage of the disease in which *T. pallidum* circulate in the blood and may potentially affect every organ. In addition to cutaneous manifestations, which is the hallmark of secondary syphilis, patients may develop constitutional flulike symptoms which precede or accompany the first skin signs. These symptoms of secondary syphilis are very variable, transient, and seldom severe. They include low-grade fever, malaise, headache, muscular aches, sore throat, hoarseness, and generalized anthralgia. With these constitutional symptoms, generalized lymphadenopathy is frequently present. Lymph nodes are characteristically discrete, nontender, have a hard rubbery feel, and may remain palpable for several weeks. Also, about this time some patients may have an enlarged liver and/or spleen.

Anemia is not an uncommon finding as well as elevated white blood cell count and sedimentation rate.[18] The liver may be enlarged due to hepatitis,[19,20] with noticeable jaundice and elevated alkaline phosphatase which is out of proportion to other liver function tests.[21] Immune complex depositions due to glomerulonephritis have been described[22] as well as proteinuria, nephrotic syndrome, and hemorrhagic nephritis.[23] About one third of patients with secondary syphilis have changes in the cerebrospinal fluid (CSF) and meningitis, although some authors report that as many as about 60% of patients with secondary syphilis may have abnormal CSF.[24] Cranial nerve palsies, transverse myelitis, and cerebral arterial thrombosis, although very rare, may occasionally occur.[25] Conditions such as myositis, synovitis, periostitis, arthritis, and anterior uveitis have been occasionally reported in association with secondary syphilis.

Although constitutional symptoms and other signs may be present, the diagnosis of secondary syphilis is suspected primarily on the basis of the skin and mucous membrane lesions. The skin rashes that occur in the secondary stage have certain common characteristics which help to distinguish them from skin rashes occurring in other common skin diseases. However, the diagnosis of secondary syphilis must not be made on clinical ground only and should be confirmed by serologic tests or, if they are not available, by demonstration of *T. pallidum* in skin or mucous membrane lesions.

Types of Skin Lesions

Macular Rash (Roseola syphilitica).   The earliest cutaneous expression of secondary syphilis is a macular (roseolar) rash which appears about 5–8 weeks after the primary chancre. It is first seen on the side of the trunk and later spreads over the chest, abdomen, and shoulders (Figure 8.12). The limbs are frequently affected, with the flexor surfaces being the sites of predilection. The macular eruption may be localized only to the trunk or be generalized, but the palms, soles, and face are usually spared except for a few lesions around the mouth. The individual spots are round or oval, with discrete margins averaging 0.5–1 cm in diameter, and are rose-pink in color. This condition is best observed in patients with a pale complexion or after physical activity or a warm bath. Since the macular rash may be very discrete, it should be seen in natural daylight or with oblique artificial illumination. It usually disappears within a few days, but in rare instances it may persist and develop into a papular rash. In pigmented patients the roseolar rash may leave a

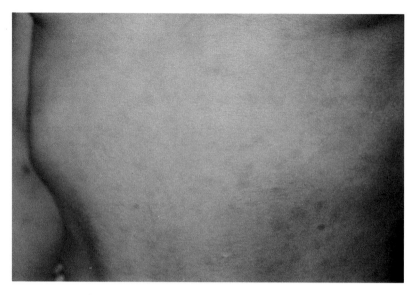

Figure 8.12. Secondary syphilis macular rash.

slight postinflammatory pigmentation resembling pityriasis versicolor which lasts for only a few days. Also, following the disappearance of macular exanthema, a patchy area lacking pigmentation has been observed.

Maculopapular Rash.   Maculopapular rash is the usual textbook description of the rash of early secondary syphilis and appears to be the most common type of skin lesion in this stage of the disease (Figure 8.13)[26,27]; it usually appears 2–4 months after infection. This eruption is generalized, involving the face, trunk, flexor surfaces of arms, and to a lesser extent, the lower extremities. The involvement of the palms and soles is very characteristic for secondary syphilis (Figures 8.14 and 8.15). In these locations the papular lesions remain flat or are only slightly elevated because of the pressure and the tough, horny character of the epithelium. Slight scaling may be present.

Papular Rash.   The papular rash along with maculopapular eruptions are the commonest and most characteristic cutaneous expressions of secondary syphilis. In general, the papular lesions are fewer in number (Figure 8.16), larger, and in contrast to the rose-pink color of the macular rash, tend to be darker dusky-red to brown in color. The individual papule can be flat or acuminate, small or large, with a smooth or scaly surface. They feel indurated when palpated with the finger. The papules may be widely distributed over the trunk, arms, legs, palms, and soles as well as the skin of the face. The lesions may be isolated or grouped, forming annular or arcuate lesions. The latter are more common in black patients and have rolled raised borders with the centers characteristically darker. The annular lesion commonly called ''nickle and dimes'' frequently occurs on the face (Figure 8.17) and also has been found on the skin of the scrotum, the vulva, and the hands. Papules which develop along the hairline may look like a crown and are called ''corona veneris.'' Besides that there are many varieties of papular lesions. Fre-

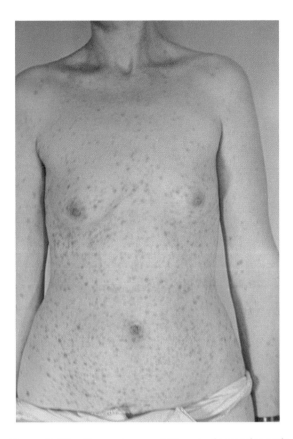

Figure 8.13. Secondary syphilis maculopapular rash.

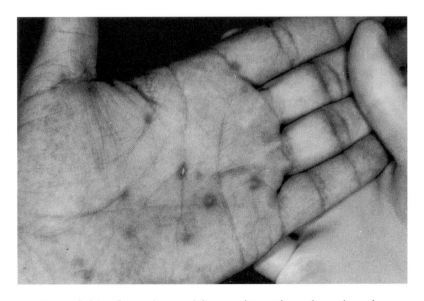

Figure 8.14. Secondary syphilis maculopapular rash on the palm.

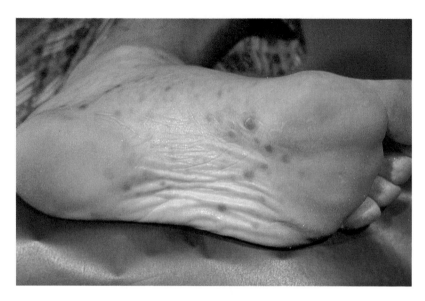

Figure 8.15. Secondary syphilis maculopapular rash on the side of the foot.

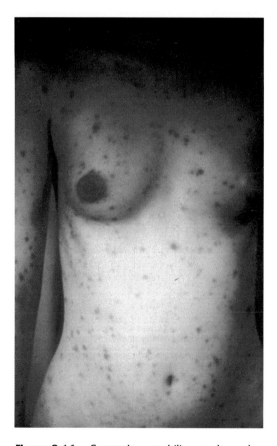

Figure 8.16. Secondary syphilis papular rash.

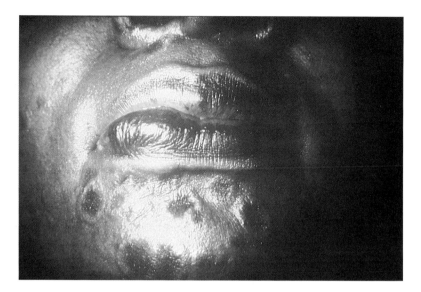

Figure 8.17. Secondary syphilis "nickel and dime" lesions on the face.

quently the papular rash resembles other skin diseases and is described as lichenoid, psoriasiform (Figure 8.18), pityriasiform, etc. Follicular, papular rash is uncommon in secondary syphilis and appears to be the only type of syphilitic lesion that is known to be pruritic; however, even with the follicular rash pruritus is never really severe. Although generally skin rashes of secondary syphilis are considered nonpruritic, in one study pruritus was reported by almost 42% of patients.[26]

In moist and warm (intertriginous) areas of the body where skin surfaces are opposed, maceration of papules may occur. Moist papules may become eroded or fissured and can be called "split papules" or may become elevated and condylomatous. Condyloma lata are hypertrophic, broad based, exuberant papules with flat, moist tops (Figure 8.19). These lesions are whitish to grayish in color. They may remain as separate lesions or may form round fleshy masses covered by a thick mucoid secretion teeming with spirochetes. These lesions are considered the most contagious of secondary syphilis. Typically, condylomata lata appear on the labia in women (Figure 8.20, p. 184), around the anus and between the buttocks in men and women, and on the lateral surfaces of the scrotum in men. They also have been found on the inner aspect of the thigh, in the groin (Figure 8.21, p. 185), and around the mouth but rarely in other parts of the body.

Pustular Rash. Pustular rash is much less common and accounts for less than 2% of all secondary syphilis.[26] It usually follows maculopapular or papular lesions. Occasionally, pustular lesions may be seen among the spots of papular or even maculopapular rash. Pustular lesions are most common on the face and scalp but can be seen elsewhere on the body as well.[28] Infrequently, the pustular lesions may be generalized, in which case it is usually associated with diminished resistance on the part of the patients. These types of pustular rash have been observed in malnourished patients, and in those with other debilitating diseases, such as AIDS (Figure 8.22, p. 185).

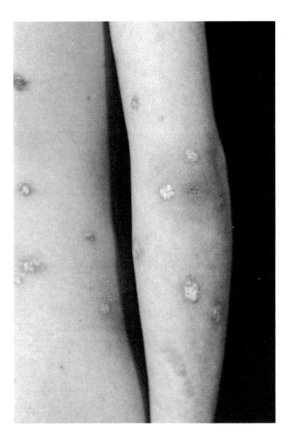

Figure 8.18. Psoriasiform lesion in secondary syphilis.

Mucous Membrane Lesions

Mucous membrane lesions occur in about one third of cases of secondary syphilis. The soft palate may be reddened before the skin rash appears; however, the most typical lesions are the so-called "mucous patches" (Figure 8.23). These lesions appear at the same time as the papular rash and can be found on the inner side of the lips and cheeks and on the tongue as well as on the fauces, tonsils, pharynx, and larynx. The typical mucous patch is usually a rounded, flat or slightly raised, greyish white or glistening patch bordered by a dull-red areola. On the soft palate and fauces the lesions may be grouped, forming an elongated ulceration, the so-called "snail-tract ulcer." On the dorsum of the tongue the mucous patches may appear as rounded dull-pink smooth spots due to the destruction of the filiform papillae by the necrotic process. Mucous patches have also been found in the nose and larynx, giving rise to the husky voice characteristic of secondary syphilis. Mucous patches may also appear on the mucous membranes of the genitals, where the vulva, glans of the penis, and the inner side of the prepuce are most commonly affected. They usually present an eroded appearance and thus are sharply defined against the background of normal mucous membranes. Mucous patches are usually painless unless secondarily infected. The mucous membrane lesions of sec-

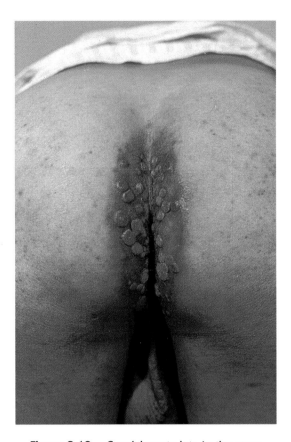

Figure 8.19.   Condylomata lata in the anus.

ondary syphilis are highly infectious, since their exudate is usually teeming with spirochetes. They are also more liable than skin lesions to recur in case of relapse following treatment.

Syphilitic Alopecia

During secondary syphilis, there may be a temporary loss of hair. It is present later during the course of secondary syphilis, usually after 6 months. The hair loss is almost invariably patchy (numerous, small discrete areas of hair loss), giving rise to a characteristic "moth-eaten" appearance (Figure 8.24, p. 186). Hair loss occurs mainly on the sides and back of the head. At times a diffuse thinning of the scalp hair may occur. Syphilitic alopecia may also affect the eyelashes, lateral third of the eyebrows, and occasionally, the body hair. The hair loss is temporal, and regrowth of hair occurs regardless of whether the patient was treated.

Syphilitic Leukoderma (Collar of Venus)

As the macular or maculopapular rash fades, small, numerous, patchy areas of hypopigmentation may persist. This is more frequently seen in women, especially those of dark complexion, and is best seen on the neck and back, giving rise

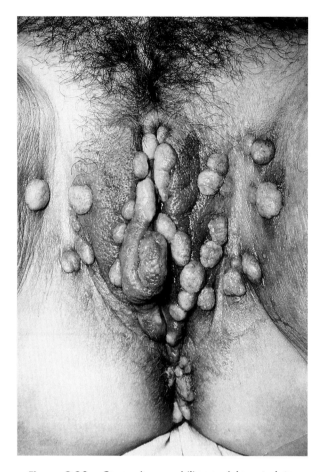

Figure 8.20. Secondary syphilis condylomata lata.

to the term "collar of venus" (Figure 8.25). The duration of the hypopigmentation is variable.

Generalized Lymphadenopathy

Generalized lymphadenopathy is a common feature of secondary syphilis. The lymph nodes have the same characteristic as the regional lymphadenopathy of primary syphilis but they are usually less prominent. The nodes are nontender discrete, freely mobile, and firm to palpation. The inguinal, axillary epitrochlear, anterior and posterior cervical, and suboccipital regions are commonly involved. All of them or only certain groups may be enlarged.

Early Latent Syphilis

Early latent syphilis is a subclinical stage of the disease characterized by positive serologic tests in the blood and negative spinal fluid examination including spinal fluid reagin test to rule out asymptomatic neurosyphilis. According to the Centers for Disease Control (CDC), "early latent syphilis" is classified as syphilis of

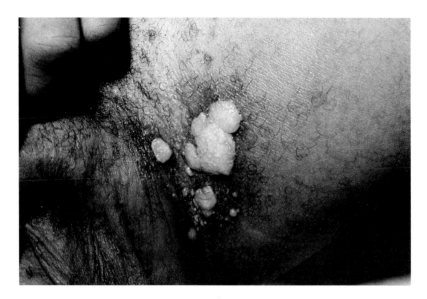

Figure 8.21. Secondary syphilis condylomata lata.

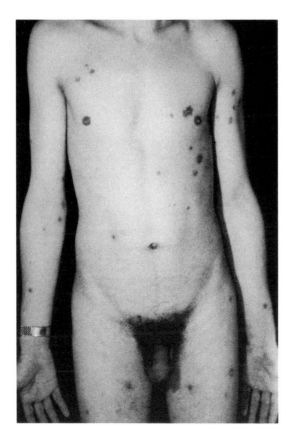

Figure 8.22. Secondary syphilis pustular rash in HIV-positive patient.

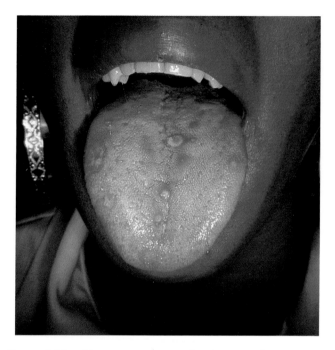

Figure 8.23.   Mucous patches at the dorsum of the tongue.

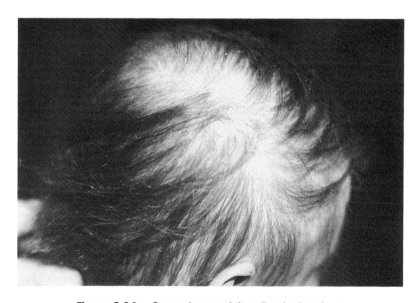

Figure 8.24.   Secondary syphilis—Patchy hair loss.

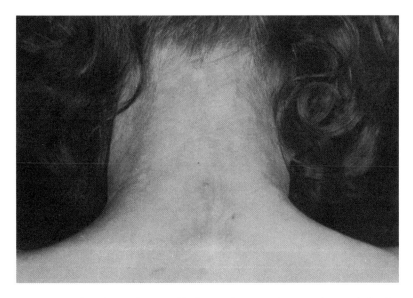

Figure 8.25. Syphilitic leukoderma: this hypopigmentation on the neck is also called "collar of Venus."

less than 1 year's duration. Latent infection may be interrupted one or more times by the appearance of symptoms or signs of secondary syphilis. Not infrequently, patients with very discrete skin rashes or inapparent lesions on mucous membranes may be misclassified as having latent infections. Early latent syphilis is considered as being potentially infectious sexually because of the possibility of recurrence of infectious lesions of secondary disease or the presence of inapparent skin or mucous membrane lesions.

Diagnosis

The diagnosis of secondary syphilis can be made with certainty if the patient presents with characteristic skin or mucosal lesions in which *T. pallidum* can be identified by dark-field microscopy. Clinical diagnosis should be supported by positive cardiolipin (VDRL, rapid plasma reagin [RPR]) or treponemal tests. In secondary syphilis all serologic tests are almost always positive and of high titers. Diagnosis of early latent disease is based on a positive cardiolipin or treponemal test in the blood. However, one should keep in mind the possibility of false-positive test results, especially those of low titer. Therefore, every positive cardiolipin test result should be verified by one or more treponemal tests.

Differential Diagnosis

Secondary syphilis should be suspected in any patient with generalized skin eruption, especially when the condition is chronic, recurrent, and nonpruritic. All these patients should have syphilis serologic tests done as soon as possible to rule out or confirm the disease. The following can be mistakenly diagnosed:

- *Macular rash* can be mistaken for measles, rubella, tinea versicolor, adverse drug reactions, seborrheic dermatitis, infectious mononucleosis, typhoid fever, and erythema multiforme.
- *Papular rash* can be mistaken for pityriasis rosea, lichen planus, psoriasis, parapsoriasis, urticaria pigmentosa. Annular lesions may mimic erythema multiforme, ringworm, granuloma annulare, and annular lichen planus.
- *Hairline lesions* can be mistaken for psoriasis and contact dermatitis (from the use of hair dyes).
- *Palmar lesions* can be mistaken for contact dermatitis, pustular psoriasis, dyshidrosis, and erythema multiforme.
- *Plantar lesions* can be mistaken for tinea pedis, dyshidrosis, pustular psoriasis, and keratoderma blenorrhagica associated with Reiter's syndrome.
- *Pustular rash* can be mistaken for acne, rosacea, chicken pox, and drug eruptions due to bromides and iodides.
- *Mucous membrane lesions* in the mouth and throat can be mistaken for aphthous ulcers, viral exanthemas, strep throat, Vincent's angina, lichen planus, Stevens-Johnson syndrome, leukoplakia, pemphigus, Behçet's disease, and herpes labialis. Mucous membrane lesions on the genitalia can be mistaken for genital herpes, balanitis, Behçet's syndrome, erythroplasia of Queyrat, genital warts, lichen planus, psoriasis and scabies.
- *Condylomata lata* can be mistaken for hemorrhoids, genital warts, and squamous cell carcinoma.
- *Alopecia syphilitica* can be mistaken for alopecia areata, traumatic alopecia, and ringworm of the scalp.

TERTIARY SYPHILIS

Clinical Features

The first manifestations of tertiary syphilis (late) may appear as early as 3–4 years after the primary stage, but in the majority of cases it takes many more years for the tertiary lesions to develop. Adequate treatment of earlier stages usually prevents development of late syphilis. In the untreated disease, only about one third of cases will develop symptoms and signs of late syphilis, whereas more than half of the patients never suffer any further effects. Although lesions of tertiary syphilis may appear anywhere in the body, the following forms of late syphilis are the most common: mucocutaneous, osseous, cardiovascular, neural, and visceral. They may occur singly or in combination, e.g., mucocutaneous plus osseous lesions or cardiovascular lesions with neurosyphilis.

In the majority of cases late syphilis is not contagious, and attempts to demonstrate *T. pallidum* from the lesions of tertiary syphilis are usually unrewarding.

Mucocutaneous Lesions

There are two main forms of mucocutaneous lesions of tertiary syphilis: nodular or noduloulcerative and gummas. They may appear singly or may coexist.

Nodular and Noduloulcerative Lesions. Nodular and noduloulcerative lesions usually show up no earlier than 5–10 years and as long as 20 years after the infection. They may appear on any part of the skin and may be solitary or more often multiple. They consist of small, painless nodules which develop very slowly and regress even more slowly. The lesions vary in size from a few millimeters to several centimeters. They are dull-red in color and, unlike skin lesions in secondary syphilis, localized and asymmetrical. They tend to be arranged in groups and take on a characteristic configuration: polycyclic or round semicircles or a horseshoe configuration (Figure 8.26). All lesions are usually hard and indurated, deep rooted in the dermis, and frequently involve the whole thickness of the skin. They may be small or may cover large areas of the skin. The surface of the nodule is usually smooth and clean, but some may have a slight scale resembling psoriasis. The nodules have a predilection for the face, extremities, or scapular and interscapular areas. Over the course of several months some nodules heal while new ones appear, usually at the periphery. There is a tendency to heal at the center, so the lesion spreads peripherally, resulting in a characteristic circular or serpiginous appearance which is pathognomonic for this stage of the disease. After healing, visible pigmentation may remain or there may be a scar which usually retains the configuration of the original lesion. The scars are superficial, atrophic, and thin so-called "tissue paper" scars.

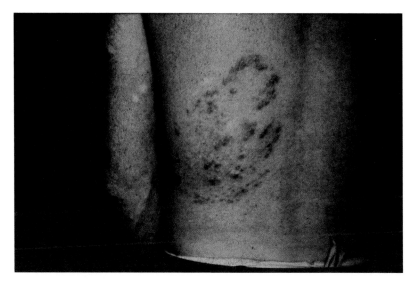

Figure 8.26.   Noduloulcerative lesions of tertiary syphilis.

Gummas. These lesions originate in the subcutaneous tissue and involve the skin secondarily. Unlike nodular and noduloulcerative lesions, gummas tend to be solitary. A gumma starts off as a painless nodule which frequently develops at the point of trauma. At the beginning of the process, the skin over the nodule is not attached and shows no change in color. Gradually the nodule increases in size, becomes attached to the skin which is then dusky red, softens, and breaks down to form a characteristic punched-out ulcer, which discharges gummy material. The edge of the ulcer is indurated, and the granulomatous floor of it may be covered with yellow, adherent wash-leather slough. The granulomatous ulcer may extend peripherally or may heal spontaneously. The lesions are very indolent and heal very slowly, leaving an atrophic scar with stippling pigmentation. Predilection sites are the skin over the sternum (Figure 8.27) and sternoclavicular joints, the legs below the knees, and the face, scalp, and buttocks. If the gumma extends or has its origin in the periosteum, the floor of the lesion may be formed by a bone. In that case the gumma, which is usually painless, may become painful.

Gummas of the Mucous Membranes. Gummatous lesions of mucous membranes usually start in the submucous tissue. May be localized or diffuse, and are most likely to involve the mouth, tongue, and soft or hard palate. The throat, larynx, and nasal septum may be also involved. Gummatous lesions originate in the submucosa but involve not only mucous membranes but deeper tissues as well. Involvement of the soft palate and uvula leads to deformity and destruction of the tonsils that may cause extensive scarring on healing. The hard palate may perforate as a result of gummatous infiltration of the roof of the mouth or the floor of the nose. Destruction of the cartilage of the nasal septum leads to a characteristic deformity of the nose, and a gummatous process affecting the laryngeal cartilage may cause significant deformity of this organ, including stenosis. As a result, the voice may be weak and hoarse.

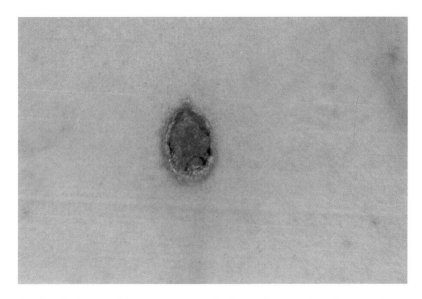

Figure 8.27. Tertiary syphilis gumma: punched-out ulcer on the skin over the sternum.

In late syphilis the tongue is a frequent target. Gummatous ulceration may appear on the tongue, but superficial glossistis is a more common sign of tertiary syphilis of the tongue. It results from diffuse gummatous perivascular infiltration of the blood vessels of the tongue. At the beginning of the process, there is painless enlargement of the tongue (macroglossia), but as healing occurs, interstitial fibrosis appears which leads to irregular fissures of the surface of the tongue and atrophy of its musculature. As a result of ischemia there is a marked loss of papillae. Chronic inflammation of the surface of the tongue is a common process which, in association with decreased blood supply, creates environment for development of leukoplakia, which is considered a precancerous lesion. Leukoplakia may appear not only on the tongue; any part of the mouth may be involved (inner cheeks, lips). Since almost half of the cases of syphilitic leukoplakia may undergo malignant changes, patients who develop this kind of lesion should be followed medically for the rest of their lives. An increase in pain, bleeding, or sudden enlargement or induration are warning signs. Biopsy should be performed immediately and appropriate treatment instituted. Otherwise the prognosis is poor.

Diagnosis.   The diagnosis of late mucocutaneous syphilis is basically dependent on the clinical feature of skin and/or mucosal lesion aided by positive serologic tests. The nontreponemal tests are positive in the majority of cases; however, negative results do not entirely rule out tertiary syphilis. The treponemal test should be positive in all cases. Evidence of syphilis elsewhere in the body and a history of genital ulceration or lesions suggestive of secondary syphilis may aid in diagnosis. At times biopsy may be necessary. Since mucocutaneous lesions may coexist with other forms of tertiary syphilis, cerebrospinal fluid as well as x-ray examination should be performed to rule out such a possibility.

Differential Diagnosis.   Depending upon the sites affected, the following conditions should be considered:

- *Skin lesions* should be distinguished from tuberculosis, sarcoidosis, leprosy, granuloma annulare, sporotrichosis, histoplasmosis, basal cell carcinoma, squamous cell carcinoma and skin manifestations of some reticuloses.
- *Facial lesions* may resemble lupus erythematosus, sarcoidosis, seborrheic dermatitis, leprosy, and rhinophyma.
- *Palmar lesions* may mimic granuloma annulare, hand eczema, infections caused by dermatophytes, tuberculosis, or psoriasis.
- *On legs,* varicose ulcers, various dermatophytoses, erythema nodosum, periarteritis nodosa, nodular vasculitis, erythema induratum, ulcus rodens, and Weber-Christian disease.
- *Mucosal lesions* should be distinguished from tuberculosis, carcinoma, infections caused by streptococci, and Vincent's organisms.
- *Interstitial glossitis* may resemble geographic tongue, scrotal tongue, and macroglossia resulting from acromegalism or hypothyroidism.
- *Leukoplakia* of the tongue should be distinguished from moniliasis, lichen planus, and hairy leukoplakia, which occur in HIV infection.

Osseous Lesions

Bone lesions of tertiary syphilis are mostly found 5–10 or more years after the infection. They may be confined either to the periosteum or involve deep structures of the bones, causing osteitis or osteomyelitis. In rare instances, periostitis and osteitis may occur together in the same bone. The bones most commonly affected are the bones of the skull, clavicle (particularly at its sternal end), sternum, humerus, femur, tibia (very often), and fibula. Occasionally, the bones of the forearm or joints may be involved.

Although tertiary osseous syphilis may be asymptomatic, patients with bone lesions commonly complain of deep-seated, gnawing, or boring pain which usually gets worse at night and is localized in the region of the bone lesion. Periostitis produces bony proliferation due to deposits of new bones. In long bones such as the tibia, subperiosteal bone tissue may be deposited on the anterior surface of this bone, producing clinically palpable and radiologically evident thickening. This produces forward bowing of the bone, causing the phenomenon called "sabre tibia." At times at the surface of the tibia irregular palpable tumors may be present or there may be pits or holes felt on palpation. If the bone is underneath the skin, the patient develops a smooth, irregular, tender swelling which is connected with the bone and can be easily palpated. The overlying skin becomes fixed to the bone, turns red, and may break down and ulcerate.

Osteitis and osteomyelitis are less common than periostitis. This destructive process usually involves flat bones, especially those of the skull. In the vault of the skull this process first involves the outer table and then may spread to the inner table. The syphilitic process may also penetrate to the dura mater and, infrequently, the brain. On the x-ray of the skull, round multiple areas of osteoporosis surrounded by sclerosis give a characteristic worm-eaten appearance. This condition may produce painful local swelling or may be symptomless and be discovered on radiologic examination only.

If the bone of the nose or nasal septum are affected, there is usually nasal discharge associated with pain. In neglected cases, perforation of the nasal septum may occur, resulting in the collapse of the nasal bridge with subsequent deformity. Involvement of the skin of the nose may produce widespread ulceration and cause severe deformation of the affected part of the face. If the syphilitic process involves the hard palate, perforation is almost a rule (Figure 8.28). This usually results in a change in voice (nasal voice) and regurgitation of fluid on drinking. Joints are rarely the sites of tertiary syphilis except "Charcot's joints," which is in fact a neurogenic arthropathy and will be discussed further in this chapter.

Diagnosis. The diagnosis of osseous lesions of tertiary syphilis is made based on clinical and radiologic features of affected bones and supported by positive treponemal or nontreponemal serologic tests. Since asymptomatic involvement of more than one bone is frequent, examination of other bones likely to be involved in the syphilitic process is advised.

Differential Diagnosis. The following conditions should be included in differential diagnosis: primary and metastatic carcinoma, tuberculosis, pyogenic osteomyelitis,

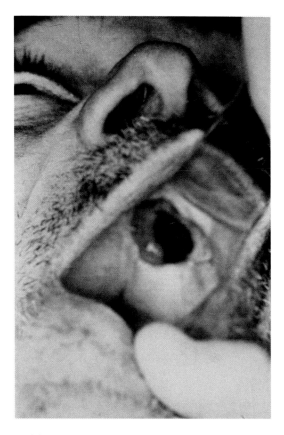

Figure 8.28.   Perforation of the hard palate in tertiary syphilis.

Ewing's tumor, myeloma, Paget's disease, eosinophilic granuloma and in areas where leprosy is endemic—leprosy.

Cardiovascular Lesions

Since the advent of antibiotics, there has been a considerable decline in the incidence of cardiovascular syphilis. About 10–15% of untreated patients may develop this complication, which usually becomes evident 10–20 years after contracting the infection. The condition is more prevalent in middle age persons, with men more frequently affected than women. Cardiovascular syphilis usually manifests as a syphilitic aortitis, stenosis of coronary ostiae, aortic incompetence, and aneurysm of the aorta.

Uncomplicated Aortitis.   Uncomplicated syphilitic aortitis is often asymptomatic. However, some patients may present with a history of substernal discomfort or aching substernal pain. Ausculation may reveal a systolic murmur at the aortic area or/and a loud tambourlike or bell-like second aortic sound. Radiologic examination may be normal or may show widening or irregularity of the aorta and its calcification.

Stenosis of Coronary Ostiae.   The symptoms of angina pectoris, resulting from stenosis or occlusion of the coronary ostiae, is most commonly found in association with aortic incompetence. The symptoms are similar to that resulting from coronary sclerosis. The cardiac pain is usually precipitated by exertion or emotion, but sometimes, especially in more advanced cases, may also occur when the patient is at rest, particularly at night. Unlike in coronary sclerosis, administration of nitrites may not produce immediate relief. Electrocardiogram shows depression of the S-T segment and flattening or inversion of the T-wave. Coronary insufficiency may develop, resulting in myocardial ischemia. Although it may occur, cardiac infarction is a rare complication.

Aortic Incompetence.   Arotic incompetence is commonly asymptomatic in the early stages. The first symptoms usually occur along with the early signs of heart failure. These include dyspnea on exertion and paroxysmal nocturnal dyspnea due to pulmonary edema from left-side heart failure. As the condition progresses, right-side heart failure may supervene, with edema of the feet and ankles, marked dyspnea and cyanosis, engorged neck veins, ascites, and liver enlargement.

The typical sign of aortic incompetence is a distinct diastolic murmur heard immediately after the aortic second sound. It is soft and blowing and best heard at the second right intercostal space close to the sternum (Erb's point). Occasionally, concomitant systolic apical murmur with or without middiastolic Austin-Flint murmur may be heard. The systolic blood pressure is increased with normal or low diastolic pressure, and the common reading would be about 180/60. The pulse is collapsing in type or the so-called "waterhammer pulse," where the wave of the pulse rises sharply during systole followed by a rapid recession. It is best felt by palpating the radial artery with the arm raised above the level of the heart. The capillary pulsation (pulse of Quincke) may be demonstrated by a gentle pressure on the fingernail or by flashing a light under the fingertips. Radiologic examination and cardioscopy may reveal enlargement of the left ventricle, dilation of the aorta, and an increased pulsation of the aortic arch. Electrocardiogram may show left axis deviation, depression of the S-T segment, and changes in the T-wave. However, in early stages the ECG is usually not diagnostic.

Aneurysms of the Aorta.   Aortic aneurysms may be fusiform, with diffuse dilatation, or saccular, characterized by localized bulging of the aortic wall. Many aneurysms produce neither symptoms nor signs, and the diagnosis is often made at autopsy, thus radiologic examination is strongly recommended for all patients with late syphilis. Symptoms and signs, if present, depend upon the size of the aneurysm and its location.

ANEURYSM OF ASCENDING AORTA. The proximal ascending aorta is the most common site of aneurysm due to syphilis. Aneurysms of the ascending aorta are frequently silent or produce few symptoms. They may bulge laterally into the right lung and anteriorly against the chest wall, producing dullness on percussion and pulsating mass that can be felt or observed in the second and third right intercostal spaces. Occasionally the aneurysm may extend medially or posteromedially, producing pressure symptoms in the left upper chest or even displacing the trachea, pressing on the pulmonary artery. Ausculation may reveal a loud aortic systolic murmur best heard in the aortic area or on the aneurysm. An aneurysm of the ascending aorta can be the cause of sudden death from rupture.

ANEURYSM OF THE ARCH OF THE AORTA. Aneurysms of the aortic arch produce symptoms by pressing on the superior mediastinum. Pressure on the trachea and major bronchi causes stridor and a brassy, nonproductive cough. Dysphagia may result from compression of the esophagus, and pressure on the recurrent laryngeal nerve may produce hoarseness and aphonia. Extension of the aneurysms upward and backward may create pressure on the cervical sympathetic nerve, resulting in miosis, enophthalmos, ptosis, and impaired sweating on the same side (Horner's syndrome). Pressure on the phrenic nerve may cause paralysis of the diaphragm, and pressure on the vena cava may cause cyanosis, edema, and distention of veins of the neck and upper chest. The systolic blood pressure may be unequal in both arms. Compression on bones or nerve roots may cause severe pain. Chest x-ray combined with a barium swallow may be helpful in the diagnosis of aneurysm of the aortic arch since it may show a compressed esophagus.

ANEURYSMS OF THE DESCENDING AORTA. These kinds of aneurysms are rare and usually asymptomatic. They may be present for a considerable time without producing symptoms and become large in size. However, some patients may experience dull pain in the back. Pressure on the thoracic vertebrae may cause erosions of the corresponding vertebrae.

ANEURYSMS OF THE ABDOMINAL AORTA. Abdominal aneurysms resulting from syphilis are much less common than in the thorax. It is a common belief that nearly all abdominal aneurysms are due to arteriosclerosis rather than other causes. They are usually asymptomatic and frequently found on palpation of the abdomen for other reasons.

DIAGNOSIS. The diagnosis of cardiovascular syphilis is based on the presence of symptoms and signs confirmed by radiologic examination, electrocardiogram, and serologic tests. Diagnosis of aneurysms is largely radiologic, and frequently x-rays in various positions are required to confirm the site affected. In some cases, angioradiography may be helpful.

Neurosyphilis

Neurosyphilis has become rare since the introduction of antibiotics to syphilis treatment. Its incidence in developed countries is low, and according to some authors, the clinical picture has changed in favor of atypical cases.[29-31] Neurosyphilis may occur in untreated cases or as a sequelae of inadequately treated early or late disease.[32-34] A precise classification of neurosyphilis is very difficult because of an overlap of clinical manifestations and occurrence of combinations of different forms. However, neurosyphilis has been divided into several categories that make it easier to describe its great variety of clinical manifestations. The following categories have been identified: asymptomatic neurosyphilis, acute meningitis, chronic meningovascular syphilis, and parenchymatous syphilis (general paresis and tabes dorsalis).

Asymptomatic Neurosyphilis Asymptomatic neurosyphilis is defined as the presence of disease identifiable by positive serologic tests in blood and cerebral spinal fluid (CSF) as well as the presence of various abnormalities in CSF with the absence of clinical signs and symptoms of the disease in the central nervous system. Because of the generalized dissemination of *T. pallidum,* more than 30% of patients with secondary syphilis demonstrate CSF abnormalities such as increased cell count, increase in total protein, and reactive serologic tests. In the majority of patients this does not cause symptoms, or they are so nonspecific (headache, malaise, low-grade fever) that the patients do not attribute them to syphilis.

Acute Meningitis Acute syphilitic meningitis may be found during the secondary stage, usually within the first 2 years of infection. Its clinical picture is essentially similar to any acute meningitis except that there is a greater variability in the intensity of symptoms and signs. Fever is usually moderately high, and the patient complains of headache, neck stiffness, nausea and vomiting, and attacks of vertigo. Generalized convulsions and coma may occur, or the patient may become stuporous with periods of alertness and agitation. Ocular palsies and occasionally papilledema may be present. Other signs include cervical rigidity and positive Kernig's and Brudzinski's signs. Depending upon the areas affected, various cranial nerves may be involved, with the third nerve most frequently involved. The pressure of CSF is raised and the cell count as well as the protein level increased. Serologic tests in blood and CSF are strongly positive.

Chronic Meningovascular Neurosyphilis Chronic meningovascular neurosyphilis may occur within the first 2 years after primary infection, but in many instances the symptoms and signs appear much later. They vary according to the degree of involvement of the blood vessels of the brain, cord, and meninges as well as the cranial nerves. The blood vessels show proliferative endarteritis and perivascular infiltration with lymphocytes, plasma cells, and fibroblasts.

Impairment of the blood supply caused by reduction of the lumen or thrombosis results in marked ischemia of the nerve tissue and/or its necrosis. Any of the vessels may be affected, but most frequently the middle cerebral and posterior cerebral arteries and their branches are involved. Other frequently involved vessels include the anterior cerebral artery and the arteries of the brain stem. General symptoms include frequent headaches, gradual intellectual and emotional deterioration, and weakening of the muscles. Other neurologic signs depend on the arteries involved.

The meningeal involvement may cause headache, nausea, and vomiting. The skull may be tender on percussion, and neck stiffness may appear; however, the latter is more characteristic for acute meningitis. The signs are very variable and depend upon the areas involved. The cranial nerves may be involved, with the 3rd, 6th, 7th, and 8th nerves most commonly affected. Argyll Robertson pupils can be found as well as papilledema and secondary optic atrophy. If the eighth nerve is affected, vertigo and deafness may occur. Lumbar puncture may reveal increased fluid pressure and elevated blood cell count (lymphocytosis), elevated total protein, and positive serologic tests.

Parenchymatous Neurosyphilis

GENERAL PARESIS. General paresis (GP) is a progressive disease of the brain leading to mental and physical deterioration. The clinical manifestations usually appear about 15–20 years after primary infection and they consist of both psychiatric and neurologic symptoms in varying proportions (Table 8.3). The earliest symptoms are frequently subtle and indeterminate and are manifested by a change in personality. The patients tend to become irritable, forgetful, and may have difficulties with concentration. Impairment of intellectual function and memory as well as a lack of judgement may be apparent. Carelessness about personal appearance may occur in individuals who have never shown such characteristics before. Patients may become moody and aggressive and, as their mental status deteriorates, their violent behavior may bring them into conflict with the law. Insomnia, headache, fatigability, or states of anxiety are not uncommon. With progression of the disease, memory becomes progressively worse: the patient becomes more and more disoriented. In this stage hallucinations or delusions frequently occur.

Clinical examination, especially in the early stage of the disease, reveals tremors of the hands, lips, and tongue. The latter may take the form of a backward-forward movement of the tongue, "trombone tremor," when the patient is asked to protrude the tongue. There may be a lack of facial expression (flattening of the facial lines) or a characteristic fatuous smile. Pupillary abnormalities are very common. The pupils are small, fixed, and unequal, sluggishly reacting to strong light. In late cases, true Argyll Robertson pupils may be present. Speech is usually indistinct in the early stage of disease, followed by dysarthria with faulty enunciation and slurring of words. As the disease progresses, dysnomia or total aphasia may occur. Handwriting is impaired, with omission of letters and misspelled words. The con-

TABLE 8.3. Symptoms and Signs of General Paresis

Symptoms	Signs
Irritability	Pupillary abnormalities including Argyll Robertson pupils
Personality changes	
Failure of memory	Tremor (tongue, hands)
Poor concentration	Dysarthria
Carelessness in appearance	Dyslexia
Intellectual deterioration	Lack of facial expression (masked face)
Decreasing efficiency	Pyramidal signs
Defective judgement	Convulsions
Insomnia	Incontinence of urine and feces
Changes in mood (euphoria, depression, agitation)	
Delusions	
Hallucinations	
Seizures	
Confusion and disorientation	

tents of sentences are frequently meaningless. Epilepsylike seizures are not uncommon and at times may be the initial symptom of the disease, bringing medical attention to a patient who has never shown mental problems before.[35] They may occur in the form of localized convulsion without loss of consciousness, as a partial seizure, or as generalized grand mal attacks. Transient ischemic attacks and apoplectiform attacks may also occur, followed by hemiparesis or hemiplegia, monoplegia, with aphasia, apraxia, or hemianopia.

In some patients with GP, deep tendon reflexes in the lower limbs may be absent, and in cases associated with tabes dorsalis (taboparesis) the signs of impairment of posterior column conduction may become apparent. As the disease progresses and mental status deteriorates, incontinence of urine and feces may occur.

The psychotic manifestations of general paresis can be classified into several forms:

- *Simple dementia of GP* appears to be the most common form of psychosis. In this form, patients usually pass rapidly from a state of moodiness and irritability through a phase of forgetfulness and defective judgment into a state of apathy. These kinds of patients frequently lie in bed without any signs of mental activity, indifferent to environment and family, not wanting to eat, soiling themselves and ultimately dying of intercurrent diseases.

- The *expansive or euphoric form of GP* is characterized by the presence of delusions of grandeur. The patients are usually euphoric ("have never felt so good") and have delusions of power, wealth, or position. Psychomotor hyperactivity is apparent, but at the same time mental deterioration progresses.

- In the *agitative form of GP*, the patients may be aggressive and destructive. If not institutionalized they may be dangerous since they are capable of committing serious crimes, including homicide. These patients should be hospitalized promptly.

- In the *depressive form of GP*, unlike in the agitative or expansive forms, the patients are slow and melancholic. They have delusions of poverty or typical hypochondriac delusions. They have tendencies to self-accusation and self-condemnation or self-punishment and frequently express guilt feelings.

Diagnosis of GP is based on typical symptoms and signs supported by CSF examination and positive syphilis serologic tests. Both nontreponemal and treponemal serologic tests in the blood are positive in over 95% of cases.[35,36] The CSF abnormalities include lymphocytic pleocytosis, increases total protein, increased globulin concentration, characteristic colloidal gold curve (Lange's curve), and positive treponemal and nontreponemal serologic tests.

TABES DORSALIS. Tabes dorsalis (TD) is a form of neurosyphilis characterized by degeneration of the dorsal or posterior columns as well as the posterior nerve roots of the spinal cord. Since the introduction of penicillin in the treatment of syphilis, the total incidence of neurosyphilis in developed countries declined dramatically, including the incidence of tabes dorsalis. However, in the preantibiotic era, TD was the most common form of neurosyphilis, accounting for about 30 percent of all forms of neurosyphilis. Even in the 1950s and 1960s in certain countries, TD was

TABLE 8.4. Symptoms and Signs of Tabes Dorsalis

Symptoms	Signs
Lightning pains	Grayish pallor of skin
Ataxia	Tabetic facies
Paresthesias and hyperesthesias	Abnormal pupils (including Argyll Robertson pupils)
Bladder disturbances	Optic Atrophy
Impotence	Ataxia
Visceral crises	Positive Romberg's sign
Failing vision	Hypotonia
	Impaired tendon reflexes
	Impaired touch and pain sense
	Diminished vibration sensibility
	Impaired or absent deep pain sensibility
	Charcot's arthropathy
	Atonic bladder
	"Mal perforans"

the most common form of neurosyphilis, comprising from 43 to over 60 percent of cases.[37,38] The introduction of antibiotics into modern medicine not only reduced the number of late sequelae of syphilis but also changed their clinical pattern and severity.[37,38]

Symptoms occur in untreated patients long after primary infection, usually after more than 20 years. This means that the majority of patients will be in their forties or fifties. The disease produces a wide variety of symptoms (Table 8.4), of which the earliest and most characteristic are the so-called "lightning pains" chiefly restricted to the legs but which may occur in any part of the body. These are sudden and usually intense stabbing pains occurring in paroxysms. The attacks may last for a few seconds or a few minutes but frequently return, and the bouts may last for several days or even weeks. It is believed that lightning pains can be precipitated by changes in barometric pressure and thus are frequently mistaken for severe rheumatic pains. Other mentioned precipitating factors are infections and constipation. The lightning pain varies in severity from slight discomfort to agonizing pain causing the patient to cry or even to consider suicide. Between the attacks there are periods of freedom without any pains, but local paresthesias or hyperesthesia may be present. Remissions may last for days or months and they usually tend to grow longer as time passes.

Another cardinal finding in TD is ataxia; it is due to the deep sensory loss. At the beginning of the process, the patients notice difficulty in maintaining balance. This is usually first noticed in the dark or when they close their eyes. When the patients watch their feet and the ground they are usually able to compensate for the unsteadiness. The problem begins at night or when they attempt to walk with their eyes closed. They gradually assume a broad base while walking with the feet apart. Even when not moving, the patients try to hold to fixed objects to help maintain balance. As the disease progresses, patients develop a characteristic stamping type of gait, raising their feet too high off the ground and bringing them down forcibly to stimulate the remaining deep sensibility. Later the length of the steps becomes irregular, the patient frequently staggering from side to side or falling; eventually walking becomes possible only when assisted with one or even two canes.

Paresthesias and *hyperesthesias* are common symptoms among tabetics. Some of them complain of numbness or aching sensations of the extremities or other parts of the body. The paresthesia is most referred to the feet, and the patient describes the feeling like walking on a thick, soft carpet, foam rubber or snow. Muscle cramps are frequently reported, and some patients observe that certain parts of their bodies are hyperesthetic or anaesthetic.

Involvement of the sacral roots may result in *bladder disturbances* and/or *impotence.* Overdistention of the bladder before micturition is frequent as the patient loses the sensory nerve supply to the bladder and is unaware that the bladder is full. Many patients complain of such difficulties of micturition as slowness in starting or inadequate, feeble, or intermittent stream. The amount of residual urine increases, leading to frequent ascending infections. Incontinence of urine is not uncommon. Impotence has been also reported as an early symptom of the involvement of sacral roots.

Constipation may occur as a result of loss of tone of the lower gut and muscles of the pelvic floor. Incontinence of feces has been also reported.

Because of the involvement of the autonomic nervous system, patients with TD develop a painful disorder which is characterized by paroxysms of pain usually associated with other symptoms called *tabetic crises.* Gastric crises begin suddenly with upper abdominal pain, nausea, and vomiting. The pain may be so severe that it can be confused with perforated peptic ulcer, and persistent vomiting may result in electrolyte imbalance. The attack may end abruptly or may remain for a few hours or even days. Recrudescences are frequent.

Rectal crises are characterized by prolonged rectal pain and tenesmus. Renal crises resemble renal colic, and laryngeal crisis may result in stridor, cough, or attacks of severe dyspnea.

Failing vision is due to optic atrophy. It is often progressing and may lead to blindness.

Tabetic patients are usually thin, with *greyish pallor* of the skin. Flabby facial muscles, dropping of the upper eyelids, together with wrinkling of the forehead which results from compensatory overaction of the frontalis muscles give the so-called ''tabetic facies.''

Pupillary changes are common but not always of Argyll Robertson type (pinpoint pupils, often irregular in outline which do not react to light but react to convergence-accommodation; they do not react to atropine nor do they dilate on painful stimuli). Some patients develop *optic atrophy,* which is characterized by a pale, well-defined optic disc. On ophthalmologic examination, attenuation of the retinal artery may be found. There is a change in visual field which usually shows concentric constriction. There also may be central or peripheral scrotoma. Syphilitic optic atrophy can be part of tabes dorsalis or may occur as an isolated manifestation of neurosyphilis.[39]

Diminished or absent tendon reflexes are frequent signs of TD. Usually ankle jerk is affected earliest, followed by knee jerk. The tendon reflexes in the upper limbs and abdominal reflexes also may be lost, especially in the more advanced cases when hypotonia of the abdominal muscles occurs. At times, the atony of the muscles is so prominent that hyperextension of the joints may be demonstrated. Plantar responses are flexor in type while the abdominal reflexes may be abnormally brisk or even normal.

Ataxia usually starts in the lower limbs. It can be demonstrated by the heel-to-shin test or Romberg's test. Ataxia of the upper limbs can be detected by the finger-to-nose test, which is characteristically worse with the eyes closed. Abnormal gait was described earlier in this chapter.

Sensory disturbances or sensory loss is common, varies in extent and degree, and can be detected early in the course of the disease. Symptoms include *loss or diminution of sensation to pin prick and light touch,* diminution of appreciation or *loss of vibration sense* mainly in the lower limbs, and loss of position sense in the toes. Deep pain sensations in the Achilles tendons are often diminished or absent. Similarly, *pain sensibility* may be lost in the testicles.

As a result of sensory changes and hypotonia, *Charcot's arthropathy* may occur. Large joints such as the knee are most commonly affected; however, other joints, particularly the hip, ankle, and spine joints, may be involved as well. The affected joint is usually swollen, frequently with fluid in the joint space. Osteophytic formations, destruction of artricular cartilage, along with altered calcification at the end of the bones results in the joint's deformation (Figure 8.29). Dislocations and pathological fractures are common. X-ray examination shows widening of the joint space, thin joint cartilage, osteophytic outgrowths, and sclerosis of the ends of the

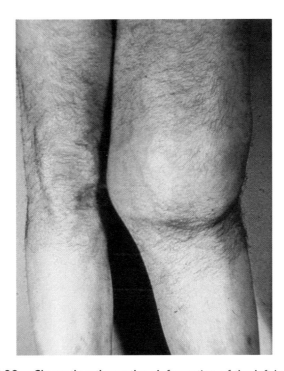

Figure 8.29. Charcot's arthropathy: deformation of the left knee joint.

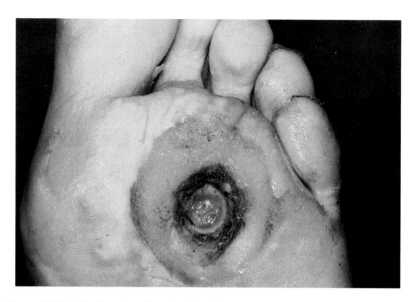

Figure 8.30.   Perforating ulcer (mal perforans) on the sole in tertiary syphilis.

bone. If the spine is involved, the symptoms may be absent, minimal, or nonspecific, and early detection of Charcot's spine arthropathy depends almost exclusively on radiologic examination.

Atonic bladder may occur as a result of interruption of the afferent fibers in the sacral nerve roots. Distention of the bladder is painless, and examination of the lower abdomen frequently reveals dull percussion extending even up to the level of the umbilicus.

Perforating ulcers (mal perforans) usually develop on the upper surface of the ball of the big toe. They are due to the loss of deep pain sense coupled with repeated trauma at the pressure points. They start as cornlike patches on the skin of a toe or a pressure point of the sole and develop into painless indolent ulcers (Figure 8.30). The ulcers may penetrate and erode the underlying bones. Secondary bacterial infection may result in osteomyelitis or pyogenic destruction of adjacent joints.

The diagnosis of tabes dorsalis depends on clinical features and a history of syphilitic infection. Unlike general paresis, serologic tests of blood and cerebrospinal fluid may be normal in up to 30 percent of cases.[40] CSF may show an increased number of lymphocytes and protein, although total protein is frequently normal. The colloidal gold curve of Lange is of the syphilitic type, with the high number in the middle tubes. It should be emphasized that the changes in CSF in the tabetic patient vary, and it is not uncommon for the patient with obvious physical signs of tabes dorsalis to have normal fluid.

SEROLOGIC TESTS

Treponemal infections, including *Treponema pallidum*, evoke a humoral antibody response that can be detected by a wide variety of serologic tests. According to

the antigens employed, these tests can be divided into nontreponemal and treponemal tests.

Nontreponemal Tests

Nontreponemal tests detect the presence of a heterogeneous group of anticardiolipin antibodies which are produced during treponemal infection. Almost all
contemporary nontreponemal tests use cardiolipin-lecithin antigens usually
derived from beef hearts. Anticardiolipin antibodies which belong to gamma
globulins can be detected by two types of tests: complement fixation test, which has
a rather historical value and is very rarely used, and several flocculation tests, of
which the VDRL test is the most widely performed.

Flocculation Tests

All flocculation tests depend on the ability of serum containing antibodies to
cause aggregation of a colloidal suspension of lipoid particles into visible flocculation, which, depending on the test, can be seen under a microscope or with the
naked eye.

The Venereal Disease Research Laboratory (VDRL) test uses purified cardiolipin-lecithin-cholesterol antigen. It can be performed as a slide test or a tube test,
and both versions can be adapted to quantitative estimations by serial dilution of
serum. In the quantitative test, the titer is recorded as the greatest serum dilution
that produces a reactive result.

In recent years, the VDRL slide test has been most widely used. In this test
antigen suspension is mixed with inactivated serum (or cerebrospinal fluid) on a
glass slide and rotated mechanically. The result is read after few minutes and
depends on the presence of microscopically observed flocculation.

Other frequently used tests are the rapid plasma reagin (RPR) card test, in
which VDRL antigen suspension is mixed with finely divided carbon particles as a
marker, and its automated version, the automated reagin test (ART); the unheated
serum reagin (USR) test; and the reagin screen test (RST).[41-44]

At present in the United States, the VDRL slide test and RPR card test are most
commonly used.

The sensitivity of the VDRL test and other flocculation tests depends on the
stage of syphilis. VDRL becomes positive between the fifth and seventh week of
infection and is positive in 59–87 percent of cases of primary syphilis. It is almost
100 percent positive in secondary syphilis and 37–94 percent positive in late
syphilis.[17] In secondary and early latent syphilis all serologic tests are strongly
positive because of the maximal antibody production. In this stage, though, very
rarely false-negative results may occur in flocculation tests due to antibody excess
(prozone phenomenon). This, however, can be resolved by serum dilutions and
reexamination of the specimen. VDRL as well as other cardiolipin tests are not as
specific as treponemal tests and occasionally may be reactive in persons without
treponemal infection. In the general population the nonspecificity of these tests is
about 1 percent,[45,46] but in selected groups of patients with certain diseases or in the
elderly the probability of false-positive results is much higher.[47-49]

Treponemal Tests

Treponemal tests detect antibodies directed toward *T. pallidum* and unfortunately toward other treponemes as well. The antigen for these tests is *T. pallidum* extracted from lesions in experimentally infected rabbit testes.

Fluorescent Treponemal Antibody Absorption Test

The fluorescent treponemal antibody absorption test is FTA-ABS, presently the most commonly used treponemal test. Tested sera are mixed with a sorbent prepared from nonpathogenic Reiter's treponemes or other appropriate material which absorbs the cross-reacting antibodies to human commensal treponemes. The sera are subsequently layered on slides containing *T. pallidum* antigens and incubated. Fluorescein-labeled antibody to human gamma globulin is added, and after further incubation the slides are examined by fluorescence microscopy. The fluorescence of the treponemes indicates the presence of specific, antitreponemal antibodies in the tested serum. The preliminary ''absorption phase'' is necessary to eliminate group-reactive antibodies which react with both pathogenic and commensal treponemes present at lower titers in many normal sera. Without the absorption phase, FTA-ABS would give false-positive results in a high percentage of cases (28 percent).[50]

The FTA-ABS test is more specific than cardiolipin tests, relatively easy to carry out, and has become one of the most popular tests used in the detection of syphilis. It is also the most sensitive test in primary syphilis and becomes positive before any test, even when the primary chancre is still present. It is positive in 86–100 percent of cases in the primary stage, 99–100 percent in cases in the secondary stage, and 96–100 percent of cases in late syphilis.[17] FTA-ABS is currently performed in many laboratories as a confirmation test of the diagnosis of syphilis. Even though the FTA-ABS test is highly specific, false-positive results have been noticed in autoimmune diseases,[51-53] genital herpes,[54] narcotic addiction, and several other conditions.[55,56]

The FTA-ABS-IgM test detects one class of immunoglobulin antibodies. This test was developed as a diagnosis test for congenital syphilis and has been performed in infants to differentiate neonatal syphilis from passive transfer of maternal antitreponemal antibodies that belong to the IgG fraction of immunoglobulins.[57] The detection of a specific IgM class of antitreponemal antibodies in neonates speaks in favor of a diagnosis of congenital syphilis since immunoglobulins of the IgM class should not cross the placenta. Unfortunately the sensitivity and specificity of this test are unacceptably low, and its value is seriously questioned.

Hemagglutination Tests

The microhemagglutination test for *T. pallidum* (MHA-TP) or the hemagglutination treponemal test for syphilis (HATTS) measures antibodies which agglutinate erythrocytes coated with *T. pallidum*. Sheep erythrocytes are used as the carrier for the *T. pallidum* antigen in the MHA-TP test, and turkey erythrocytes are used in the HATTS test.[46] The MHA-TP test was initially described as the *T. pallidum* hemagglutination test (TPHA), but its less costly micromethod made the test more widely used. The MHA-TP test is highly specific but appears to be slightly less sensitive in primary syphilis than FTA-ABS. It can be quantified and automated (AMHA-TP),[58] which makes it attractive for many laboratories. The specificity of the MHA-TP test appears to be similar to that of the FTA-ABS.[59,60] False-positive results also have been reported.[61,62] The *T. pallidum*–specific IgM hemagglutination test [TP(IgM)HA], which uses erythrocytes sensitized with antiserum to human IgM to separate IgM from IgG in serum, was recently studied. The authors concluded that the TP(IgM)HA test, which easily detects treponemal IgM, can be useful especially in monitoring the treatment of syphilis.[63]

Treponema pallidum *Immobilization Test*

The *Treponema pallidum immobilization* (TPI) test, the first specific test for syphilis, was described by Nelson and Mayer in 1949.[64] It was used extensively as a confirmatory test in the 1950s and 1960s and was later replaced by FTA-ABS and MHA-TP. It is still used in certain countries and in a few research laboratories in the United States. TPI measures different antibodies than other tests called the immobilizing antibodies. In this test, live virulent *T. pallida* are incubated with patient's serum in the presence of complement. If 50 percent or more of the treponemes are immobilized, the test is reported positive. Immobilization of 20 percent or less is regarded as negative, and if between 20 and 50 percent, then the result is considered to be doubtful. TPI is highly specific, and positive results are obtained only in patients with syphilis or suffering from other treponematoses. Unfortunately, this test is time consuming, complicated to perform, expensive, and even hazardous to laboratory personnel since it uses virulent treponema. It is basically used to verify other tests and also in the diagnosis of certain cases of late syphilis. A positive result from TPI speaks in favor of syphilis past or present but does not indicate current activity of the disease. Negative results, with the exception of first 6–8 weeks of infection and of some cases of tabes dorsalis, make diagnosis of treponemal infection rather unlikely. TPI becomes positive after 5–8 weeks of infection and with the exception of promptly treated primary syphilis may remain positive for life, irrespective of treatment.

Other Techniques

In recent years several new techniques to detect antitreponemal antibodies have been developed.[65-70] Some of them are very sensitive and specific and are capable of detecting antibodies to certain molecules of *T. pallidum*.[69,70] However, they are still being studied, and until now VDRL, FTA-ABS, and MHA-TP tests and their variants are the most widely used tests in the serodiagnosis of syphilis in the United States and elsewhere.[71]

Interpretation of Serologic Tests

All standard serologic tests for syphilis remain negative for about 3–5 weeks after infection, although IgG and IgM antibodies to certain molecules of *T. pallidum* can be detected before the development of a primary chancre.[72] In the case of primary syphilis the FTA-ABS test is the first to become positive, followed by MHA-TP and VDRL and after 1–3 weeks by TPI. The antibodies increase rapidly in titer for the next several weeks and reach their maximum in secondary syphilis. In untreated cases high titers remain positive for about 2 years and then gradually decrease. In some untreated patients (accidental cure with antibiotics taken for other reasons cannot be ruled out), they may disappear "spontaneously," but in the majority of cases they remain positive for life. In treated cases seroreactivity varies with the duration of infection and the type of test performed. If treatment starts before antibodies are detectable in the serum, it may never become positive, and the patient will remain seronegative. In primary seropositive and secondary syphilis antibodies usually disappear or at least drop in titer within a few months of the start of treatment.

In adequately treated primary syphilis, the cardiolipin tests become negative in 6–12 months, whereas in secondary and early latent syphilis seronegativity occurs usually after 12–18 months. Antitreponemal antibodies even in adequately treated cases may remain positive for many years or for life; however, a significant drop in titer is usually sufficient to declare the patient cured. These persistent antibodies are presumably of the immunoglobulin G (IgG) class whereas IgM antibodies reportedly disappear within 12–24 months after treatment.[67,69,73,74] The persistence of weakly positive serologic tests after treatment must not be an indication for treatment.

In patients treated for late syphilis, the antibodies may be present for life, although they usually show a slow, fluctuating drop in titer. If any of the tests become negative, they are usually those which use cardiolipin antigens. Treponemal tests usually remain positive for the rest of the patient's life or at least for a very long time.

For practical reasons all patients treated for syphilis should have quantitive pretreatment and posttreatment serologic evaluations. Periodic (3, 6, 12, and 24 months) posttreatment tests showing a significant drop in titer will document the adequacy of treatment.

False-positive Reactions

In small groups of people tested for syphilis, a false-positive reaction may occur. This means that a positive test occurs in an individual who has never been infected. False-positive reactions can be divided into two categories: (1) biological false-positive (BFP) reactions and (b) technical false-positive reactions. They are most common in nontreponemal tests; therefore, anytime BFP is considered, one of the treponemal tests, usually FTA-ABS, should be performed to rule out or confirm syphilis. In studies in which nontreponemal tests have been used to screen the general population for syphilis, the rate of false positive results was about 1 percent.[45,46] However, among patients with certain medical problems, the rate may be much higher.[47,48,74-78] Nontreponemal BFP reactions have been reported in a wide variety of conditions, including lupus erythematosus,[75] infectious mononucleosis,[76] leprosy,[78] aging,[49,79] and many others (see Table 8-5).

BFP reactions which occur in nontreponemal tests have become less common since the introduction of well-purified cardiolipin-lecithin-cholesterol antigen[80] and more frequent use of the VDRL test owing to the expense of the complement

TABLE 8.5. Causes of Biological False-positive Nontreponemal Tests

Acute viral infections	Leprosy (LL)
Addison's disease	Lupus erythematosus
Aging (per se)	Lymphatic leukemia
Atopic dermatitis	Lymphosarcoma
Bacterial pneumonia	Malaria
Brucellosis	Metastatic carcinoma
Cirrhosis of liver	Myeloma multiplex
Cryoglobulinemia	Pemphigus vulgaris
Dermatomyositis	Periarteritis nodosa
Diabetes mellitus	Pernicious anemia
Dysproteinemia	Pregnancy (?)
Erythema nodosum	Rheumatic fever
Glomerulonephritis	Rheumatoid arthritis
Hashimoto's thyroiditis	Sarcoidosis
Hemolytic anemia	Scleroderma
Histoplasmosis	Subacute bacterial endocarditis
Idiopathic thrombocytopenic purpura	Tuberculosis
Intravenous drug abuse	Vaccinations

fixation test.[81] Moreover, in the majority of cases their titer is low, usually no more than 1 : 8; however, among intravenous drug users the titer may be as high as 1 : 64 or even 1 : 128.[82] Whether the pregnancy per se can be the cause of BFP is still not clear, and many authors suggest rather that syphilis or other illnesses which may occur during pregnancy are responsible for positive serology in these women.[71,83,84] BFP reactions can be transient (acute), lasting a few weeks or months (usually less than six), or chronic (of more than 6 months' duration). All of them are usually of low titer with the exception of drug addicts[82] and can be verified with more specific treponemal tests. Treponemal tests may also give false-positive results. However they are less common than in the nontreponemal test. The FTA-ABS test, which is the most commonly performed treponemal test, can give BFP results in genital herpes,[54] certain autoimmune and connective tissue diseases,[53,85] and in drug addicts.[48] Lyme disease, which is caused by a spirochete, *Borrelia burgdorferi*, and is a tick-borne disease occurring in certain regions in the United States, can be the cause of false-positive FTA-ABS test.[86] If Lyme disease is suspected, the MHA-TP or even RPR test (nontreponemal) is recommended to differentiate it from syphilis.[87] However, the greatest FTA-ABS specificity problems have not been with BFP results but rather with technical false-positive results in cases with 1 + and 2 + gradations of fluorescence.[55,88,89] One must remember that FTA-ABS test is read qualitatively and the results depend a great deal on factors such as quality of reagents used and the experience of the technicians performing the test.

The MHA-TP test is probably less prone to either technical or biologic false-positive reactions; nevertheless, the BFP reaction may also occur.[16,59] Given that biological false-positive reactions may occur in many conditions, syphilis is still a disease which is the most common cause of a positive serologic test. Consequently, any positive result should be interpreted as evidence of current treponemal infection until proved otherwise. In geographic regions where endemic treponematoses (yaws, pinta) occur, the interpretation of syphilis serologic tests may be difficult. In both instances the venereal syphilis and the nonvenereal, endemic treponematoses syphilis serologic tests are positive, and none of the specific tests is capable of differentiating between these conditions. Other factors such as medical records, scar after skin lesion, or the titer of treponemal and nontreponemal tests (high titer will make syphilis a more likely diagnosis) may help to establish the diagnosis.

Technical false-positive reactions result from human error. Improperly collected or misslabeled specimens, outdated or low-quality reagents, and mistakes in performance or in recording should not, but can be, the cause of the false-positive result. Therefore, all positive results which have no confirmation in clinical findings or medical history should be verified by testing other specimens from the same patient with a different test.

Syphilis Serologic Test and AIDS

It has been known that patients infected with the human immunodeficiency virus (HIV) respond abnormally to a variety of antigenic stimuli. Hence they may also fail to develop a serologic response to treponemal infection. There is a danger that patients with AIDS and concomitant syphilis may have false negative serologic test results. This phenomenon may lead to an incorrect diagnosis with all of its medical and epidemiologic consequences and, in the case of a patient with mucous or skin lesions, to unnecessary and fruitless evaluation for opportunistic infection. A recent report of a case of secondary syphilis (proven by clinical picture and skin biopsy revealing spirochetes) with negative VDRL and FTA-ABS tests proves that these fears are not unfounded.[90] Clinicians treating HIV-infected patients, a group whose incidence of syphilis exceeds that of the general population, should be aware of the problems of serologic diagnosis of syphilis. In the case of an HIV-infected patient with skin or mucous membrane lesions suspected to be of syphilitic origin, a negative serologic test does not rule out the diagnosis of syphilis. Other diagnostic methods such as dark-field examination or skin biopsy with silver staining which reveals *T. pallida* may be necessary to confirm or rule out syphilis.

CONGENITAL SYPHILIS

Congenital syphilis is a disease which is transmitted from the infected mother to her unborn child. The term "congenital syphilis" is inaccurate since the disease is not inherited: the infection is passed from infected mother through the placenta into the fetus. The syphilitic father is not capable of transmitting the infection to the child without intermediate infection of the mother.

Mode of Infection

Treponema pallidum passes from the maternal circulation into the fetal circulation through placental capillaries. It was considered to happen only in the second trimester of pregnancy, since it has been supposed that Langhan's layer provides a barrier against infection of the fetus. However, in one study *T. pallidum* was demonstrated in fetuses of 9 and 10 weeks' gestation with Langhan's cell layer intact.[8] Even though the spirochetes may probably cross the placenta before the second trimester of pregnancy, the pathologic changes take place not sooner than before the fetus becomes capable of an inflammatory response, which occurs between 18 and 20 weeks of gestation.

The impact on the fetus and the outcome of pregnancy depends on how recently the mother was infected. In general, the more recent the infection in the mother, the more destructive the changes to the fetus. Kassowitz's law says that in untreated women infected with syphilis, early pregnancies should result in miscarriages and stillbirths followed by deliveries of living children but with congenital syphilis. After a period of years, the same mother may deliver a healthy child without any clinical or serologic evidence of the disease. In fact, this law has been rarely "obeyed" and exceptions are common. Miscarriages may alternate with stillborn, syphilitic, and healthy children.

Epidemiology

With the advent of penicillin four decades ago, the incidence of congenital syphilis in developed countries fell dramatically. However, the resurgence of syphilis in groups of child-bearing age seen recently may result in an increased incidence of congenital syphilis. In the United States the number of reported cases of congenital syphilis in patients younger than 1 year of age rose in the period 1978–1987 from 108 to 449 cases (Figure 8.31), reflecting an increased incidence of primary and secondary syphilis in women of child-bearing age.[91,92] In developing countries, congenital syphilis remains a serious problem, as indicated from some African countries.[2,93-95] In both developing and developed countries, two main factors contribute to the incidence of the disease: the prevalence of syphilis among young women and the inadequacy of prenatal care.[2,95,96]

Congenital syphilis is absolutely a preventable disease, since the administration of penicillin to infected women during pregnancy precludes delivery of a syphilitic child.

Clinical Features

Clinical manifestations of congenital syphilis traditionally have been categorized into three groups: early congenital syphilis, late congenital syphilis, and stigmata.

Early Congenital Syphilis

With the exception of bullous eruption, the lesions of early congenital syphilis resemble in many ways those of secondary syphilis in adults. Frequently, at birth the syphilitic infant appears healthy and may not develop clinical signs for a few weeks. When they appear the skin lesions can be macular, maculopapular and papular, or papulosquamous. They are usually widespread and symmetrical, with a

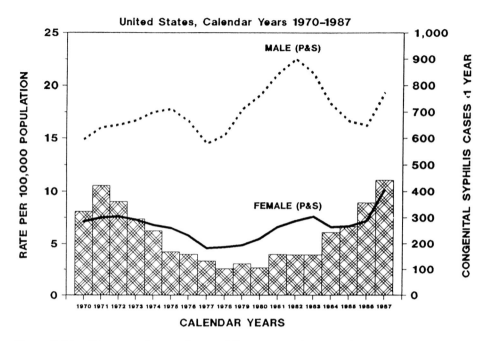

Figure 8.31. Primary and secondary syphilis case rates by sex and congenital syphilis (< 1 year) cases. From *Sexually Transmitted Disease Statistics, Calendar Year 1987.* US DHHS PHS, Center for Disease Control, No 136. 1988.

predilection for the face (around the mouth and nose), the napkin area, and the palms and soles. In moist areas the lesion may erode and become moist; if the rash is exposed to friction, the skin between the lesions may become reddened and has a glazed appearance. At mucocutaneous junctions, similarly to acquired syphilis, hypertrophic papules (condylomata lata) may be present. Dehydration and weight loss may produce wrinkling of facial skin, giving "the old man look." Commonly the whole skin has a yellowish brown color, the so-called "cafe-au-lait" tint. There may be patchy loss of hair chiefly on the sides and back of the scalp. Syphilitic alopecia may also affect eyelashes and eyebrows, this feature being very character-istic for congenital syphilis. The remaining hair may be brittle and sparse. The nails may be loosened and shedding (onychia), and paronychia may cause the newly growing nails to be irregular, atrophic and narrow, or even clawlike.

Mucous membranes are frequently involved. The mucous patches may be found in the nose and mouth, on the lips, and in the throat and larynx. In the nasal cavity they cause a discharge, giving rise to syphilitic rhinitis, a nasal obstruction that causes the infant to make a bubbling sound known as "syphilitic snuffles." At times the obstruction may be so severe that it interferes with nourishing, causing subsequent weight loss. The nasal discharge which is loaded with spirochetes may be an outward manifestation of serious destructive changes in the nasal supporting tissue, leading to perforation of the nasal septum and depression of the nasal bridge. Mucous patches in the larynx may cause aphonia or a thin or hoarse cry or cough. The lesions around the mouth, at the nasolabial folds, and around the anus may become fissured and produce radiating scars (rhagades) which often remain for the rest of the patient's life.

Vesiculobullous eruptions are characteristic of congenital syphilis and practically are never seen in acquired syphilis. They are located usually on the palms and soles and occasionally on other parts of the body. The fluid in the bullae may be hemorrhagic or contain seropurulent fluid teeming with spirochetes. Bullous rash can be the earliest type of lesion, present even at birth; prognosis in such cases is poor despite treatment.

In congenital early syphilis, there may be generalized lymphadenopathy which is usually less marked than in the secondary stage of acquired syphilis. The abdomen may be distended owing to the enlargement of the liver and spleen. Infants who died of early congenital syphilis were also found to have infiltration of the lungs, the so-called "white pneumonia." Although asymptomatic neurologic involvement with changes in CSF is more common, acute syphilitic meningitis with bulging of fontanellas, neck rigidity, positive Kernig's sign, convulsions, and alterations of the level of consciousness have been observed. Unfortunately, this condition frequently has been fatal.

The bone structure may be affected in various ways, frequently in the first few weeks of life. Osteochondritis or epiphysitis usually occur within the first 6 months of life. The ends of the long bones are swollen, painful, and tender. The sites commonly affected are the distal ends of radius, ulna, and the upper end of the tibia. Movements of the nearby joint can be very painful, causing the infant to hold the affected limb immobile, which gives the impression that the limb was paralyzed—the so-called "pseudoparalysis of Parrot." X-ray of the long bones may reveal enlarged epiphysis, broadened and irregular epiphyseal line, and thickening of the zone of provisional calcification of the distal end of the metaphysis, giving it an irregular "saw toothed" appearance. Patchy decalcification of the bone of the cranial vault also has been observed. An "onion-peel" periosteum, which results from irregular thickening of the bones due to syphilitic periostitis, occurs usually after the age of 6 months. Osteoperiostitis of the proximal phalanges (dactylitis) may appear in the second year of life. One digit or several may be involved, causing painless swelling in the affected area. Fingers are more frequently involved than toes.

Ocular involvement (chorioretinitis, glaucoma, and uveitis) is probably more common than thought but frequently overlooked. Syphilitic chorioretinitis produces "salt and pepper" pigmentary patches at the periphery of a granular fundus.[97] This can be found later in life as a stigma of congenital syphilis. Typical glaucoma and uveitis are rare conditions.

In general a child with early congenital syphilis is much more severely sick than an adult in the same stage of acquired syphilis. Constitutional symptoms may be severe, and these infants are more prone to intercurrent infections such as pneumonia or gastroenteritis. Anemia, thrombocytopenia, leukocytosis, and jaundice are common,[95,98,99] and their presence carries a bad prognosis. It was also observed that the younger the infant, the more likely was jaundice to occur and the higher was the incidence of mortality.[95]

Late Congenital Syphilis

The manifestations of late congenital syphilis occur after the second year of life and are most common between the ages of 7 and 15 years. About 80 percent of children with congenital syphilis pass through the early years of life undetected,[96]

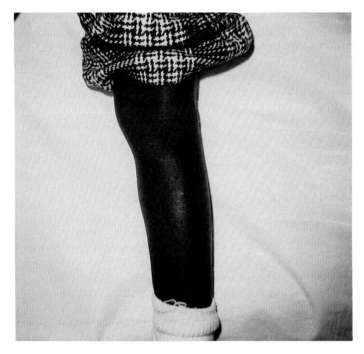

Figure 8.32. Late congenital syphilis "sabre shin."

and frequent administration of antibiotics for intercurrent diseases in early child-hood modifies the classic symptoms so that typical manifestations of late syphilis are rarely seen. In general the clinical manifestations of late congenital syphilis are identical with the tertiary stage of acquired syphilis.

Gummatous lesions are rarely seen before the age of 5 years. They tend to occur in the skin, subcutaneous tissue, and muscles but are more frequent in the nasal septum and the palate. Gummata in the nasal septum may produce septal perforation. Occasionally a gummatous process of the nasal septum may spread out, causing partial or complete destruction of the supporting structure and col-lapse of the nose: "saddle nose." Gummata of the hard and soft palate may result in palate perforation, causing regurgitation of food and a nasal voice. Periostitis of the long bones may occur, and osteoperiostitis of the tibia produces the so-called "sabre shin" (Figure 8.32), where as a result of thickening of the middle third of the tibia, a characteristic bowing of the legs occurs. Another, although rare, sign of congenital syphilis is Higoumenakis sign, which is a thickening of the sternal end of the clavicle.

Clutton's joints is a painless hydrarthrosis of the knee joints, although other joints can also be involved. There is no history of injury, and in most cases there are signs of joint effusion without evidence of inflammation. It is believed to be a hypersensitivity reaction, since administration of antibiotics neither prevents nor cures the condition. This syndrome appears rarely before 10 years of age; the onset is insidious and the course is chronic usually over several months. When the condition resolves, the patient is left with normal joints without any deformities. X-ray examination shows increased joint space but no changes in the bone structure. The joint fluid contains a few lymphocytes but no polymorphonuclear cells.

Symptomatic neurosyphilis is rare, and its occurrence is usually delayed until adolescence; asymptomatic involvement of the central nervous system is more common. As in acquired syphilis, the lesions can be meningeal, vascular, or parenchymatous. The syphilitic meningitis may result in cranial nerve palsies and occasionally blindness, hydrocephalus, mental deficiency, and/or seizure disorders. The vascular lesion may cause monoplegia, hemiplegia, hemianopia, or sensory loss. Parenchymatous neurosyphilis may result either in a junvenile form of general paresis or juvenile tabes dorsalis. Both forms usually follow the same pattern as in acquired syphilis.

Eight-nerve deafness may start at any stage of congenital syphilis, but it usually occurs around the age of 10 years. It is frequently preceded by tinnitus and vertigo or it may be manifested as a bilateral, progressive loss of hearing. On examination the tympanic membrane is normal, and sometimes only audiometry can detect the impairment of hearing, mainly in the high-frequency range, while the usual hearing tests are normal. Discrimination of speech may be difficult or impossible. The nerve deafness does not react dramatically to antisyphilitic therapy but can be modified by administration of corticosteroids.

Interstitial keratitis appears to be one of the most common lesions of late congenital syphilis. It usually starts in one eye with pain, photophobia, lacrimation, and blurred vision. There is injection of the slcera at the margin of the cornea, and invasion of deep layers of the cornea by small blood vessels produces dull-pink areas called "salmon patches." As a result of cellular infiltration the cornea becomes opaque, loses its normal transparent appearance, and becomes hazy ("ground glass" appearance). In many instances, vascularization of the cornea is less intense, so it can be detected only with the corneal microscope and the slit lamp. Changes in the cornea may mask chorioretinitis, which is frequently overlooked. Antitreponemal treatment has no effect on the course of interstitial keratitis, but it can be stopped by systematic steroids.

Depending on the extent of corneal changes, the impairment of vision may be minimal or the eye lesions may result in complete blindness. Some changes persist for life as stigmata of the disease (corneal scarring, ghost vessels). Interstitial keratitis along with eight-nerve deafness and "Hutchinson's teeth" forms "Hutchinson's triad," which is very characteristic for late congenital syphilis. Although cardiovascular manifestations may occur, they are extremely rare in late congenital syphilis.

Stigmata. The stigmata of congenital syphilis are the residual effects resulting from damage done to developing parts of the body in utero or during the early or late stages of syphilitic infection (see Table 8.6). They appear with different frequencies depending on the population studied.[100,101] Some of them were described before. Dental changes characteristic for late syphilis which remains for life include Hutchinson's teeth (Figure 8.33) and "Moon's" or "mulberry molars." These abnormalities are due to the effect of treponemal infection on the developing teeth buds shortly before and after birth. Both changes are found in the permanent teeth only. In Hutchinson's teeth the middle denticle is damaged by the syphilitic process and the teeth develop only from lateral denticles which expand to fill the gap. The central incisors are widely spaced and smaller than normal. Frequently there is also a lack of parallelism. The teeth are changed in that the sides are rounded (barrel shaped) and the cutting edge may be narrow like a screwdriver and may show a

TABLE 8.6. Stigmata of Late Congenital Syphilis

Saddle nose
Bulldog jaw (relative protuberance of the mandible)
Short maxilla
Frontal bossing
Gothic palate (high palatal arch)
Rhagades
   Interstitial keratitis ⎫
   Eight-nerve deafness ⎬ Hutchinson's triad
   Hutchinson's teeth ⎭
Mulberry (Moon's) molars
Saber shins
Clutton's joints
Scaphoid scapulae
Higoumenakis sign (sternoclavicular thickening)
Choroid scarring ("pepper and salt" fundus)
Optic atrophy

semilunar notch. Upper central incisors are most commonly affected, but the upper lateral and lower incisor may be also involved.

Moon molars are less common than Hutchinson's teeth. The first lower molars, which develop at the same time as the incisor teeth, are most frequently affected. Their biting surfaces are dome shaped, with badly developed cusps producing a mulberrylike surface. These teeth are poorly enamelized and are highly prone to decay.

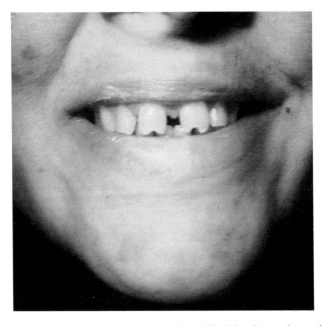

Figure 8.33. Stigma of congenital syphilis: Hutchinson's teeth.

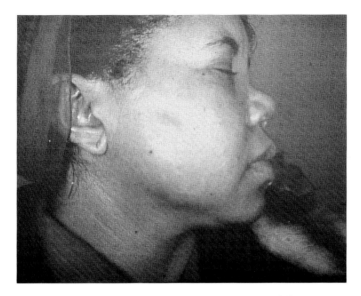

Figure 8.34.   Stigma of congenital syphilis: saddle nose.

Facial disfigurement is caused by localized thickening due to periostitis and chondritis. The most common is frontal bossing, which results from thickening of the frontal and parietal bones of the skull. Other deformities include "Olympian" or "beetle brow" (supraorbital thickening) or a "tower skull." Involvement of the nasal cavities may cause the nose deformity "saddle nose" (Figure 8.34), and pathologic changes in the maxilla may produce a high-arched palate called "gothic palate." The failure of the maxilla to develop makes the jaw look very prominent, giving the appearance of "bulldog jaw."

Other stigmata described before include rhagades (Figure 8.35), the linear scars around the mouth and/or anus; corneal opacities resulting from interstitial keratitis; "pepper and salt" fundus attributed to chorioretinitis; gummatous scars or perforations of the hard palate or nasal septum; depression of the vertebral border of the scapulae (scaphoid scapulae); eight-nerve deafness; and optic atrophy.

Diagnosis*

The definite diagnosis of congenital syphilis can be made by finding *T. pallidum* on dark-field examination, immunofluorescence, or in biopsy specimens. The specimens for these tests can be obtained from mucous or skin lesions and/or nasal discharge, autopsy material, placenta, or the umbilical cord.[102]

The blood test results from the umbilical cord taken at birth are very helpful in establishing the diagnosis. However, they must be interpreted with caution, since the positive results in a newborn may be due to passive transfer of maternal antibodies, which usually disappear within the first 6 weeks of life. On the other hand,

---

*Detailed information can be found in *MMWR* 37(S-1):1–13, 1988.

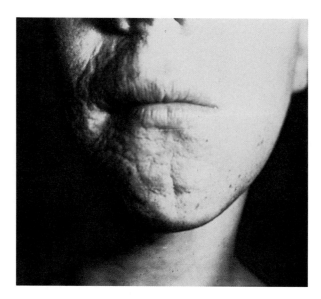

Figure 8.35. Stigma of congenital syphilis: rhagades—linear scars around the mouth.

the negative tests at births do not exclude syphilis. In the case of congenital syphilis they may become positive within several weeks after the birth; therefore, if negative at birth they should be performed after 3 weeks, 6 weeks, 3 months, and 6 months. If negative after 6 months and the baby has no clinical signs of congenital syphilis or the titers of passively transferred antibodies have declined, the diagnosis of congenital syphilis may be ruled out.

As maternal IgM does not cross the placenta, it is assumed that increased serum IgM levels represent a neonatal response to infection. The FTA-ABS (IgM) test and the flagellum ELISA (IgM) test are capable of distinguishing between antibodies produced by the neonate and those passively transferred from the mother[95]; however, these tests are not always reliable. FTA-ABS (IgM) test can be false-positive in a small proportion of cases and was reported to be false-negative in about 30 percent of cases of delayed onset of the disease.[103] Similarly, the flagellum ELISA (IgM) test has failed to detect IgM antibodies in several premature babies with highly suspicious features of congenital syphilis.[95]

Until the current methods of serodiagnosis are improved or new, more sensitive and specific tests are developed, the following serologic features might be helpful in interpretation of serologic tests for congenital syphilis:

1. Higher titer of antibodies in the infant than in the mother
2. Fourfold rise in the titer during a 3-month period
3. Development of a positive treponemal antibody test after birth
4. Seropositivity which does not revert to nonreactivity within 4 months

All aforementioned serological features with or without the presence of clinical signs speak in favor of the diagnosis of congenital syphilis.

Differential Diagnosis

The skin lesions in congenital syphilis may pose a problem; however, if supported by positive serologic tests and medical history, they should make the diagnosis of congenital syphilis relatively easy.

The following skin conditions can be mistaken for lesions of congenital syphilis in the infant.

- Diaper rash, insect bites, scabies, and atopic dermatitis all are itchy conditions that have a characteristic distribution or causative agent that can be identified in the skin lesions.
- Bullous eruption should be distinguished from toxic epidermal necrolysis, bacterial sepsis, staphylococcal scaled skin syndrome, herpes simplex, cytomegalovirus infection, varicella or vaccinia inoculata, and candidiasis.
- Rarely, hereditary skin diseases can be the cause of bullous or vesiculobullous eruption in the infant. These include epidermolysis bullosa, dermatitis herpetiformis, urticaria pigmentosa, porphyria, Letterer-Siwe disease, and chronic bullous dermatosis of childhood.

TREATMENT*

Acquired Early Syphilis

Acquired early syphilis (primary, secondary, and latent syphilis of less than 1 year's duration) should be treated with *benzathine penicillin G*, 2.4 million units IM, given in a single dose. Those allergic to penicillin should be given *tetracycline* 500 mg by mouth 4 times daily for 15 days or *doxycycline,* 100 mg orally 2 times a day for 14 days. Those who cannot tolerate tetracycline should be given *erythromycin,* 500 mg by mouth 4 times daily for 14 days. (Tetracycline and doxycycline are contraindicated in pregnant women.)

Comment: In many countries other forms of penicillin are preferred over benzathine penicillin G, especially procaine penicillin G. It is recommended in the treatment of primary, secondary, and early latent syphilis of less than 2 year's duration in doses ranging from 0.6 million units IM daily for 10–12 days in Great Britain, to 0.6–1.2 million units IM daily for 14 days in the Federal Republic of Germany, to 1.2 million units IM daily for 20–30 days in Poland.

Latent Syphilis of More than 1 Year Duration, Gummas and Cardiovascular Syphilis

Latent syphilis of more than 1 year's duration (except neurosyphilis) gummas and cardiovascular syphilis should be treated with *Benzathine penicillin* G, 2.4 million units IM once a week for 3 consecutive weeks for a total dose of 7.2 mil-

---

*Treatment recommendations for syphilis are based on the CDC's treatment guideline for STDs. For detailed information, see *MMWR* 38(S-8):5–15, 1989.

TABLE 8.7. Indications for CSF Examination in Adults with Latent Syphilis Present for More Than 1 Year*

Neurologic signs or symptoms
Treatment failure
Serum nontreponemal titer ≥1:32
Other evidence of active syphilis (aortitis, gumma, iritis)
Non-penicillin therapy planned
Positive HIV antibody test

*CDC Sexually Transmitted Diseases Treatment Guidelines. MMWR 38(S-8):5–15, 1989.

lion units. Those allergic to penicillin should receive *doxycycline,** 100 mg orally 2 times a day for 4 weeks, or *tetracycline** 500 mg by mouth 4 times daily for 4 weeks. Those who cannot tolerate tetracycline should be given *erythromycin,** 500 mg by mouth 4 times daily for 30 days. (This regimen can be recommended only if compliance and serologic follow-up can be assured.)

Cerebrospinal Fluid Examination. All patients with syphilis of greater than 1 year's duration should ideally have a CSF examination; however, performance of lumbar puncture can be individualized. (For indications for CSF examination see Table 8.7.)

Treatment of Syphilis in HIV-Infected Patients

Treatment of early syphilis (of any duration) in HIV positive patients creates special problems since their damaged immune system may be unable to cope with treponemal infection in the same manner as in HIV-negative patients.

No change in therapy for early syphilis HIV-coinfected patients is recommended. However, experts disagree on this issue; some authorities advise CSF examination and/or treatment with a regimen appropriate for neurosyphilis for all patients coinfected with syphilis and HIV, regardless of the clinical stage of syphilis. In all cases careful follow-up is necessary to ensure adequacy of treatment.

Penicillin regimens should be used whenever possible for all stages of syphilis in HIV-infected patients. Patients allergic to penicillin should have their allergy confirmed and the method of treatment should be carefully chosen in consultation with an expert. A desensitization procedure should be considered also.

Follow-up of HIV-Positive Patients Treated for Syphilis. HIV-infected patients treated for syphilis should be followed clinically and with quantitative nontreponemal serologic tests (VDRL, RPR) at 1, 2, 3, 6, 9, and 12 months after treatment. Patients with early syphilis whose titers fail to decrease fourfold within 6 months should undergo CSF examination and be retreated. In such patients, CSF abnormalities could be due to HIV-related infection, neurosyphilis, or both. STD clinics and others providing STD treatment should ensure adequate follow-up.

---

*Since efficiency of these drugs in syphilis is not adequately documented, CSF examination is recommended before therapy with this regime. Tetracycline and doxycycline are contraindicated in pregnancy.

Neurosyphilis

Patients with neurosyphilis should be treated with

Aqueous crystalline penicillin G, 12–24 million units IV per day (2–4 million units every 4 hours) for 10–14 days.

or

Procaine penicillin G, 2.4 million units IM daily, plus probenecid 500 mg by mouth 4 times daily, both for 10–14 days.

Many authorities recommend the addition of benzathine penicillin, 2.4 million units IM weekly, for three doses after completion of these neurosyphilis treatment regimens.

Syphilis in Pregnancy

All pregnant women should have serologic tests for syphilis at the first prenatal visit. If possible, the test should be repeated during the third trimester, especially in those patients who might be at high risk for STDs.

Women for whom adequate treatment for syphilis in the past is documented need not be retreated unless there is clinical, serologic or epidemiologic evidence of reinfection.

For pregnant women with syphilis who are not allergic to penicillin, penicillin should be used in dosage schedules appropriate for the stage of syphilis recommended for the nonpregnant patients (see above). Tetracycline and doxycycline are contraindicated in pregnancy. Erythromycin should not be used because of the high risk of failure to cure infection in the fetus. Pregnant women with a history of penicillin allergy should first be carefully questioned and then skin tested and either treated with penicillin or referred for desensitization. Women who are treated in the second half of pregnancy are at risk for premature labor and/or fetal distress if their treatment precipitates a Jarisch-Herxheimer reaction. They should be advised to seek medical attention following treatment if they notice any change in fetal movements or have any contractions.

Follow Up. Women who have been treated for early syphilis during pregnancy should have monthly quantitative serologic tests for the remainder of the current pregnancy. Those who do not show a fourfold decrease in titer within a 3-month period as well as those who show a fourfold rise in titer should be retreated.

Congenital Syphilis*

For symptomatic and asymptomatic infants, administer 100,000–150,000 units/kg of *aqueous crystalline penicillin* G daily (administered as 50,000 units/kg IV every 8 to 12 hours) or 50,000 units/kg of *procaine penicillin* daily (administered once IM) for 10 to 14 days. If more than 1 day of therapy is missed, the entire

---

*For detailed information please see *1989 STD Treatment Guidelines* MMWR 38(S-8):5–15, 1989.

course should be restarted. Asymptomatic infants, whose mothers were treated adequately with a penicillin regimen during pregnancy, do not require treatment if follow up can be ensured; however, if the follow up cannot be ensured, many consultants choose to treat the infant with *benzathine penicillin,* 50,000 units/kg IM in a single dose.

Infants born to mothers whose treatment was unknown or inadequate or did not include penicillin, or if adequate follow up of the infant cannot be ensured, should be treated at birth. Infants with congenital syphilis should have a CSF examination before treatment to provide a baseline for follow-up as well as ophthalmologic examination.

Jarish-Herxheimer Reaction

The Jarish-Herxheimer reaction is a self-limited phenomenon following administration of the first dose of drug used in the treatment of syphilis. It was seen in the past after administration of mercury, arsenic, or bismuth, and presently it is seen after administration of penicillin or other antibiotics. The mechanisms of the Jarish-Herxheimer reaction is unknown. Several theories have been suggested, including host reaction to the products of disintegrated treponemes, reaction to endotoxins, and even an allergic mechanism, but none of them has been well documented nor fully convincing.

The reaction occurs more frequently (55 percent in seronegative primary patients to 95 percent in seropositive patients) and with greatest severity in cases of early syphilis. It is less common (about 25 percent) in late syphilis with the exception of general paresis, in which it occurs in over 75 percent of cases.[104-106] The Jarish-Herxheimer reaction has been observed in congenital syphilis, occurring more commonly in children treated during the first 6 months of life.[107] The reaction usually occurs within 4–6 hours after administration of penicillin (it may be delayed up to 12 hours if an antibiotic other than penicillin is used), reaches its peak at about 8 hours, and subsides usually within less than 24 hours. Clinical manifestations include fever of 38.5°C (101.3°F) or above, chills, malaise, headache, myalgia, and arthralgia. There may be leukocytosis with lymphopenia and exacerbation of the skin and mucosal lesion.[105]

The primary chancre may become swollen and rashes of secondary syphilis may become more prominent. There may be worsening of lymphadenopathy with slight tenderness of involved lymph nodes. The peak of the reaction is followed by peripheral vasodilation with flushing and sweating and occasionally a slight drop in blood pressure.[108] Some patients treated for neurosyphilis may experience transient worsening of their neurologic and psychiatric symptoms because of this reaction. The Jarish-Herxheimer reaction is usually of no consequence unless an unwarned patient seeks medical advice in a hospital emergency room or, frightened by its severity, ceases to attend for further treatment. The reaction appears only after the administration of the first dose of penicillin or other antibiotics and does not reappear with subsequent treatment.

In cases in whom the Jarish-Herxheimer reaction might be dangerous, e.g., in general paresis, syphilitic aortitis, or other serious conditions, it is advisable to prevent it or diminish its severity. This may be achieved by administration of prednisone, 30–40 mg daily in divided doses given 2–3 days prior to administration of penicillin. Administration of prednisone should be discontinued gradually 2–4 days after the start of antisyphilitic therapy. Steroids appear to reduce the febrile component of the reaction, but its effect on local inflammatory response is questionable.[109,110]

Follow Up

All patients treated for early syphilis and congenital syphilis should be encouraged to return for follow up quantitative tests at least at 3, 6, and 12 months after treatment. Patients with syphilis of more than 1 year's duration should also have serologic tests 24 months after treatment or longer if necessary. Patients with neurosyphilis should have periodic serologic testing and clinical evaluation at 6-month intervals, for at least 3 years. If an initial CSF pleocytosis was present, CSF examination should be repeated every 6 months until the cell count returns to normal level. If it has not decreased within 6 months nor returned to normal value by 2 years retreatment should be considered.

HIV-infected patients should have follow-up serologic testing at 1, 2, 3, 6, 9, and 12 months.

In patients treated for early syphilis the quantitative nontreponemal test titers usually decline to nonreactive or low titer reactive within a year following treatment with penicillin. Patients treated for syphilis of more than 1 year's duration should become seronegative or low titer reactive in up to 2 years. In general, the serologic test results decline more slowly in patients treated for syphilis of longer duration. Retreatment should be considered when: 1) clinical signs or symptoms of syphilis persist or recur; 2) there is a four-fold increase in the titer of a nontreponemal test; or 3) an initially high-titer nontreponemal test fails to decrease four-fold within a year.

All syphilis patients should be encouraged to be counseled and tested for HIV.

MANAGEMENT OF SEX PARTNERS

All patients who have been exposed to infectious syphilis within the preceding 3 months should be treated as for early syphilis.

REFERENCES

1. Cumberland MC, Turner TB: The rate of multiplication of *Treponema pallidum* in normal and immune rabbits. *Am J Syph Gon Vener Dis* 33:201–221, 1949.
2. *Report of a WHO Scientific Group: Treponemal infections.* Geneva, WHO, 1982, WHO Tech Rep Series No. 674.
3. Thirumoorthy T, Lee CT, Lim KB: Epidemiology of infectious syphilis in Singapore. *Genitourin Med* 62:75–77, 1986.
4. Morton RS: Control of sexually transmitted diseases today and tomorrow. *Genitourin Med* 63:202–209, 1987.

5. Hart G, Adler M, Stapinski A, et al: STD control in industrialized countries, in Holmes K, Mardh P-A, Sparling PF, Wiesner PJ (eds), *Sexually Transmitted Diseases* (2nd ed). New York, McGraw-Hill. In press.

6. Continuing increase in infectious syphilis in the USA. *MMWR* 37:35–38, 1988.

7. Progress toward achieving the national 1990 objectives for sexually transmitted diseases. *MMWR* 36:173–176, 1987.

8. Harter CA, Benirschke K: Fetal syphilis in the first trimester. *Am J Obstet Gynecol* 124:705–711, 1976.

9. Chapel TA: The variability of syphilitic chancres. *Sex Transm Dis* 5:68–70, 1978.

10. Chapel TA, Prasad P, Chapel J, et al: Extragenital syphilitic chancres. *J Am Acad Dermatol* 13:582–584, 1985.

11. Starzycki Z: Primary syphilis of the fingers. *Br J Vener Dis* 59:169–171, 1983.

12. Chapel TA: Primary and secondary syphilis. *Cutis* 33:47–53, 1984.

13. Donofrio P: Unusual location of syphilitic chancre: Case report. *Genitourin Med* 62:59–60, 1986.

14. Drusin LM: Syphilis and other sexually transmitted diseases. *Cutis* 27:286–306, 1981.

15. Lejman K, Starzycki Z: Syphilitic balanitis of Follmann developing after the appearance of the primary chancre. *Br J Vener Dis* 51:138–140, 1975.

16. Technique for Direct Immunofluorescent Identification of *Treponema pallidum* in Body Fluids and Tissue Secretions. Venereal Disease Research Laboratory, Centers for Disease Control, Atlanta 1971.

17. Jaffe HW: Management of reactive serology, in Holmes K, Mardh P-A, Sparling PF, Weisner PJ (eds), *Sexually Transmitted Diseases.* New York, McGraw-Hill, 1984, p. 313.

18. Fowler W: The erythrocyte sedimentation rate in syphilis. *Br J Vener Dis* 52:309–312, 1976.

19. Lee RV, Thornton GF, Conn HO: Liver disease associated with secondary syphilis. *N Engl J Med* 284:1423–1425, 1971.

20. Feher J, Somogyi T, Timmer M, et al: Early syphilitic hepatitis. *Lancet* 2:896–899, 1975.

21. Campisi D, Whitcomb C: Liver disease in early syphilis. *Arch Intern Med* 139:365–366, 1979.

22. Gamble CN, Reardan JB: Immunopathogenesis of syphilis glomerulonephritis: Elution of antitreponemal antibody from glomerular immune-complex deposits. *N Engl J Med* 292:449–454, 1975.

23. Bhorade MS, Carag HB, Lee HJ, et al: Nephropathy of secondary syphilis: A clinical and pathological spectrum. *JAMA* 216:1159–1166, 1971.

24. Lowhagen G-B, Andersson M, Blomstrand C, et al: Central nervous system involvement in early syphilis. Part I Intrathecal immunoglobulin production. *Acta Derm Venereol* (Stockh) 63:409–417, 1983.

25. Wetherill JH, Webb HE, Catterall RD: Syphilis presenting as an acute neurological illness. *Br Med J* 1:1157–1158, 1965.

26. Chapel TA: The signs and symptoms of secondary syphilis. *Sex Transm Dis* 7:161–164, 1980.

27. Hira SK, Patel JS, Bhat SG, et al: Clinical manifestations of secondary syphilis. *Int J Dermatol* 26:103–107, 1987.

28. Noppakun N, Dinehart SM, Solomon AR: Pustular secondary syphilis. *Int J Dermatol* 26:112–114, 1987.

29. Hooshmand H, Escobar MR, Kopf SW: Neurosyphilis: A Study of 241 patients. *JAMA* 219:726–729, 1972.

30. Joyce-Clarke N, Moltena ACB: Modified neurosyphilis in the Cape Peninsula. *S Afr Med J* 53:10–14, 1978.

31. Rosenhall U, Lowhagen G-B, Roupe G: Oculomotor dysfunction in patients with syphilis. *Genitourin Med* 63:83–86, 1987.

32. Short DH, Knox JM, Glicksman J: Neurosyphilis: The search for adequate treatment. *Arch Dermatol* 93:87–91, 1966.

33. Wilner E, Brody JA: Prognosis of general paresis after treatment. *Lancet* 2:1370–1371, 1968.

34. Eijk van RVW, Wolters ECh, Tutuarima JA, et al: Effect of early and late syphilis on central nervous system: Cerebrospinal fluid changes and neurological deficit. *Genitourin Med* 63:77–82, 1987.

35. Dawson-Butterworth K, Heathcote PRM: Review of hospitalized cases of general paralysis of the insane. *Br J Vener Dis* 46:295–302, 1970.

36. Heathfield KWG: The decline of neurolues. *Practitioner* 217:753–762, 1976.

37. Aho K, Sievers K, Salo OP: Late complications of syphilis: A comparative epidemiological and serological study of cardiovascular syphilis and various forms of neurosyphilis. *Acta Derm Venereol* (Stockh) 49:336–342, 1969.

38. Towpik J, Nowakowska E: Changing patterns of late syphilis. *Br J Vener Dis* 46:132–134, 1970.

39. Hahn RD: Tabes dorsalis with special reference to primary optic atrophy. *Br J Vener Dis* 33:139–148, 1957.

40. King A, Nicol C, Rodin P: Neurosyphilis, in *Venereal Disease,* London, Bailliere Tindol, 1980, Chap. 5, p. 81.

41. Centers for Disease Control: *Manual of Tests for Syphilis.* 1969, Washington, DC, U.S. Dept of Health, Education, and Welfare, USDHEW publication (CDC) 78-8347.

42. March RW, Stiles GE: The reagin screen test: A new reagin card test for syphilis. *Sex Transm Dis* 7:66–70, 1980.

43. Pettit DE, Larsen SA, Pope V, et al: Unheated serum reagin test as a quantitative test for syphilis. *J Clin Microbiol* 15:238–242, 1982.

44. McGrew BE, DuCros MJF, Stout GW, et al: Automation of a flocculation test for syphilis. *Am J Clin Pathol* 50:52, 1968.

45. Cohen P, Stout G, Ende N: Serologic reactivity in consecutive patients admitted to a general hospital. *Arch Intern Med* 124:364–367, 1969.

46. Wentworth BB, Thompson MA, Peter CR, et al: Comparison of a hemagglutination treponemal test for syphilis (HATTS) with other serologic methods for the diagnosis of syphilis. *Sex Transm Dis* 5:103–111, 1978.

47. Catterall RD: Presidential address to the MSSVD: Systematic diseases and the biologic false positive reaction. *Br J Vener Dis* 48:1–12, 1972.

48. Kaufman RE, Weiss S, Moore JD, et al: Biological false positive serological tests for syphilis among drug addicts. *Br J Vener Dis* 50:350, 1974.

49. Carr RD, Becker SW, Carpenter CM: The biological false-positive phenomenon in elderly men. *Arch Dermatol* 93:393–395, 1965.

50. Goldman JN, Lantz MA: FTA-ABS and VDRL slide test reactivity in a population of nuns. *JAMA* 217:53–55, 1971.

51. Kraus SJ, Haserick JR, Lantz MA: Atypical FTA-ABS test fluorescence in lupus erythematosus patients. *JAMA* 211:2140–2141, 1970.

52. Shore RN, Faricelli JA: Borderline and reactive FTA-ABS results in lupus erythematosus. *Arch Dermatol* 113:37–41, 1977.

53. Monson RAM: Biologic false-positive FTA-ABS test in drug induced lupus erythematosus. *JAMA* 224:1028–1030, 1973.

54. Wright JT, Cremer AW, Ridgway GL: False positive FTA-ABS results in patients with genital herpes. *Br J Vener Dis* 51:329–330, 1975.

55. Dans PE, Judson FN, Larsen SA, et al: The FTA-ABS test: A diagnostic help or hindrance. *South Med J* 70:312–315, 1977.

56. Peter CR, Thompson MA, Wilson DL: False-positive reactions in the rapid plasma reagin-card, fluorescent treponemal antibody-absorbed and hemagglutination treponemal syphilis serologic tests. *J Clin Microbiol* 9:369–372, 1979.

57. Johnston NA: Neonatal congenital syphilis. Diagnosis by the absorbed fluorescent treponemal antibody (IgM) test. *Br J Vener Dis* 48:464–469, 1972.

58. Cox PM, Logan LC, Norins LC: Automated quantitative microhemagglutination assay for *Treponema pallidum* antibodies. *Appl Microbiol* 18:485–489, 1969.

59. Lesinski J, Krach J, Kadziewicz E: Specificity, sensitivity and diagnostic value of the TPHA test. *Br J Vener Dis* 50:334–340, 1974.

60. Larsen SA, Hambie EA, Pettit DE, et al: Specificity, sensitivity and reproducibility among the fluorescent treponemal-absorption test, the microhemagglutination assay for *Treponema pallidum* antibodies and the hemagglutination treponemal test for syphilis. *J Clin Microbiol* 14:441–445, 1981.

61. Garner MF, Backhouse JL, Daskalopoulos G: The *Treponema pallidum* haemagglutination (TPHA) test in biological false positive and leprosy sera. *J Clin Pathol* 26:258–260, 1973.

62. Jaffe HW, Larsen SA, Jones OG, et al: Hemagglutination test for syphilis antibody. *Am J Clin Pathol* 70:230–233, 1978.

63. Sato T, Kubo E, Yokota M, et al: *Treponema pallidum* specific IgM haemagglutination test for serodiagnosis of syphilis. *Br J Vener Dis* 60:364–370, 1984.

64. Nelson RA, Mayer MM: Immobolization of *Treponema pallidum* in vitro by antibody produced in syphilitic infection. *J Exp Med* 89:369–393, 1949.

65. Moyer NP, Hudson JD, Hausler WJ: Evaluation of the Bio-EnzaBead test for syphilis. *J Clin Microbiol* 25:619–623, 1987.

66. Lindenschmidt E-G, Muler F: A treponema-specific soluble antigen for an IgM and IgG-TP-ABS-ELISA and its application for the serodiagnosis of syphilis. *WHO-VDT-Res* 81:369, 1981.

67. Schmidt BL: Solid-phase hemadsorption: A method for rapid detection of *Treponema pallidum*-specific IgM. *Sex Transm Dis* 7:53–58, 1980.

68. Moskophidis M, Muller F: Molecular analysis of immunoglobulins M and G immune response to protein antigens of *Treponema pallidum* in human syphilis. *Infect Immun* 43:127–132, 1984.

69. Baker-Zander SA, Roddy RE, Handsfield HH, et al: IgG and IgM antibody reactivity to antigens of *Treponema pallidum* after treatment of syphilis. *Sex Transm Dis* 13:214–220, 1986.

70. Van Eijk RVW, Van Embden JDA: Molecular characterization of *Treponema pallidum* antigens involved in the human immune response to syphilis (meeting report). *Sex Transm Dis* 10:166, 1983.

71. Hart G: Syphilis tests in diagnostic and therapeutic decision making. *Ann Intern Med* 104:368–376, 1986.

72. Baker-Zander SA, Hook EW III, Bonin P, et al: Antigens to *Treponema pallidum* recognized by IgG and IgM antibodies during syphilis in humans. *J Infect Dis* 151:264–272, 1985.

73. Shannon R, Booth SD: The pattern of immunological responses at various stages of syphilis. *Br J Vener Dis* 53:281–286, 1977.

74. Merlin S, Andre J, Alacoque B, et al: Importance of specific IgM antibodies in 116 patients with various stages of syphilis. *Genitourin Med* 61:82–87, 1985.

75. Harvey AM, Shulman LE: Connective tissue diseases and the chronic biologic false-positive test for syphilis (BFP reaction). *Med Clin North Am* 50:1271–1279, 1966.

76. Hoagland RJ: False-positive serology in mononucleosis. *JAMA* 185:783–785, 1963.

77. Tuffanelli DL: Narcotic addiction with false-positive reaction for syphilis: Immunologic studies. *Acta Derm Venereol* (Stockh) 48:542–546, 1968.

78. Murray KA: Syphilis in patients with Hansen's disease. *Int J Lepr Mycobact Dis* 50:152–158, 1982.

79. Tuffanelli DL: Ageing and false positive reactions for syphilis. *Br J Vener Dis* 42:40–41, 1966.

80. Cabrera HA, Carlson J: Biologic false-positive reaction and infectious mononucleosis. *Am J Clin Pathol* 50:643–645, 1968.

81. British Cooperative Clinical Group: Acute and chronic biological false positive reactors to serological tests for syphilis, ABO blood groups and other investigations. *Br J Vener Dis* 50:428–434, 1974.

82. Cherubin CE, Millian SJ: Serologic investigations in narcotic addicts. I. Syphilis, lymphogranuloma venereum, herpes simplex, Q fever. *Ann Intern Med* 69:739–742, 1968.

83. Salo OP, Aho K, Nieminen E, et al: False-positive serological tests for syphilis in pregnancy. *Acta Derm Venereol* (Stockh) 49:332–335, 1969.

84. Manikowska-Lesinska W, Linda B, Zajac W: Specificity of the FTA-ABS and TPHA tests during pregnancy. *Br J Vener Dis* 54:295–298, 1978.

85. Kraus SJ, Haserick JR, Lantz MA: Fluorescent treponemal antibody-absorption test reactions in lupus erythematosus: Atypical beading pattern and probable false-positive reactions. *N Engl J Med* 282:1287–1290, 1970.

86. Hunter EF, Russell H, Farshy CE, et al: Evaluation of sera from patients with Lyme disease in the fluorescent treponemal antibody-absorption test for syphilis. *Sex Transm Dis* 13:232–236, 1986.

87. Russell H, Sampson JS, Schmidt GP, et al: Enzyme-linked immunosorbent assay and indirect immunofluorescence assay for Lyme disease. *J Infect Dis* 149:465–470, 1984.

88. Burns RE: Spontaneous reversion of FTA-ABS test reactions. *JAMA* 234:617–618, 1975.

89. Larsen SA, Farshy CE, Pender BJ, et al: Staining intensities in the fluorescent treponemal antibody-absorption (FTA-ABS) test: Association with the diagnosis of syphilis. *Sex Transm Dis* 13:221–227, 1986.

90. Hicks ChB, Genson PM, Lupton GP, et al: Seronegative secondary syphilis in a patient infected with the human immunodeficiency virus (HIV) with Kaposi sarcoma: A diagnostic dilemma. *Ann Intern Med* 107:492–495, 1987.

91. Congenital syphilis—United States, 1983–1985. *MMWR* 35:625–628, 1986.

92. Centers for Disease Control: *Sexually Transmitted Disease Statistics, 1987,* U.S. Dept. of Health and Human Services, Public Health Service. Atlanta, 1988, No. 136.

93. Hira SK, Ratnam AV, Sehgal D, et al: Congenital syphilis in Lusaka. I. Incidence in a general nursery ward. *East Afr Med J* 59:241–246, 1982.

94. Ratnam AV, Din SN, Hira SK, et al: Syphilis in pregnant women in Zambia. *Br J Vener Dis* 58:355–358, 1982.

95. Hira SK, Bhat GJ, Patel JB, et al: Early congenital syphilis: Clinico-radiologic features in 202 patients. *Sex Transm Dis* 12:177–183, 1985.

96. Kaufman RE, Jones OG, Blount JH, et al: Questionnaire survey of reported early congenital syphilis. *Sex Transm Dis* 4:135–139, 1977.

97. Contreras F, Pereda J: Congenital syphilis of the eye with lens involvement. *Arch Ophthalmol* 96:1052–1053, 1978.

98. Whitaker JA, Sartain P, Shaheedy M: Hematological aspects of congenital syphilis. *J Pediatr* 66:629–636, 1965.

99. Frieman I, Super M: Thrombocytopenia and congenital syphilis in South African Bantu infants. *Arch Dis Child* 41:87, 1966.

100. Fiumara NJ, Lessell S: Manifestations of late congenital syphilis. *Arch Dermatol* 102:78–83, 1970.

101. Fiumara NJ, Lessell S: The stigmata of late congenital syphilis: An analysis of 100 patients. *Sex Transm Dis* 10:126–129, 1983.

102. Guidelines for the prevention and control of congenital syphilis. *MMWR* 37:1–13, 1988.

103. Kaufman RE, Olansky DC, Weisner PJ: The FTA-ABS (IgM) test for neonatal congenital syphilis: A critical review. *J Am Vener Dis Assoc* 1:79–84, 1974.

104. Putkonen T, Salo OP, Mustakallio KK: Febrile Herxheimer reaction in different phases of primary and secondary syphilis. *Br J Vener Dis* 42:181–184, 1966.

105. Aronson IK, Soltani K: The enigma of the pathogenesis of the Jarish-Herxheimer reaction. *Br J Vener Dis* 52:313–315, 1976.

106. Heyman A, Sheldon WH, Evans LD: Pathogenesis of the Jarish-Herxheimer rection: A review of clinical and experimental observatons. *Br J Vener Dis* 28:50–60, 1952.

107. Putkonen T: The febrile Herxheimer reaction to penicillin in congenital syphilis. *Dermatologica* 101:313–317, 1950.

108. Bryceson ADM: Clinical pathology of the Jarish-Herxheimer reaction. *J Infect Dis* 133:696–704, 1976.

109. Gudjonsson H, Skog E: The effect of prednisolone on the Jarish-Herxheimer reaction. *Acta Derm Venereol* (Stockh) 48:15–18, 1968.

110. Kleinhans D, Knoth W: High dose methylprednisolone as prophylaxis against Jarish-Herxheimer reaction in syphilis. *Z Hautkrh* 50:601–615, 1975.

9

CHANCROID

Chancroid is an ulcerative disease of the genitals caused by *Haemophilus ducreyi,* a small gram-negative bacillus. Characteristic inguinal lymphadenopathy or buboes often accompanies the genital lesions, but systemic spread does not otherwise occur. Synonyms for chancroid are soft chancre, soft sore, ulcus molle, and chancre mou.

EPIDEMIOLOGY

Chancroid infection is almost invariably transmitted by sexual contact,[1] but the clinical disease is encountered more often in males than in females, who usually constitute a small fraction of reported cases. (Women may be inapparent carriers or have asymptomatic infection.[2,3]) The disease has been reported primarily from African and Asian countries, but within the last 10–20 years small outbreaks of chancroid were observed in Europe, Greenland, and Canada,[4–7] and recently in the United States.[8–11] Prostitutes have been frequently incriminated as an important reservoir of infection, and in almost all outbreaks a high proportion of patients reported them as source contacts.[7,9,12,13]

Since the last few years the number of reported cases of chancroid in the United States has been increasing, reaching in 1987, 4,998 cases. Several outbreaks of chancroid have recently occurred in New York City and in the Gulf States of the United States, including New Orleans, Louisiana.[14]

CLINICAL FEATURES

The incubation period is usually between 3 and 7 days (range 1–35 days). No prodromal symptoms have been observed. The typical lesion appears at the site of inoculation as a small, tender red papule or pustule which rapidly (1–2 days) breaks down to form an ulcer. Individual ulcers are sharply demarcated and have ragged undermined edges and sloughing bases frequently covered with a grayish

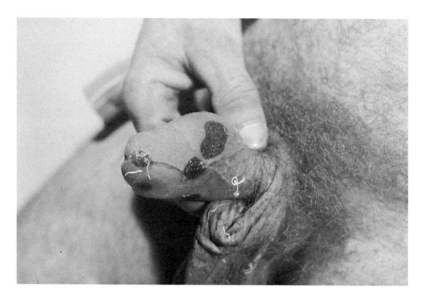

Figure 9.1. Multiple chancroidal ulcers on the skin of the penis.

necrotic exudate. Upon removal of this exudate, there appears an uneven, purulent, granulation tissue. The size of the individual ulcer ranges from a few millimeters to 2 cm. It is soft and nonindurated to the touch and will change its shape when squeezed.

Multiple ulcers are frequent (Figure 9.1), and several ulcers may either remain separate or, more commonly, merge to form rosette, serpiginous, or giant lesions. The lesions are usually quite painful but may be painless as well. Painful lesions have been observed more often in men, whereas chancroid ulcers in females are more often painless, causing that many females with chancroid to be unaware of their disease.

There is a wide variety of clinical appearance of chancroid, and several clinical forms have been described (Table 9.1 and Figures 9.2–9.6).[2,3]

The genital sites commonly affected are those subjected to sexual trauma, such

TABLE 9.1. Clinical Types of Ulceration Caused by *H. ducreyi*

1. Single, sharply demarcated ulcer with undermined ragged edges.
2. Multiple shallow ulcers resembling genital herpes.
3. "Transient chancroid": small ulcer which resolves within a few days and is followed by regional lymphadenopathy.
4. "Giant chancroid": extensive ulceration produced by peripheral extension of a single lesion or merging of several small ulcers.
5. "Phagedenic ulcer" (ulcus molle gangrenosum): an ulcer that rapidly becomes large and destructive with widespread necrosis of tissue (superinfection with anaerobes).
6. Ulcus molle serpiginosum: rapidly spreading, superficial ulcers which are usually long and narrow.
7. "Dwarf chancroid": small shallow ulcers resembling folliculitis or pyogenic infection.

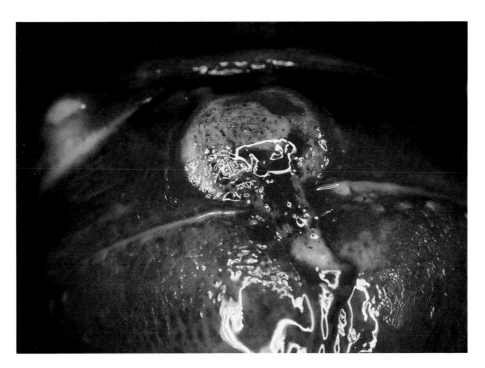

Figure 9.2. Painful ulcer on the frenulum extending to the glans of penis. (Courtesy of Dr. A.R. Ronald.)

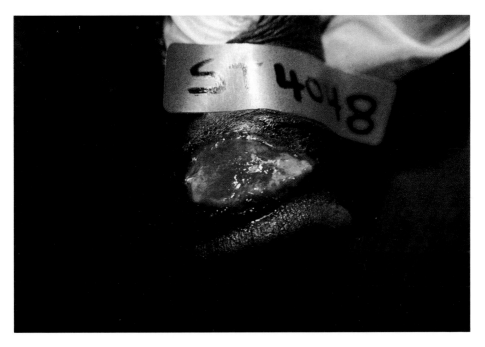

Figure 9.3. A large ulcer on the corona sulcus with ruptured bubo in the groin. (Courtesy of Dr. A.R. Ronald.)

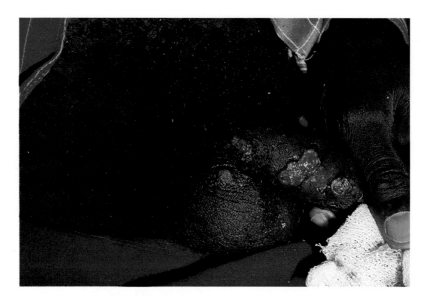

Figure 9.4. Multiple painful ulcerations on the skin of the penis and scrotum.

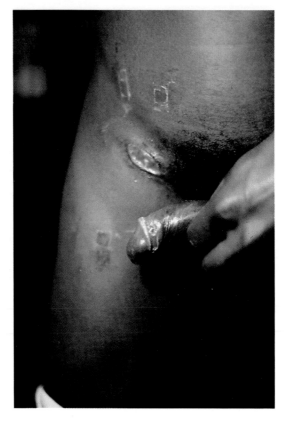

Figure 9.5. Chancroidal ulcers in the coronal sulcus and in the groin (presumably due to autoinoculation).

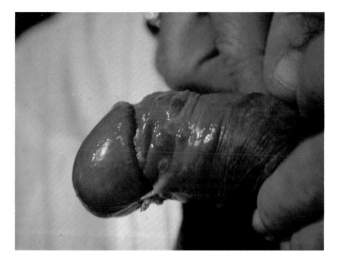

Figure 9.6. Multiple shallow ulcers with a tendency to coalesce.

as the prepuce, frenulum, coronal sulcus, and glans and shaft of the penis and the fourchette, labia, vestibule, and clitoris. Although the majority of lesions in females are at the entrance to the vagina (Figure 9.7), they also may be present on the cervix and perineum.

Extragenital lesions are rare, and they have been described within the mouth and on the fingers, the breasts, and the thighs.[3,15] In rare cases, *H. ducreyi* may cause

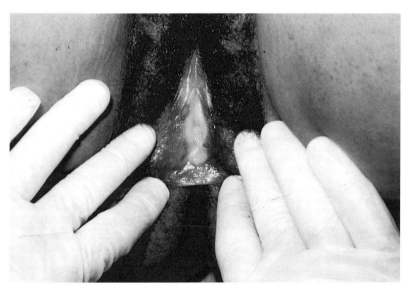

Figure 9.7. Chanroid in woman: single, painful, irregular ulcer at the entrance to the vagina.

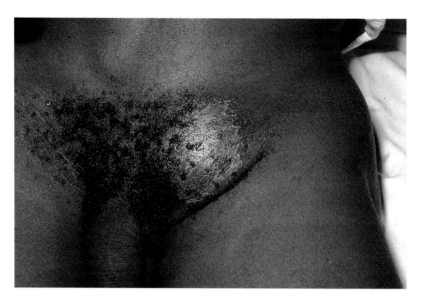

Figure 9.8.   Unilateral, painful lymphadenopathy accompanying lesion on the penis. Suppuration is common.

urethritis: it was isolated from the urethra of men who presented with genital ulceration and simultaneous symptoms and signs of urethritis.[16]

If untreated, chancroid may be complicated by adenitis and bubo formation. Lymphadenitis appears approximately 1 week after the ulcer and is quite characteristic. The typical chancroid bubo is usually unilateral, unilocular, spherical, and painful. It is often associated with redness of the overlying skin (Figure 9.8). Suppuration commonly occurs, and the bubo becomes fluctuant with spontaneous rupture (Figure 9.9). The pus oozing from the ruptured bubo is usually thick and viscous. A large ulcer may form in the groin with subsequent destruction of skin and soft tissue. Both inguinal adenitis and bubo occur in about 50% of patients but are less common in females.

Constitutional symptoms may accompany the genital lesions but are usually mild and non-specific. Systemic infection or spread to distant sites have not been reported as yet.

Patients with chancroid do not develop immunity. New lesions may develop by autoinoculation or reinfection shortly after cure.

COMPLICATIONS

If one or more ulcers appears on the margin of the prepuce they may result in phimosis or paraphimosis. Destructive lesions on the glans of the penis may cause urethral fistulas, and a phagodenic type of ulceration may affect and destroy large areas around the genitals. Rectovaginal fistulas have also been reported. Secondary infection with fusospirochetes or other bacilli may lead to rapid tissue destruction and permanent scars. Recalcitrant serpiginous ulceration may persist for several months without healing.[2,3]

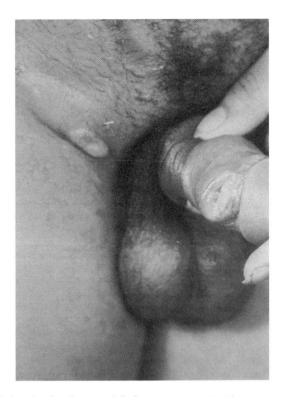

Figure 9.9. Penile chancroidal ulcer accompanied by ruptured bubo.

DIAGNOSIS

Although diagnosis of chancroid is often made on the clinical presentation (short incubation period and highly erosive, soft, painful, often multiple lesions associated with painful inguinal adenopathy), an attempt should be made to demonstrate *H. ducreyi* by cultures and/or smears.

It is very important to exclude other STDs associated with similar findings such as primary syphilis, genital herpes, lymphogranuloma venereum and Donovanosis. Present data show that the clinical diagnosis of genital ulcers is often inaccurate and unreliable and that definite diagnosis requires laboratory confirmation wherever possible.[17,18]

Gram stains of exudate from skin lesions are of little value because of massive contamination with other gram-negative rods and the low percentage of cases in whom *H. ducreyi* can definitely be identified.[19-21] *H. ducreyi* is a facultative anaerobe and requires hemin (X factor) for growth. Successful demonstrations of *H. ducreyi* have been obtained using enriched chocolate agar medium made selective by the addition of 3 μg/ml vancomycin hydrochloride.[22] Scrapings from cleaned ulcers or bubo aspirates should be inoculated onto culture plates and incubated at 33°C in a "candle jar" in a water-saturated environment. Colonies appear after 48–72 hours, and *H. ducreyi* is identified in a gram-stained smear. *Haemophilus ducreyi* is very susceptible to changes in temperature, CO_2 concentration, and humidity, and even small deviations from these requirements may cause difficulties in isolating the microorganism.

Presumptive identification can be made by demonstrating short, gram-negative bacilli occasionally arranged in chains or long parallel rows and performing porphyrin test. Confirmation can be made by demonstration of hemin (X factor) requirement for growth and the absence of requirement for NAD (V-factor) on enriched media. Isolation of *H. ducreyi* is not easy, and the isolation rate can be improved by the use of more than one culture medium. In recent studies the positive yield was increased from 81 to 93 percent by simultaneous use of gonococcal agar supplemented with bovine hemoglobin (GcHbS) and Mueller-Hinton agar (MHHb).[23,24]

The histopathology of chancroid is not very specific and should be reserved for clinically ambiguous cases or when malignancy is suspected.

Several non-culture methods have also been developed including monoclonal antibodies specific for *H. ducreyi*[25,26] and enzyme-linked immunosorbent assay (ELISA) which detects serum IgG antibodies to *H. ducreyi*.[27]

The use of a DNA probe in polymerase chain reactions is currently under investigation[28] and as soon as the specificity of this test is improved it may become a valuable method of detection of *H. ducreyi* in patients with chancroid.

DIFFERENTIAL DIAGNOSIS

Since in many clinics the diagnosis is still made based on clinical appearance, the differentiation should be made very carefully. However, one must bear in mind that as many as 50 percent of genital ulcers may be incorrectly diagnosed if laboratory confirmation is not done.

- *Primary syphilis:* longer incubation period (2–3 weeks); hard, indurated, painless ulcer which does not change its shape upon squeezing; positive dark-field examination; FTA-ABS or RPR test may be positive; painless adenopathy without bubo formation: mixed chancre (ulcus mixtum) may be seen when both syphilis and chancroid are present.
- *Genital herpes* (Condition most often mistakenly diagnosed as chancroid): history of recurrences, positive Tzanck smear, positive viral culture, positive direct immunofluorescence or other tests.
- *Lymphogranuloma venereum:* primary lesion is transient and often missed, positive test for *Chlamydia trachomatis.*
- *Donovanosis:* huge boggy ulcer with chronic course, Donovan bodies found in smear or in histopathology.
- *Bacterial infection:* ruled out with bacterial culture.
- *Trauma:* history, negative culture.
- *Squamous cell carcinoma:* history of long-lasting lesion, older age of patients, positive biopsy.

TREATMENT

The susceptibility of *H. ducreyi* to antimicrobial agents differs among geographic regions, and this should be taken into account when selecting therapy.[29-32]

Systemic Antimicrobials

In the United States the following regimens are recommended:

Erythromycin, 500 mg by mouth 4 times a day for 7–10 days
Or
Ceftriaxone, 250 mg IM in a single dose[32,33]
Alternative Regimen
Trimethoprim-sulfamethoxazole, one double-strength (160/800 mg) dose by mouth twice daily for at least 7 days
Or
*Ciprofloxacin,** 500 mg orally 2 times a day for 3 days* (not evaluated in the United States)
Or
Amoxicillin, 500 mg, plus *clavulanic acid,* 125 mg orally 3 times daily for 7–10 days[34] (not evaluated in the United States)

Comment: If the patient is treated with antibiotics capable of masking incubating syphilis, a serologic blood test should be performed prior to the initiation of therapy and for a minimum period of 3 months after treatment. Should this be impossible or impractical (e.g., poor patient cooperation), it is recommended that a full antisyphilitic dose be given, namely *erythromycin,* 500 mg 4 times a day for 15 days.

Local Measures

Local therapy is a helpful adjunct to the systemic antimicrobials. Patients should be treated with topical cleansing and soaks of the ulcer and with measures to reduce edema if it occurs. Retraction of the foreskin is not recommended in the presence of preputial edema, and if circumcision is required, it should be postponed until after effective antibiotic therapy.

Most patients with small buboes respond to antimicrobial therapy, but some authors believe that the frequent aspiration (not incision) of fluctuant nodes may prevent spontaneous drainage, with subsequent scarring and deformity.

---

*Not recommended in pregnant women and children less than 16 years of age.

FOLLOW-UP

Effectively treated ulcers are almost invariably clinically improved within 5–7 days. If they are not, an alternative regimen should be considered along with antimicrobial susceptibility testing on isolated microorganisms. Clinical resolution of lymph nodes is slower and may require needle aspiration (through healthy, adjacent skin), even during successful therapy, to prevent spontaneous rupture or fistula formation.[35]

MANAGEMENT OF SEX PARTNERS

All sexual contacts of patients with chancroid should be treated with the regimen effective for the index patient.[36,37] Individuals with chancroid and their sex partners have a high risk of acquiring other sexually transmitted diseases and thus should be tested and treated for all diagnosed STDs prevalent in the community.

CONTROL AND PREVENTION

Since prostitution was recognized as an important epidemiologic factor in the outbreaks of chancroid in the United States and Canada as well as in Africa, widespread treatment of prostitutes, those with genital ulcers and those named as sex partners of men with chancroid, is strongly advisable. Since chancroid, along with other diseases causing genital ulcerations, may increase the risk of acquisition of the AIDS virus,[38-40] these measures should not be considered too harsh. Similar to other sexually transmitted diseases, the use of condoms significantly reduces the chance of acquisition of chancroid.

REFERENCES

1. Handsfield HH, Totten PA, Fennel CL, et al.: Molecular epidemiology of *Haemophilus ducreyi* infections. *Ann Intern Med* 95:315–318, 1981.
2. Felman MY, Nikitas JA: Chancroid. *Cutis* 26:464–478, 1980.
3. Hart G: *Chancroid, Donovanosis, Lymphogranuloma Venereum.* U.S. Dept. of Health, Education and Welfare, 1975, DHEW Publication (CDC) No. 75–8302, p. 7.
4. Nayyar KC, Stolz E, Michel MF: Rising incidence of chancroid in Rotterdam: Epidemiological, clinical, diagnostic and therapeutic aspects. *Br J Vener Dis* 55:439–441, 1979.
5. Hafiz S, Kinghorn GR, McEntegart MG: Chancroid in Sheffield: A report of twenty-two cases diagnosed by isolating *Haemophilus ducreyi* in a modified medium. *Br J Vener Dis* 57:381–386, 1981.
6. Lykke-Olesen L, Larsen L, Pedersen TG, et al.: Epidemic of chancroid in Greenland, 1977–78. *Lancet* 1:654–655, 1979.
7. Hammond GW, Slutchuk M, Scatliff J, et al.: Epidemiologic, clinical, laboratory and therapeutic features of an urban outbreak of chancroid in North America. *Rev Infect Dis* 2:867–879, 1980.

8. Chancroid—California. *MMWR* 31:173–175, 1982.

9. Blackmore CA, Limpakarnjanarat K, Rigau-Perez JG, et al.: An outbreak of chancroid in Orange County, California: Descriptive epidemiology and disease-control measures. *J Infect Dis* 151:840–844, 1985.

10. Schmidt GP, Sanders LL, Jr., Blount JH, et al: Chancroid in the United States, reestablishment of an old disease. *JAMA* 258:3265–3268, 1987.

11. Becker TM, DeWitt W, vanDusen G, et al.: *Haemophilus ducreyi* infection in South Florida: A rare disease on the rise. *South Med J* 80:182–184, 1987.

12. Plummer FA, D'Costa LJ, Nsanze H, et al.: Epidemiology of chancroid and *Haemophilus ducreyi* in Nairobi, Kenya. *Lancet* 2:1293–1295, 1983.

13. Plummer FA, D'Costa LJ, Nsanze H, et al: Clinical and microbiologic studies of genital ulcers in Kenyan women. *Sex Transm Dis* 12:193–197, 1985.

14. David H. Martin—unpublished data.

15. Brandt R, Sanderson ES, Hicks DV: Extragenital chancroid: A case report. *Vener Dis Info* 22:89, 1941.

16. Kinimoto DY, Plummer FA, Namaara W, et al.: Urethral infection with *Haemophilus ducreyi* in men. *Sex Transm Dis* 15:37–39, 1988.

17. Chapel TA, Brown WJ, Jeffries CH, et al.: How reliable is the morphological diagnosis of penile ulcerations? *Sex Transm Dis* 4:150–152, 1977.

18. Fast MV, D'Costa LJ, Nsanze H, et al.: The clinical diagnosis of genital ulcer disease in men in the tropics. *Sex Transm Dis* 11:72–76, 1984.

19. Sehgal VN, Prasad ALS: Chancroid or chancroidal ulcers. *Dermatologica* 170:136–141, 1985.

20. Borchardt KA, Hoke AW: Simplified laboratory technique for diagnosis of chancroid. *Arch Dermatol* 102:188–192, 1970.

21. Chapel T, Brown WJ, Jeffries CH, et al: The microbiological flora of penile ulcerations. *J Infect Dis* 137:50–56, 1978.

22. Hammond GW, Lian CJ, Wilt JC, et al.: Determination of the hemin requirement of *Haemophilus ducreyi:* An evaluation of the porphyrin test and media used in the satellite growth test. *J Clin Microbiol* 7:243–246, 1978.

23. Nsanze H, Plummer FA, Maggwa ABN, et al.: Comparison of media for the primary isolation of *Haemophilus ducreyi*. *Sex Transm Dis* 11:6–9, 1984.

24. Dylewski J, Nsanze H, Maitha G, et al.: Laboratory diagnosis of *Haemophilus ducreyi:* Sensitivity of culture media. *Diag Microbiol Infect Dis* 4:241–245, 1986.

25. Hansen EJ, Loftus TA: Monoclonal antibodies reactive with all strains of *Haemophilus ducreyi*. *Infect Immun* 44:196–198, 1984.

26. Schalla WO, Sanders LL, Schmid GP, et al: Use of dot-immunobinding and immunofluorescence assay to investigate clinically suspected cases of chancroid. *J Infect Dis* 153:879–887, 1986.

27. Museyi K, van Dyck E, Vervoort T, et al: Use of an enzyme immunoassay to detect serum IgG antibodies to *Haemophilus ducreyi*. *J Infect Dis* 157:1039–1043, 1988.

28. Risi GF, Martin DH, Cohen JC: Use of Polymerase Chain Reaction to detect *Haemophilus ducreyi* in clinical specimens. in press.

29. Kraus SJ, Kaufman HW, Albritton WL, et al.: Chancroid therapy: A review of cases confirmed by culture. *Rev Infect Dis* 4(Suppl):S848–S856, 1982.

30. Handsfield HH: Problems in the treatment of bacterial sexually transmitted diseases. *Sex Transm Dis* 13:179–184, 1986.

31. Fast MV, Nsanze H, D'Costa LJ, et al: Antimicrobial therapy of chancroid: An evalua-

tion of five treatment regimens correlated with in vitro sensitivity. *Sex Transm Dis* 10: 1–6, 1983.

32. Taylor DN, Pitarangsi C, Echeverria P, et al: Comparative study of ceftriaxone and trimethoprim-sulfamethoxazole for treatment of chancroid in Thailand. *J Infect Dis* 152:1002–1006, 1985.

33. Bowmer MI, Nsanze H, D'Costa LJ, et al: Single dose ceftriaxone for chancroid. *Antimicrob Agents Chemother* 31:67–69, 1987.

34. Fast MV, Nsanze H, D'Costa LJ, et al: Treatment of chancroid by clavulanic acid with amoxycillin in patients with beta-lactamase-positive *Haemophilus ducreyi* infection. *Lancet* 2:509–511, 1982.

35. Felman YM, Nikitas YA: Update on chancroid. *Sex Transm Dis* 31:602–615, 1983.

36. Roland AR: Chancroid: Recent advances in treatment and control. *Int J Dermatol* 25: 31–33, 1986.

37. D'Costa LJ, Bowmer I, Nsanze H, et al.: Advances in diagnosis and management of chancroid. *Sex Transm Dis* 13:189–191, 1986.

38. Piot P, Plummer FA, Rey MA, et al: Retrospective seroepidemiology of AIDS virus infection in Nairobi populations. *J Infect Dis* 155:1108–1112, 1987.

39. Greenblatt RM, Lukehart SA, Plummer FA, et al: Genital ulceration as a risk factor for human immunodeficiency virus infections. *AIDS* 2:47–50, 1988.

40. Simonsen JN, Cameron DW, Gakinya MN, et al: Human immunodeficiency virus infection in men with sexually transmitted diseases. *N Engl J Med* 319:274–278, 1988.

10

LYMPHOGRANULOMA VENEREUM

Lymphogranuloma venereum (LGV) is a systemic disease caused by *Chlamydia trachomatis* immunotypes* L_1, L_2, and L_3.[1,2] It is characterized by a transitory genital lesion followed by involvement of the lymphatic channels and nodes of the genitalia, the pelvis and the rectum. Synonyms for LGV are tropical (climatic) bubo, Durand-Nicholas-Favre disease, lymphogranuloma inguinale, poradenitis inguinalis, and fourth venereal disease.

EPIDEMIOLOGY

The disease is sporadic in Europe and North America (303 cases reported to the Centers for Disease Control [CDC] in 1987) and is rarely the cause of inguinal adenopathy in the United States. It is prevalent in many tropical countries in Southeast Asia, India, East and West Africa, and South and Central America. Most of the cases in nonendemic areas occur in military personnel, sailors, or travelers returning from endemic areas.[3] LGV is acquired by sexual contact, and it is reported more frequently in men than in women by a ratio of approximately 5:1.[4] As with other STDs, lymphogranuloma venereum is more common in urban populations, among the sexually promiscuous, and in low socioeconomic classes.[5] In the past it was endemic in blacks of lower socioeconomic status in the southeastern parts of the United States.

CLINICAL FEATURES

The incubation period varies from 3 days to 3 weeks (average 10–14 days), and the disease can be divided into three clinical stages: primary lesion, lymphatic dissemination, and late complications.

---

*Other *Chlamydia trachomatis* serotypes have been isolated from specimens obtained from patients who had symptoms compatible with LGV.[1,2]

Primary Lesions

The primary lesion usually develops on the external genitalia and rarely at other sites. It appears as a small, painless, vesiculating papule, ulcer, or herpetiform erosion which is transient and frequently overlooked (Figures 10.1 and 10.2). The most common locations in men are the coronal sulcus, prepuce, glans of the penis, and the urethra. In women the posterior vaginal wall, the fourchette, the cervix, and the vulva are common locations. In homosexual men and in women practicing anal or oral sex, the site of primary inoculation may be the rectum and/or mouth. In men the primary lesion may be followed by lymphangitis of the dorsal penis and formation of "bubonulus." The latter is a large, tender node which may rupture, with subsequent formation of sinuses, fistulas, or deforming scars at the base of the penis.[6]

Regional Lymphadenitis/Lymphadenopathy

Regional lymphadenitis (Figure 10.3) appears usually 7–30 days following the disappearance of the primary lesion. It is the second stage of LGV but can be the first evidence of the disease. Lymphadenitis develops in the nodes draining the site of primary lesion, and the infection disseminates further via the lymphatic system.

If the primary lesion is on the penis, vulva, or anus, the superficial inguinal nodes will be involved, with partial involvement of the deep iliac nodes. Primary inoculation of the vagina or cervix will result in adenopathy in the deep iliac, perirectal, retrocrural, and lumbosacral nodes. Rectal inoculation will produce perirectal and/or deep iliac adenopathy. Oral primary lesion will result in submaxillary and cervical adenopathy.[7,8] Involvement of supraclavicular, mediastinal, as well as multiple nodes has also been reported.[9-11]

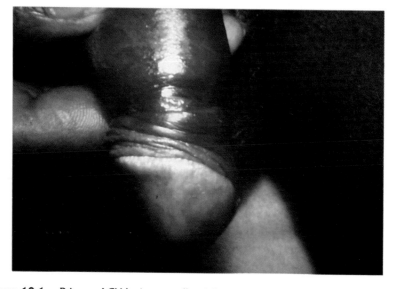

Figure 10.1. Primary LGV lesion: small painless erosion on the shaft of the penis.

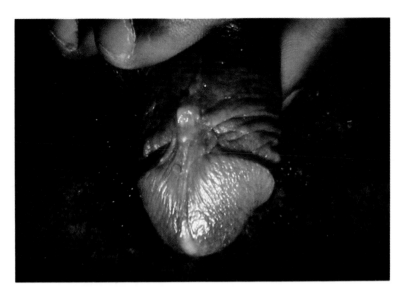

Figure 10.2. Primary LGV lesion on the frenulum.

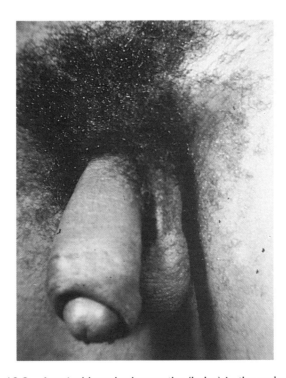

Figure 10.3. Inguinal lymphadenopathy (bubo) in the early stage.

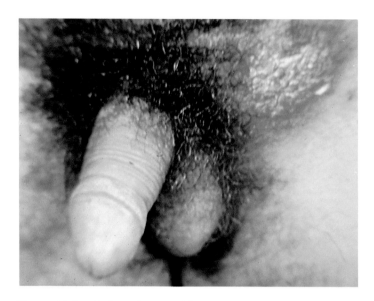

Figure 10.4.   Unilateral inguinal lymphadenopathy (bubo) in LGV.

Inguinal lymphadenopathy is the most common manifestation of LGV lymphatic dissemination (Figure 10.4).[12] It is unilateral in about two thirds of cases. The horizontal group of inguinal nodes is most commonly affected, but in some cases the vertical nodes and even the femoral nodes may be involved. Enlargement of glands above and below Poupart's ligament gives the characteristic LGV "groove sign" (Figure 10.5). The onset is gradual, with tenderness in the groin. The nodes are initially hard and firm. Within 1–2 weeks they become fixed to the skin and subcutaneous tissue. The overlying skin is reddened, with a characteristic viola-

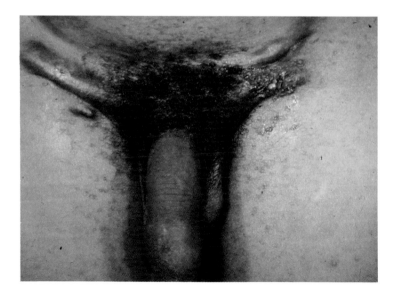

Figure 10.5.   Inguinal adenopathy divided by the inguinal ligament "sign of the groove."

ceous hue, and fluctuation may be felt in the abscess below it. As the bubo enlarges, it becomes painful. The nodes eventually break down, with the formation of multiple sinuses which drain from sticky yellowish fluid to thick, tenacious pus. Rupture through the skin usually relieves pain. Only about one third of inguinal buboes become fluctuant and rupture; the remaining involute and form a hard inguinal mass without suppuration.[13,14]

Constitutional symptoms are common and probably result from systemic spread of the infection, during which chlamydiae may be recovered from the blood and even the cerebrospinal fluid.[15] Systemic signs may include fever, chills, headache, meningismus, anorexia, nausea, vomiting, muscle and joint pains, and skin rashes. Hepatosplenomegaly, pericarditis, and meningitis have also been reported.[13,16]

Inguinal lymphadenopathy is comparatively rare in women and occurs in 20–30 percent of cases. About one third of them may have symptoms and signs (lower abdominal and/or back pain) suggesting involvement of the deep pelvic and lumbar nodes.[17] Spread of the infection to the perirectal lymphatics may cause involvement of the rectal wall with subsequent proctocolitis and ulceration of the rectal mucosa.

In women or homosexual men practicing anal intercourse, the rectal mucosa can be directly inoculated with LGV microorganisms. Additionally, in women the rectal mucous membrane can be infected by migration of vaginal secretions or by the spread of infection from the cervix or vagina through the lymphatic channels.[18-20] Early protocolitis is manifested by anal pruritus and passage of mucoid discharge which may become blood-stained within several days or weeks. Patients may complain of rectal pain, tenesmus, and fever.[5,13] On digital examination, the bowel wall seems to be thickened and the rectal mucosa feels granular with palpable and movable lymph nodes under the rectal wall.[21] Since the mucous membrane of the involved segment of the bowel is hyperemic and friable, the digital examination usually results in minor bleeding. Sigmoidoscopic findings are not pathognomonic, although together with histologic examination they may be helpful in establishing diagnosis.[22]

Late Complications

The late complications of LGV are both debilitating and disfiguring. The most serious, although uncommon, is elephantiasis of the genitalia, which may involve the penis, scrotum, and vulva (Figure 10.6). The latter may develop ulcerative lesions of the vulva surrounded by edema and induration, a condition that is called "esthiomene" (which is Greek for "eating away"). The chronic ulcerations are very painful, and edema may extend down to the anus and interfere with physiologic functions.[16] In men, damage to the lymphatic system may result in obstruction of lymphatic vessels, causing penile edema, distortion of the penis ("saxophone penis"), and massive enlargement of the scrotum.[23] Complications of rectal LGV include perianal abscess; rectovaginal, rectovesical, and ischiorectal fistulas; anal fistulas; and rectal stricture.[5,16]

The rectal stenosis or strictures are more common in women and homosexual men. They take the form of an annular band or tubular constriction 2–5 cm above the rectal orifice margin, where the lymphatic tissue is the richest.[21] Intermittent constipation and a passage of "pencil" stool occurs with established stenosis.

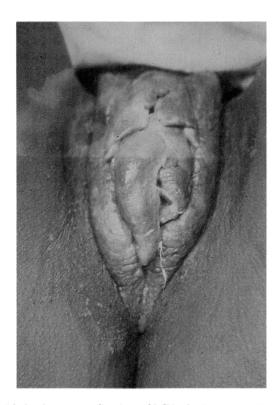

Figure 10.6. Late complication of LGV: elephantiasis of the vulva.

Complete bowel obstruction is rare, but painful ileus, distention, and bowel perforation with subsequent peritonitis can be the cause of death.[16] A higher incidence of rectal cancer in patients with LGV rectal strictures has been reported,[24,25] but the role of LGV in the development of rectal cancer has not been conclusively proved.

As a result of the obstruction of the lymphatic and venous drainage of the anal region, lymphorrhoids may develop. These anal tags are often confused with hemorrhoids and consist of dilated lymph vessels with perilymphatic inflammation.[13,14]

DIAGNOSIS

The diagnosis of LGV is usually based on the clinical picture and positive laboratory tests.

Laboratory tests include

Isolation of the microorganisms

Complement fixation test

Microimmunofluorescence test

Other procedures, including cytology, lymphangiography, and histopathology

Isolation of *Chlamydia trachomatis*

There have been several methods of isolation of *Chlamydia*, but the cell culture method (cycloheximide-treated McCoy cells) is now preferred.[26] The recovery of *Chlamydia* from clinical material obtained from bubo, genital, or rectal tissues is low (less than 30 percent)[27,28] and much lower than in nongonococcal urethritis, the disease caused by other *Chlamydia* serovars.[29]

Complement Fixation Test

The complement fixation (CF) test has become the standard test in the diagnosis of lymphogranuloma venereum. It utilizes a group-specific antigen which measures antibodies against *Chlamydia trachomatis* and *Chlamydia psittaci*. Although it is nonspecific, it can be titrated, which enhances its value. (The higher the titer, the more likely the diagnosis of LGV). The CF test is more sensitive that the previously used Frei test,* but its results should be evaluated with caution because of the cross reactivity with infections caused by other *chlamydiae*. A fourfold or higher rise in the titer in the presence of clinical symptoms should be diagnostic for chlamydial infections but not necessarily LGV strains. In general, active LGV infections have CF test titers 1:64 or greater. Titers below 1:64 should be interpreted with great caution.

Microimmunofluorescent Test

The microimmunofluorescent (micro-IF) test is more sensitive and more specific than the CF test. It has been used for typing isolates and in serodiagnosis; it may identify the specificity of the serologic response.[30,31] The titers of micro-IF in LGV are usually 1:512 or higher. The micro-IF test is not widely available and has been performed in a few specialized laboratories.

Other Diagnostic Procedures

Cytologic examination using Giemsa, iodine, or fluorescent antibody staining may visualize the elementary or inclusion bodies in infected tissues.[29] Lymphangiography may demonstrate the characteristics and the extent of involvement of the lymphatic system.[32] Histopathologic studies may reveal a characteristic pattern, but some authors believe it is not pathognomonic for LGV.

---

*The Frei intradermal test has been the standard test in LGV for many years. Recently, its sensitivity and specificity have been questioned, and it is no longer in use.

DIFFERENTIAL DIAGNOSIS

The primary lesion must be distinguished from

- *Genital herpes:* multiple, superficial, painful erosions and/or vesicles; non-suppurating lymphadenopathy; Tzanck smear may reveal multinucleated giant cells; virus can be isolated by culture; immunofluorescence or other tests would be positive
- *Primary syphilis:* single, round or oval painless ulcer with hard button-like indurated base; positive dark-field exam, positive serology, (FTA-ABS); painless non-suppurating lymphadenopathy.
- *Chancroid:* single or multiple painful ulcers which do not heal rapidly; positive culture for *Haemophilus ducreyi.*
- *Trauma* (history)

The inguinal buboes must be distinguished from

- *Chancroid bubo:* chancroidal ulcer(s) usually present at the same time; frequently unilateral; positive culture for *H. ducreyi* from material obtained from ulceration or bubo.
- *Lymphadenopathy in primary syphilis:* positive serologic tests; usually painless; does not suppurate; primary chancre frequently present; positive dark-field examination.
- *Donovanosis:* not true buboes which appear with ulcer; "Donovan bodies" present in cytoplasm of large mononuclear cells in smears of crushed material.
- *Nonvenereal causes of inguinal lymphadenopathy:* lymphoma or metastatic malignancies; cat scratch disease; infectious mononucleosis; bubonic plague; tularemia; brucellosis; actinomycosis; tuberculosis; bacterial infections of lower extremities.

Pelvic or lumbar lymphadenitis may mimic appendicitis, tuboovarian abscess, or pelvic inflammatory disease (PID). Anogenital lesions must be distinguished from hemorrhoids, polyposis, and ulcerative pyogenic granuloma. Proctitis and rectal stricture may be mistaken for Crohn's disease, ulcerative colitis, proctocolitis caused by enteric infections and rectal carcinoma.

In homosexual men the differential diagnosis of anorectal LGV should include primary and secondary syphilis, gonorrhea, ulcerative colitis, Crohn's disease, carcinomas, and also infections caused by herpes simplex virus, *Yersinia* spp., *Campylobacter* spp., and *Clostridium difficile, Shigella, Giardia lamblia, Entamoeba histolytica,* and other microorganisms which produce enteric disease.

TREATMENT

Systemic

Doxycycline, 100 mg tablets twice daily for 3 weeks
Or
Tetracycline hydrochloride, 500 mg tablets 4 times a day for 3 weeks or longer

Or

Erythromycin, 500 mg tablets 4 times a day for 3 weeks

Or

Sulfisoxazole, 500 mg by mouth 4 times a day for a minimum of 3 weeks or other sulfonamides in equivalent dosages

Local Measures

Fluctuant nodes should be aspirated before they burst, repeatedly if necessary. (Incision and drainage or excision of nodes are contraindicated.) Late sequelae (rectal stricture, fistulas), besides antimicrobial therapy, may require surgical intervention.[33] In some cases it can be the only means of improving the patient's condition.

SEX PARTNER MANAGEMENT

Sex partners of LGV patients should be treated with one of the proposed regimens.

PREVENTION

Early diagnosis and treatment, including prophylactic treatment of persons exposed to LGV, are the most effective measures. The condom provides protection against genital-anogenital transmission but has little impact on transmission between other sites. In homosexuals with anal lesions or proctocolitis, the possibility of rectal LGV should be kept in mind. Prompt treatment and appropriate epidemiologic measures (contact tracing) may prevent further spread of the disease in this environment.

REFERENCES

1. Schachter J, Meyer KF: Lymphogranuloma venereum: Characterization of some recently isolated strains. *J Bacteriol* 99:636–638, 1969.
2. Schachter J: Confirmatory serodiagnosis of lymphogranuloma venereum proctitis may yield false-positive results due to other chlamydial infections of the rectum. *Sex Transm Dis* 8:26–28, 1981.
3. Abrams AJ: Lymphogranuloma venereum. *JAMA* 205:199–202, 1968.
4. Schachter J: Lymphogranuloma venereum and other nonocular *Chlamydia trachomatis* infections, in Hobson D, Holmes KK (eds), *Nongonococcal Urethritis and Related Infections.* Washington, DC, America Society of Microbiology, 1977, p. 91.
5. Annamuthodo H: Rectal lymphogranuloma venereum in Jamaica. *Ann R Coll Surg Engl* 29:141–159, 1961.
6. Hopsu-Havu VK, Sonck CE: Infiltrative, ulcerative, and fistular lesions of the penis due to lymphogranuloma venereum. *Br J Vener Dis* 49:193–202, 1973.

7. Andrada MT, Dhar JK, Wilde H: Oral lymphogranuloma venereum and cervical lymphadenopathy. *Milit Med* 139:99–101, 1974.

8. Thorsteinisson SB, Musher DM, Min K-W, et al.: Lymphogranuloma venereum: A cause of cervical lymphadenopathy. *JAMA* 235:1882, 1976.

9. Walzer PD, Armstrong D: Lymphogranuloma venereum presenting as superclavicular and inguinal lymphadenopathy. *Sex Transm Dis* 4:12–14, 1977.

10. Sheldon WH, Wall MJ, Slade DR, et al.: Lymphogranuloma venereum in a patient with mediastinal lymphadenopathy and pericarditis. *Arch Intern Med* 82:410–416, 1948.

11. Eberhard TP: Generalized lymphogranuloma inguinale. *Ann Surg* 107:380–388, 1938.

12. Abrams AJ: Lymphogranuloma venereum. *JAMA* 205:199–202, 1968.

13. Koteen H: Lymphogranuloma venereum. *Medicine* 24:1–69, 1945.

14. D'Aunoy R, Von Haam E. Veneral lymphogranuloma. *Arch Pathol* 27:1032–1082, 1939.

15. Benson PP, Wall MJ, Heyman A: Isolation of virus of lymphogranuloma venereum from blood and spinal fluid of a human being. *Proc Soc Exp Biol Med* 62:306–307, 1946.

16. Coutts WE: Lymphogranuloma venereum: A general review. *Bull WHO* 2:545–562, 1950.

17. von Haam E, D'Aunoy R: Is lymphogranuloma inguinale a systemic disease? *Am J Trop Med Hyg* 16:527–546, 1936.

18. Torpin R, Pund ER, Greenblatt RB, et al.: Lymphogranuloma venereum in the female: A clinical study of ninety-six consecutive cases. *Am J Surg* 43:688–694, 1939.

19. Levine JS, Smith PD, Brugge WR: Chronic proctitis in male homosexuals due to lymphogranuloma venereum. *Gastroenterology* 79:563–565, 1980.

20. Miles RPM: Rectal lymphogranuloma venereum. *Postgrad Med J* 35:92–96, 1959.

21. Mathewson C Jr: Inflammatory strictures of the rectum associated with venereal lymphogranuloma. *JAMA* 110:709–714, 1938.

22. Mindell A: Lymphogranuloma venereum of the rectum in homosexual men. *Br J Vener Dis* 59:196–197, 1983.

23. Willcox RR: Lymphogranuloma venereum, in Morton RS, Harris JRW (eds), *Recent Advances in Sexually Transmitted Diseases*. London, Churchill Livingstone, 1975, p. 188.

24. Rainey R: The association of lymphogranuloma inguinale and cancer. *Surgery* 35:221–235, 1954.

25. Levin I, Romano S, Steinberg M, et al.: Lymphogranuloma venereum, rectal stricture and carcinoma. *Dis Colon Rectum* 7:129–134, 1964.

26. Ripa KT, Mardh P-A: Cultivation of *Chlamydia trachomatis* in cycloheximide-treated McCoy cells. *J Clin Microbiol* 6:328–331, 1977.

27. Schachter J, Smith DE, Dawson CR, et al.: Lymphogranuloma venereum: I. Comparison of Frei test, complement fixation test, and isolation of the agent. *J Infect Dis* 120:372–375, 1969.

28. Philip RN, Hill DA, Greaves AB: Study of chlamydia in patients with lymphogranuloma venereum and urethritis attending a venereal disease clinic. *Br J Vener Dis* 47:114–121, 1971.

29. Paavonen J: Chlamydial infections: Microbiological, clinical and diagnostic aspects. *Med Biol* 57:135–151, 1979.

30. Wang SP, Grayston JT: Immunologic relationship between genital TRIC, lymphogranuloma venereum and related organisms in a new microtiter indirect immunofluorescence test. *Am J Ophthalmol* 70:367–374, 1970.

31. Wang S-P, Grayston JT, Alexander ER, et al.: A simplified microimmunofluorescence test with trachoma-lymphogranuloma venereum (*Chlamydia trachomatis*) antigens for use as a screening test for antibody. *J Clin Microbiol* 1:250–255, 1975.

32. Osoba AO, Bettlestone C: Lymphographic studies in acute LGV infection. *Br J Vener Dis* 52:399–403, 1976.

33. Parkash S, Radhakrishna K: Problematic ulcerative lesions in sexually transmitted diseases: Surgical management. *Sex Transm Dis* 13:127–133, 1986.

11

DONOVANOSIS

Donovanosis is a chronic, slowly progressive, and mildly contagious sexually transmissible disease. It is caused by the gram-negative bacterium *Calymmatobacterium granulomatis* and is characterized by granulomatous ulcerations usually affecting the genitalia and neighboring sites. Synonyms for donovanosis are granuloma inguinale, granuloma venereum, granuloma donovani, chronic venereal sore, and granuloma inguinale tropicum.

EPIDEMIOLOGY

Donovanosis is endemic in certain tropical and subtropical areas: New Guinea, North and Central Australia, Southern India, Central and West Africa, the Caribbean, and South America.[1-6] It is very rare in Europe and North America. The number of cases reported in the United States in 1987 was 22. Donovanosis is mildly contagious, and repeated exposure is probably necessary for the development of the disease. Although sexual contact seems to be the most common mode of transmission,[7,8] the disease probably can also be acquired by close, repeated physical contact especially of the anogenital region[7] or by autoinoculation from the rectum.[9] Donovanosis is twice as common in men as in women,[8,10] with the greatest incidence in patients between 20 and 40 years of age.[10] It has been observed more frequently in blacks than in whites.[11] Hot and humid climate, low socioeconomic status, poor personal hygiene, and prostitution and sexual promiscuity play important roles in prevalence and transmission.[12]

CLINICAL MANIFESTATIONS

The incubation period is not precisely known, and estimates range from a few days to several months.[8,10,13] The disease is insidious in onset, which is marked by formation of a painless firm papule or subcutaneous module which later erodes to form an ulcer. An ulcer or ulcers are also painless and when fully developed show

250

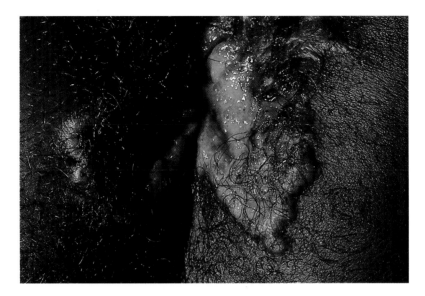

Figure 11.1. Typical beefy protuberant granulations caused by donovanosis.

variations in their morphology. They can be classified as (1) ulcerative or ulcero-granulomatous, (2) hypertrophic or verrucous, (3) necrotic, and (4) sclerotic or cicatricial.[10,14,15]

The *ulcerative* or *ulcerogranulomatous* form is characterized by the presence of a fleshy, beefy-red granulomatous lesion which is usually single, nontender, nonindurated, and bleeds profusely on touch. Multiple ulcers may be rarely encountered. Long-lasting lesions may have a tendency to spread slowly and to form raised irregular, slightly indurated margins (Figures 11.1–11.3).

The *hypertrophic* or *verrucous* variety consists of an ulcer or vegetative granulation tissue, with an elevated irregular border, that is drier than the ulcerative form and that has an elevated granulomatous base protruding above the surrounding skin (Figure 11.4). This variety occurs both in men and women and may involve extensive areas of the skin in the genital and adjacent regions.

The *necrotic* type is characterized by extensive and rapid destruction of affected tissue. These lesions may be painful and, if secondarily infected, covered with a gray foul-smelling exudate.

Sclerotic or *cicatricial* donovanosis is more common in women and results from an extensive formation of fibrous tissue and presents as a bandlike scar in affected parts of the genitalia and perineum or as a deep, nontender ulcer with a clean base and nonfriable border (Figure 11.5).

The genitalia are involved in 80–90 percent of cases.[16] The prepuce, coronal sulcus, glans, and shaft of the penis and the labia, the fourchette, and to a lesser extent, the vagina and cervix are the most commonly affected sites.[7,15,17] The inguinal region is involved in about 10 percent of cases and the anal region in 5–10 percent of cases, predominantly in homosexuals;[18] the distant lesions were observed in 1–5 percent of cases.[16] All distant site lesions were usually accompanied by primary lesions in the genitals except for the primary lesion in the oral cavity, which seemed to be the site of primary inoculation.[19]

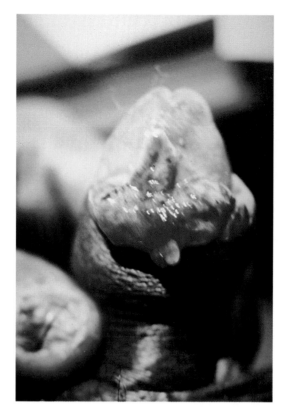

Figure 11.2.   Granulomatous lesion on the glans of the penis in donovanosis.

Oral lesions are next in frequency to donovanosis in the anogenital region. Infection of the oral cavity can be the result of direct inoculation or autoinoculation from other sites. The lips, cheeks, gums, and palate are most frequently affected. Oral ulcers caused by *C. granulomatis* are more superficial than those in the anogenital region. Similar to lesions elsewhere, oral ulcers may produce pseudo-buboes in the regional lymph nodes and, unlike genital donovanosis, the oral lesions can be painful, especially those located on the gums and around the teeth. Although a local disease, donovanosis, albeit rarely, can become systemic and involve any organ or tissue. Systemic involvement is usually associated with fever, low-grade anemia, and weight loss. The hematogenic spread is rare, but metastatic lesions in bones, liver, uterus, salpinges, ovaries,[19-22] gingiva,[23] and epididymis[24] were reported. In hematogenic spread, the bladder may be affected. Perforation into the vagina with subsequent formation of vesicovaginal fistulas or hydrone-phrosis may result from the extension of donovanosis to other organs of the genitourinary tract. Contiguous spread from the genital region into adjacent pelvic organs has also been reported.[25]

There is probably no spread through the lymphatic channels, and lesions of the inguinal regions usually involve the subcutaneous tissue. The lymph nodes are not involved, although there may be swelling in the groins resembling "suppurating

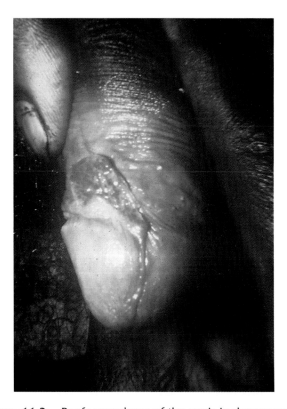

Figure 11.3. Beefy granuloma of the penis in donovanosis.

bubo," which in fact is a subcutaneous granuloma (pseudobubo) (Figure 11.6). Pseudobuboes may break down to form ulcers. Histopathologic examination reveals inflammatory changes, granulation tissue, and/or Donovan bodies.[26] The course of the disease is slowly progressive, with little or no tendency for spontaneous healing. In men long-lasting donovanosis may destroy the penis (Figure 11.7) and can be the cause of phimosis and urethral or anal stenosis. The latter occurs mainly in the sclerotic or cicatricial form of the disease. In women massive, elephantiasislike lesions (pseudoelephantiasis) or extensive ulcerations on the labia or in the vulva may cause urethral, vaginal, or anal stenosis which interferes with physiologic functions. The latter is seen more often in the sclerotic variety.[10]

An association between squamous cell carcinoma of the penis or cervix and donovanosis has been stressed by several investigators, but this is not very common.[27,28]

DIAGNOSIS

The clinical feature of donovanosis is highly suggestive of the diagnosis, but it should be confirmed by finding *C. granulomatis* in tissue smears or by biopsy.

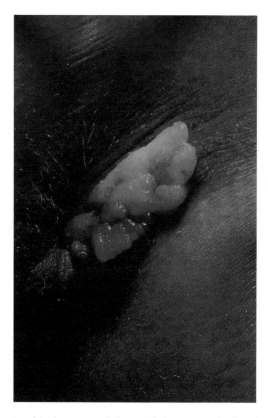

Figure 11.4. Hypertrophic (verrucous) form of donovanosis closely resembling genital warts.

Tissue Smears

It is very important to obtain a fragment of granulation tissue in order to make proper examination. Samples collected with cotton swabs or by scraping with a scalpel or glass slide are usually inadequate.

Tissue smears are best made by removing a small piece of granulation tissue with a biopsy punch, scalpel, or biopsy forceps. Specimen should be placed between two glass slides and crushed and spread throughout the slides. Giemsa's, Wright's, or Leishman's stains give the best definition of cells and microorganisms.[29]

The causative microorganisms, called "Donovan bodies," are large intracytoplasmic rods with a "safety pin" appearance due to the characteristic bipolar staining. They are found in large mononuclear cells in encapsulated and noncapsulated forms. In Wright's staining the encapsulated microorganisms are deep blue or even black and are surrounded by well-defined pinkish material. The noncapsulated form may have a varying morphology which conforms to bacillary, coccoid, or diplococcoid. The latter in particular resembles a closed safety pin. Although very important, the tissue smear should not be overemphasized, since it may be negative in very early or late lesions.[30] The same problem may be faced in necrotic or sclerotic varieties of donovanosis and in lesions resembling malignancy.[10]

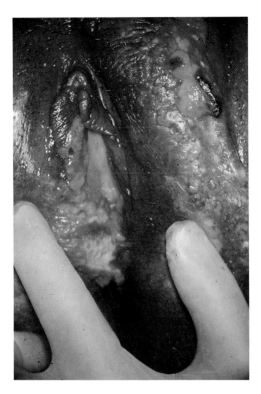

Figure 11.5.   Cicatricial lesions on the labium majoris in a woman with donovanosis.

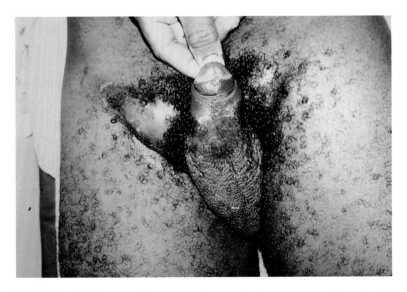

Figure 11.6.   Pseudobuboes of donovanosis are subcutaneous granulomata which eventually will rupture, producing typical beefy lesions in the groin.

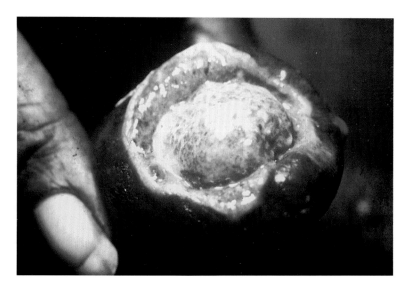

Figure 11.7. Mutilation of the penis caused by long-lasting donovanosis.

Histopathology

Biopsy is a valuable aid in the diagnosis of donovanosis as well as in excluding malignancies. The histopathologic changes may affect both the dermis and epidermis.[31,32] Dermal changes include a massive cellular reaction surcharged with plasma and mononuclear cells but with a paucity of lymphocytes and neutrophils. Histiocytes may be seen in varying numbers. Larger cells containing cystic spaces with darkly staining inclusions and nuclei shifted to the sites (cells of Greenblatt) are very conspicuous. Diffuse and/or focal polymorphonuclear leukocyte infiltration in the papillae as well as dermal blood vessel dilation and endothelial proliferation can be seen. The presence of intracellular and extracellular Donovan bodies is pathognomonic. They have different morphologic features: coccoid, coccobacillary, or bacillary and are best identified in Giemsa-stained specimens. Donovan bodies may also be visualized by electron microscopy.[33]

Epidermal changes may show discontinuity in the epidermis with ulcerations varying from mild to severe. In hypertrophic variants of donovanosis, acanthosis in the form of elongation of the rete ridges is a constant feature, while in the ulcerative form it is less frequent. Rarely is pseudoepitheliomatous hyperplasia noticed in the hypertrophic variant. Neutrophilic sprinkling of both the upper dermis and epidermis occurs very often. Rarely these may form microabscesses.[32]

Culture

Although *C. granulomatis* can be cultivated in the yolk sac, routine culturing is of no benefit and the diagnosis is usually established by the examination of tissue smears and/or by histopathologic examination of biopsy specimens.

DIFFERENTIAL DIAGNOSIS

- *Primary syphilis:* round or oval painless superficial ulcer usually with well-defined borders, an indurated base, and a raw exuding surface; painless inguinal lymphadenopathy; positive dark-field examination; FTA-ABS test may be positive; slowly resolves to latency even without treatment; quickly responds to treatment with penicillin.
- *Secondary syphilis:* condylomata lata especially in the anal area may strikingly resemble donovanosis; positive serology (high titer); positive dark-field examination; responds to penicillin therapy.
- *Chancroid:* short incubation period; ulcer, or frequently multiple ulcers, are usually small and often painful; tender unilateral lymphadenopathy; positive culture for *Haemophilus ducreyi.* Certain cases of chancroid may simulate donovanosis.[34]
- *Lymphogranuloma venereum:* initial lesion rarely noticed; unilateral or bilateral tender lymphadenopathy; sign of the groove often present; suppuration and fistulas may occur; positive CFT; positive culture for *Chlamydia trachomatis;* late manifestations of LGV due to lymphatic obstruction may closely resemble pseudoelephantiasis of donovanosis.
- *Carcinoma:* frequently misdiagnosed for penile donovanosis; both conditions produce chronic, granulomatous, and ulcerated growth; in late stages of carcinoma because of metastases of the inguinal lymph nodes, they become firm and fixed to the underlying tissue; histopathologic examination is decisive, but if not possible, therapeutic trial answers the question.
- *Cutaneous amebiasis:* distinction may be difficult in necrotic form of donovanosis, and one has to remember that in certain endemic areas two diseases may coexist; histopathologic examination may reveal trophozoites of *Entamoeba histolytica.*
- *Cutaneous tuberculosis, pyogenic granuloma:* should be excluded by histopathologic and bacteriologic examinations.
- *Filariasis, schistosomiasis,* and *leishmaniasis* should be considered in certain geographic regions.

TREATMENT

Tetracycline hydrochloride, 500 mg tablets 4 times a day for 14–21 days. In the case of tetracycline resistance or allergy, *Trimethoprim-sulfamethoxazole,* 2 tablets twice daily for a minimum of 14 days. Other antibiotics of proven efficacy are *chloramphenicol,* 500 mg tablets 3 times a day for 14–21 days* and *gentamicin,* 40 mg IM, twice daily for 14–21 days. In pregnancy: *erythromycin,* 500 mg tablets 4 times a day for 14–21 days.

---

*Toxic (bone marrow depression).

Surgical Measures

When antibiotics are not instituted in the early stage of the disease, longstanding lesions can be so extensive or mutilating that surgical intervention may be necessary. Surgical removal of granulations may also assist chemotherapy to overcome infection that is slow to respond. Occasionally patients may require plastic surgery, e.g., skin grafting or vulvectomy.

Comment: although oral administration of antibiotics allows for outpatient treatment, early hospitalization whenever possible is recommended. This allows assessment of the effectiveness of systemic therapy as well as application of local measures which consist of dressings with astringent and antiseptic lotions.

FOLLOW-UP

Since the disease sometimes tends to relapse after healing, the patient should be kept under surveillance for a few months before being discharged as cured.

MANAGEMENT OF SEX PARTNERS

Because of the long incubation period of the disease, all sex partners of patients with donovanosis must not be kept under observation but treated with the regimen effective for the index patient.

PREVENTION

Early diagnosis and treatment including prophylactic treatment of contacts seem to be the most effective way of controlling donovanosis. The use of condoms and cleansing of the genital area with antiseptics or even soap and water should in theory reduce the risk of sexual transmission. In the areas where donovanosis is endemic, more diversified control methods are required, including periodic screening of the sexually active male population.

REFERENCES

1. Maddocks I, Anders EM, Dennis E: Donovanosis in Papua New Guinea. *Br J Vener Dis* 52:190–196, 1976.
2. Hart G: Psychological and social aspects of venereal disease in Papua New Guinea. *Br J Vener Dis* 50:453–458, 1974.
3. Sehgal VN, Prasad ALS: Donovanosis. Current concepts. *Int J Dermatol* 25:8–16, 1986.
4. Bhagwandeen BS, Naik KG: Granuloma venereum (granuloma inguinale) in Zambia. *East Afr Med J* 54:637–642, 1977.
5. Stewart DB: The gynecological lesions of lymphogranuloma venereum and granuloma inguinale. *Med Clin North Am* 48:773–786, 1964.

6. Mitchell KM, Roberts AN, Williams VM, et al.: Donovanosis in Western Australia. *Genitourin Med* 62:191–195, 1986.

7. Kuberski T: Granuloma inguinale (Donovanosis). *Sex Transm Dis* 7:29–36, 1980.

8. Lal S, Nicholas C: Epidemiological and clinical features in 165 cases of granuloma inguinale. *Br J Vener Dis* 46:461–463, 1970.

9. Goldberg J: Studies on granuloma inguinale: VII. Some epidemiological considerations of the disease. *Br J Vener Dis* 40:140–145, 1964.

10. Rajam RV, Rangiah PN: *Donovanosis (Granuloma Inguinale, Granuloma Venereum)*. Geneva, World Health Organization, 1954, WHO Monograph Series, No. 24, pp. 1–72.

11. D'Aunoy R, von Haam E: Granuloma inguinale. *Am J Trop Med* 17:747–763, 1937.

12. Sowmini CN, Nair GM, Vasantha MNL: Climatic influence on the prevalence of donovanosis in India. *Indian J Dermatol Venerol Leprol* 37:111–114, 1971.

13. Anderson K: The cultivation from granuloma inguinale of a microorganism having the characteristic of Donovan bodies in the yolk sac of chick embryos. *Science* 97:560–561, 1943.

14. Subramaniam S: Sclerosing granuloma inguinale. *Br J Vener Dis* 57:210–212, 1981.

15. Sehgal VN, Prasad ALS: A clinical profile of donovanosis in a non-endemic area. *Dermatologica* 168:273–278, 1984.

16. Hart G: *Chancroid, Donovanosis, Lymphogranuloma Venereum*. U.S. Department of Health, Education and Welfare, 1975, Public Health Service (CDC); Publication no 75-8302.

17. Scrimgeour EM, Sengupta SK, McGoldrick IA: Primary endometrial and endocervical granuloma inguinale (donovanosis). *Br J Vener Dis* 59:198–201, 1983.

18. Marmell M: Donovaniosis of the anus in the male: An epidemiological consideration. *Br J Vener Dis* 34:213–218, 1958.

19. Garg BR, Lal S, Bedi BMS, et al.: Donovanosis (granuloma inguinale) of the oral cavity. *Br J Vener Dis* 51:136–137, 1975.

20. Kirkpatric DJ: Donovanosis: A rare cause of osteolytic bone lesions. *Clin Radiol* 21:101–106, 1970.

21. Kalstone BM: Granuloma inguinale with hematogenous dissemination to the spine. *JAMA* 176:530–533, 1961.

22. Pund ER, Gotcher VA: Granuloma venereum (granuloma inguinale) of uterus, tubes and ovaries. *Surgery* 3:34–40, 1948.

23. Bhaskar SN, Jacoway JR, Fleuchaus PT: Primary granuloma venereum of the gingiva. *Oral Surg* 20:535–541, 1965.

24. Jannach JR, Granuloma inguinale of the epididymis (case report). *Br J Vener Dis* 34:31–33, 1958.

25. Schneider J, O'Shea J, Finley-Jones LR, et al.: Extragenital donovanosis: Three cases from Western Australia. *Genitourin Med* 62:196–201, 1986.

26. Greenblatt RB, Dienst RB, Pund ER, et al.: Experimental and clinical granuloma inguinale. *JAMA* 113:1109–1116, 1939.

27. Goldberg J, Annamunthodo H: Studies on granuloma inguinale: VIII. Serological reactivity of sera from patients with Ca penis when tested with donovania antigens. *Br J Vener Dis* 42:205–209, 1966.

28. Stewart DB: The gynecological lesions of lymphogranuloma venereum and granuloma inguinale. *Med Clin North Am* 48:773–786, 1964.

29. Greenblatt RB, Dienst RB, West RM: A simple stain for Donovan bodies for the diagnosis of granuloma inguinale. *Am J Syph Gon Vener Dis* 35:291–293, 1951.

30. Greenblatt RB, Barfield WE: Newer methods in diagnosis and treatment of granuloma inguinale. *Br J Vener Dis* 23:123–128, 1952.

31. Pund ER, Greenblatt RB: Specific histology of granuloma inguinale. *Arch Pathol* 23: 224–230, 1937.

32. Sehgal VN, Shyamprasad AL, Beohar PC: The histopathological diagnosis of donovanosis. *Br J Vener Dis* 60:45–47, 1984.

33. Dodson RF, Fritz GS, Hubler WR, et al.: Donovanosis: A morphologic study. *J Invest Dermatol* 62:611–614, 1974.

34. Kraus SJ: Pseudogranuloma inguinale caused by *Haemophilus ducreyi. Arch Dermatol* 118:494–496, 1982.

12
ECTOPARASITE INFESTATIONS

SCABIES

Scabies is a sexually transmitted disease (STD) caused by the parasitic mite *Sarcoptes scabiei* var. *hominis*. Person-to-person spread is by means of close body contact, including sexual contact. It is characterized by an erythematous papular rash of characteristic distribution and severe itching which is worse at night. A common synonym for scabies is "the itch".

Etiology

The adult female *Sarcoptes scabiei* is a small mite just visible to the naked eye which measures about 0.3−0.4 mm. The male mite is smaller and seldom seen on the skin. The impregnated female mite burrows into the horny layer of the skin where she lays eggs. The female lives about 30 days and dies at the end of a tunnel when egg laying is complete. The eggs hatch within 3−4 days, giving rise to larvae which emerge from the tunnel and burrow into the adjacent skin where maturation stages take place. Two subsequent molts occur thereafter, and the whole development is complete in 10−14 days.[1] The mites may survive away from their host for 2−3 days at a temperature of 25°C. They are completely immobilized by the cold at 16°C and do not move actively below 20°C. Exposure to 50°C for 10 minutes proved fatal to the mites.[1]

Epidemiology

In Europe and North America, epidemics of scabies occur in 30-year cycles with a 15-year gap between them. The epidemics last about 15 years.[2,3] The disease was relatively uncommon in the 1950s, and the current worldwide epidemic dates from the mid-1960s with a sharp increase in the United States in the early 1970s.[3,4] Accurate data are not available and morbidity in the United States was estimated in 1987 at about 3,000 cases.

The reasons for resurgence of the disease are not well understood, but the following factors have been postulated: poor hygiene and poverty, overcrowding, sexual promiscuity, population movements by migration and tourism, medical misdiagnosis, and loss of immunity.[5,6] The socioeconomic characteristics of patients with scabies are representative of those of the general population, but in the United States scabies is more common in whites than blacks[7] and in males than females[8]; in recent years it has been seen frequently in sexually active male homosexulas.[6]

Scabies is contracted by direct intimate contact with an infected person. There is a general agreement that among sexually active adults sexual transmission of the disease is the most common. As with other sexually transmitted diseases, scabies is more common in men than in women and is observed more often in wartime.[7]

The disease may spread through nonsexual contact, e.g., among family members, patients in nursing homes, health workers,[9] or military personnel. It is frequent in school-age children, but school room transmission is rather unlikely.[10] Scabies may be contracted indirectly through contaminated clothing, blankets, and bed linen.

CLINICAL FEATURES

There are three cardinal clinical features characeristic of scabies:

1. Intense itching which worsens at night or when the patient is warm.
2. Typical distribution of a papular erythematous rash or pruritic nodules.
3. The presence of burrows: linear or tortuous, slightly elevated, threadlike ridges on the skin that are several milimeters long with small vesicles or papules at the end above the mite.

A history of scabies in the family or other household members or a history of casual sexual contact may help to establish diagnosis.

The disease becomes manifest 4–6 weeks after first infestation, during which time the patient may be infectious to others. The first symptom is usually itching that is often severe and worse at night or when the patient becomes warm.

Excoriations may be the first sign, and they are usually accompanied by a papular rash of characteristic distribution. Inflammatory vesicles or urticarial papules also may be present. In longer-lasting infestation dermatitis with or without secondary pyoderma or nodular lesions particularly on the penis can be found. The sites commonly affected are volar aspects of the wrists and forearms, finger webs, elbows, anterior axillary folds, abdomen (belt line and around the umbilicus), genitals, lower portion of buttocks, and around the nipples (Figures 12.1 and 12.2). When transmitted sexually, the lesions may be chiefly on or around the genitals (Figures 12.3–12.5).

The face, upper back, neck, scalp, palms, and soles are spared except in young babies or in the Norwegian form of the disease (Figure 12.6). The burrow is patho-

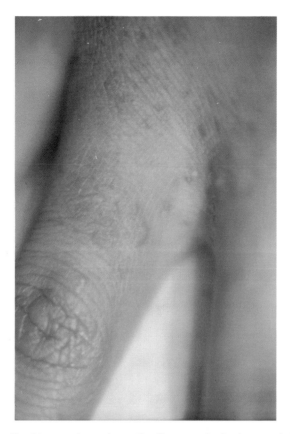

Figure 12.1. Pruritic papular rash on the finger webs is characteristic for scabies.

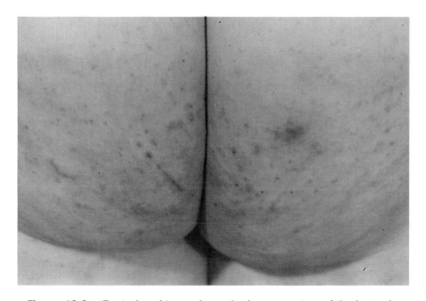

Figure 12.2. Typical scabies rash on the lower portion of the buttocks.

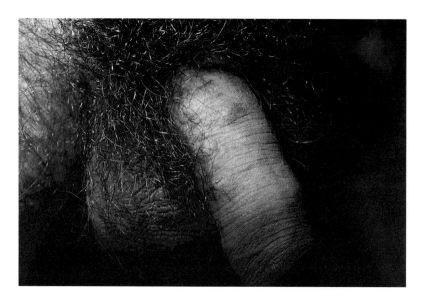

Figure 12.3. Pruritic papules and nodules on the genitalia are highly suggestive of scabies.

gnomonic. It is usually a short (several millimeters to a few centimeters), dirty-appearing line or zigzag often crossing the skin lines. The burrows are most common on the finger webs and volar aspects of the wrists.[11] The absence of burrows does not rule out diagnosis.

Special Forms of Scabies

Nodular Scabies

Nodular lesions occur most frequently on male genitalia (Figure 12.7), in groins, and in axillary regions. They are infrequent in females. The lesions are reddish brown and appear to be infiltrated. They may persist for months despite therapy or may clear spontaneously. Mites are rarely identified especially in the older lesions.[12] The nodules probably develop as a cell-mediated immune response to the mite antigens.

Norwegian Scabies

Norwegian scabies has been described chiefly in immunocompromised, mentally retarded, and physically debilitated persons. It also has been reported in patients with AIDS.[13] Pruritus is minimal, and skin lesions are characterized by extensive crusting and scaling as well as by the presence of an enormous number of mites in the exfoliated scales. The lesions are distributed mainly on the hands, feet (Figure 12.8), ears, face, and scalp. This form of scabies is highly contagious but fortunately rare.[14,15] However, with the increasing number of AIDS cases, Norwegian scabies can be seen more frequently.

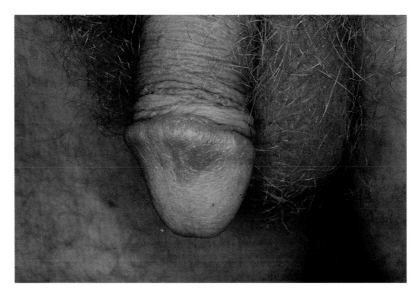

Figure 12.4. Rash on the penis caused by scabies.

Scabies in Clean Persons

Scabies seen in clean persons has become more common recently. Typical lesions may be barely observable and burrows difficult to find. The patients presumably wash out the mites during frequent bathing, and the disease can be easily misdiagnosed. Meticulous physical examination will suggest the diagnosis, which can be confirmed by mite identification.[4,15]

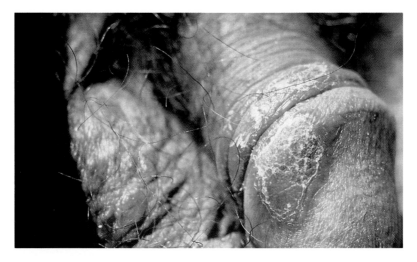

Figure 12.5. Scabies on the genitalia: note the scaly lesions on the glans and prepuce and the nodular rash on the scrotum.

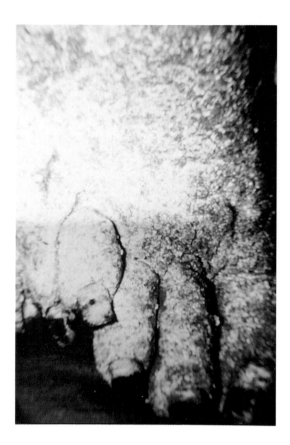

Figure 12.6. Extensive crusting and scaling is characteristic for Norwegian scabies.

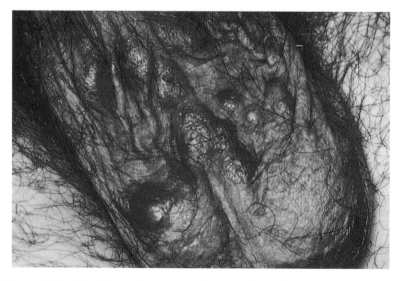

Figure 12.7. Scabies on the scrotum frequently produces nodular lesions.

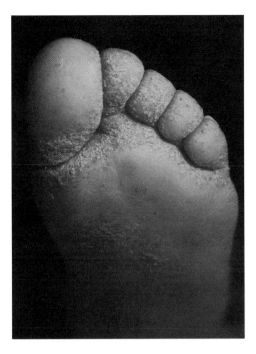

Figure 12.8. Norwegian scabies: scaly lesions on the feet in a patient with AIDS.

Scabies Incognito

With a generous administration of topical corticosteroids to any pruritic rash and easy accessibility of over-the-counter preparations containing overly potent steroids, scabies may be mistakenly treated with these drugs. This may result in atypical clinical presentations such as an unusual extent of skin involvement and atypical distribution, which in some instances may simulate other skin diseases.[4] The clinical course of scabies can be also altered in patients treated with systemic or topical corticosteroids for other reasons.[16]

Scabies in Children

The distribution of lesions is different in children than in adults. The palms, soles, head, and neck as well as the other parts of the skin may be affected. Vesicular lesions and eczematous eruptions can be found. Secondary bacterial infection is frequent, and typical burrows are difficult to find. This form of scabies is frequently misdiagnosed because of the low index of suspicion and atypical distribution.[17]

Animal-transmitted Scabies

Scabies transmitted by animals is not contagious between humans. People get infected by direct contact with infested animals (mainly dogs). Dogs infested with canine scabies (*Sarcoptes scabiei* var. *canis*) develop crusty and scaly lesions mainy on the ears and the abdomen. People are infested by petting or cuddling the animal.

The disease has a short incubation period and a different distribution pattern. The burrows are absent. It is self-limited (lasts several weeks).[18,19] The other source of animal scabies is cats infested with *Notoedres cati* (notoedric scabies). The disease was reported from Czecholovakia, Japan, and India, where outbreaks of cat scabies in people have been seen.[20,21]

Diagnosis

The diagnosis is often made on clinical grounds, but the disease can be positively confirmed by obtaining the mite from the burrow and examining it under a light microscope. A history of exposure to people with scabies or an "itchy" disease among other members of the household support the diagnosis.

Laboratory Identification of Scabies

- *Skin scrapings:* Place a drop of mineral oil on a lesion. Scrape the top of the burrow or a papule several times with sterile scalpel blade or needle. Transfer the scraped material onto a glass slide and apply a coverslip. Examine under low power magnification (10–20 objective). Diagnosis is confirmed by the presence of the mite or typical fecal pellets (Figure 12.9).[22,23]
- *Biopsy:* Shave or punch biopsy can be used to demonstrate mites or their products.[24] Histology is not characteristic. There is usually eosinophilic infiltration of the dermis and parakeratosis, spongiosis, and exocytosis in the epidermis.
- *Ink test:* Place a drop of ink on the lesion. Wipe off the surface ink with an alcohol pad. The ink should track down the mite burrow, forming a dark line crossing the skin lines.[25]

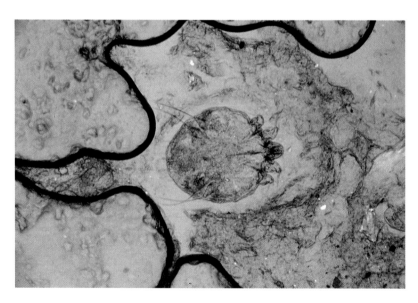

Figure 12.9. Demonstration of an adult mite in skin scrapings under the microscope is diagnostic for scabies.

Failure to demonstrate the mite on any of these laboratory methods should not preclude diagnosis. A therapeutic trial administering the usual treatment may be performed on patients with typical clinical lesions.

Differential Diagnosis

Differential diagnosis should include all pruritic dermatoses: atopic dermatitis, contact dermatitis, neurodermatitis, insect bites, papular urticaria, systemic diseases associated with itching, dermatitis herpetiformis, lichen planus, urticaria, keratosis follicularis, acarophobia, and neurotic excoriations.

Sexually transmitted disease include:

- *Secondary syphilis:* positive serology or dark-field examination; papular rash on face, palms, and soles as well as mucous membranes; no or minimal itching
- *Genital herpes:* grouped or linearly arranged vesicles; stinging instead of itching sensations; positive Tzanck test or positive culture or other tests
- *Pediculosis pubis:* pruritic rash limited to pubic region; *Maculae cerulae;* presence of lice and/or nits

Treatment

Prior to therapy the patient should take a warm soapy bath.

- *Lindane* 1% cream or lotion* (gammabenzenehexachloride, sold under the tradenames Gammexane, Kwell, Quellada, and Scabene): Apply a thin layer to the entire body from the neck down and leave on for 8 hours. Then take a shower or bath to remove thoroughly the medication. Dress in clean clothes.
- *Crotamiton 10%* (*N*-ethyl-*o*-crotonotoluidide, sold under the tradename Eurax): Apply to the entire body from the neck down nightly for two nights and wash off thoroughly 24 hours after the second application. Dress in clean clothes. (This regimen is recommended for children 2 years of age and pregnant and lactating women.)
- *Precipitated sulfur 5% in petrolatum:* Apply to the entire body nightly for three nights. Patients may bathe before reapplying and should bathe 24 hours after the final application. Dress in clean clothes.

Special considerations: In some patients pruritus may persist for several weeks after adequate therapy. A single retreatment after 1 week may be appropriate if there is no clinical improvement. Symptomatic relief may be obtained by application of a hydrocortisone preparation or lubricating or emollient agents. Secondary infection may require administration of oral or topical antibiotics.

Since the mites can be harbored under the nails[26] and be the reservoir of reinfestation, care should be given to applying the medication to the subungual area.

---

*Lindane is not recommended for pregnant and lactating women and children under 10 years of age.

Some patients may continue to have symptoms or signs probably due to a hypersensitivity reaction. In those cases oral antihistamines, antipruritics, or minor tranquilizers may be recommended. In rare instances in adults, a short course of systemic steroids may be considered.

Nodular lesions are often recalcitrant to traditional therapy and may require intralesional steroids or topical steroids under occulsion for resolution.

Note: Intimate apparel should be washed and dried by machine (hot cycles), boiled, or washed and ironed. Clothing or bed linen which may have been contaminated should be dry cleaned or washed and dried by machine (hot cycles).

Management of Sex Partners

Sex partners and close household contacts should be treated with appropriate scabicide.

Scabies and Other STDs

A diagnosis of scabies in a sexually active person should prompt a search for other sexually transmitted diseases. This is usually done routinely in venereal disease clinics but it must be remembered when the scabetic patient is seen elsewhere. Asymptomatic gonorrhea has been found among females with scabies in the 15–29-year age bracket,[27] and the primary chancre of syphilis may be sometimes seen in the scabetic lesion (chancre goleuse).[28] Norwegian scabies in a young person should prompt a physician to test for HIV antibodies since this form of scabies has been observed in patients with AIDS.

Prevention

Early diagnosis and adequte treatment of the patient and his or her sex partners as well as certain members of the household is the most effective means of prevention. Physicians should be especially alerted in cases of itchy skin among more than one member of the household, among people living in dormitories or chronic care institutions, or among military personnel.

PEDICULOSIS PUBIS

Pediculosis pubis is an infestation with the crab louse, which inhabits and attaches its eggs to the body hair. The disease is transmitted by close intimate contact. Synonyms for pediculosis pubis are phthiriasis pubis and crabs or lice.

Epidemiology

The prevalence of infestation is believed to parallel that of other STDs, and there has been a sharp increase in the frequency of pediculosis pubis infestation in the United States and Western Europe.[29-31] It was estimated that morbidity in the United States in 1987 was about 14,000.

Pediculosis pubis is one of the most contagious STDs[30] and it is very unlikely for a person to have sex with an infested partner and avoid infestation. The crab lice pass from person to person by hair-to-hair contact, usually during sexual intercourse. They also can be acquired from sleeping in the same bed with other infested persons and occasionally from towels, clothing, or toilet seats. Small children may acquire pubic lice from an infected mother or other members of the household.

As with most STDs, pediculosis pubis is most commonly seen between puberty and middle age. It is more common in women younger than 19 years of age, with the sex distribution reversed over the age of twenty.[31] More than one third of patients may have simultaneous infections with other STDS.[31,32]

Cause and Pathophysiology

Three lice are parasitic for humans: *Pediculus humanus capitis* (head louse), *Pediculus humanus corporis* (body louse), and *Phthirius pubis* (crab louse). All of them have similar anatomic features: are small (0.8–3.0mm), flattened dorsoventrally, and possess 3 pairs of legs, each of which ends in a curved claw used for grasping hairs or clothing fibers.

The pubic louse is broader than it is long (1.2 × 0.8 mm). Its almost square crablike shape contrasts with the elongated appearance of other lice. The crab louse is very sedentary but may occasionally be seen moving slowly on the skin or hairs. It moves by its four hind legs, which cling to two hairs, but do not travel more than 10 cm/day.[33] Pubic lice feed almost continuously on human blood, inserting their mouthparts into skin capillaries. The life of the lice is so dependent on human blood that they rarely survive more than a few days away from a host.

The life cycle of the pubic louse, from egg to egg, is completed in about 25 days. The female begins laying eggs about 24 hours after coitus. The individual egg (nit) is brownish and is glued to the cutaneous exit of the hair with a cementlike material. After incubating for 7–8 days, the nymph is hatched. The nymph undergoes 3 molts within 13–17 days to reach sexual maturity. The life expectancy of the adult female pubic louse is between 25 and 35 days.

Clinical Features

The incubation period is about 30 days.[31] The chief symptom is intense itching in the pubic region, although infestation may be present without the patient noticing it.[34] The mechanism of pruritus is unknown, but some authors suspect an immunologic reaction rather than a mechanical irritation from feeding lice.[35,36] Sensitivity to the effect of louse bites varies with the individual. In previously unexposed persons there may be no symptoms at all, and 5–6 days must pass before sensitization occurs.[37]

The skin lesions consist of small red pruritic papules with central puncta which soon become excoriated and impetiginized. Because of the intense itching, widespread excoriations and crusts can be present. Rarely, some patients may develop characteristic blue-gray spots (maculae ceruleae) seen on the trunk or thighs which persist for several days.[38] They are asymptomatic and do not blanch upon pressure.

Their nature is uncertain, and they are either altered blood pigments or an excretion substance from the louse's salivary glands.[35] Occasionally, scratching of pubic lice bites may lead to secondary infections, mild fever with malaise, lymphadenitis, and/or pyoderma.

The most common site affected is the pubic region, with infestation frequently extending to the hair around the anus and thighs. In hairy individuals, the lice can be found on the chest, arms, beard, and mustache. The involvement of the eyelashes, eyebrows, and periphery of the scalp occurs infrequently but mainly in children who are infested through close contact with the infested mother.[15] Infestation of the scalp by pubic lice is extremely rare, but this has been reported.[39]

Diagnosis

Itching in the pubic region confirmed by finding the motile lice or nits attached to the hair, visible to naked eye (Figure 12.10) or identified with the help of a magnifying lens, is diagnostic for pediculosis pubis. Small rust-colored specks of lice excreta, minute blood spots on the skin or underwear, as well as maculae caeruleae are also diagnostic.

At times, crab lice can escape detection since the adult lice population on an infested person usually numbers fewer than 12.[34] Numerous nits can be seen, and since they grow out with the shaft of the hair, the approximate duration of the infestation can be estimated by their distance from the surface of the skin. (Hair grows approximately 1.2 mm/week.)

Laboratory Diagnosis

Pediculosis pubis is one of the few STDs which can be diagnosed by physical examination only. However, the following laboratory procedure can be helpful.

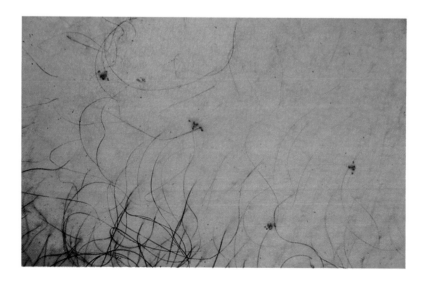

Figure 12.10. Pediculosis pubis: pubic lice attached to the hair in the pubic area.

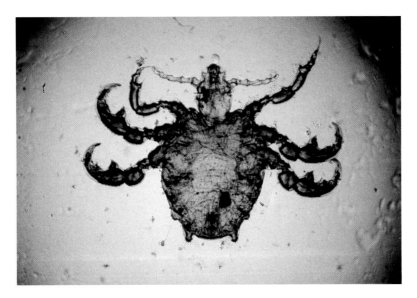

Figure 12.11. The pubic louse has almost a square, crablike appearance.

The lice or nits can be identified microscopically by plucking the hair, placing it in a glass slide containing a drop of mineral oil, covering it with a coverslip, and examining under low power. A broad, crablike body with powerful claws is characteristic for *Phthirius pubis* (Figure 12.11). Nits look like tapered barrels attached to the hair shaft (Figure 12.12).

Differential Diagnosis

- *Seborrheic dermatitis:* in addition to lesions in the pubic region and genitalia there are often scaly erythematous lesions along the hair line, eyebrows, and nasolabial folds; annular eruptions may be seen on the chest or neck

- *Contact dermatitis:* erythematous papulovesicular rash with associated pruritus; common causes of contact dermatitis in anogenital region are intimate deodorants, topical antifungals, spermicides, and hemorrhoid creams (history, patch test)

- *Atopic dermatitis and eczema:* eczematoid lesion in the other parts of the skin; previous history

- *Lichen simplex chronicus:* single, well-circumscribed, or a small number of lichenified scaly papules or plaques; very chronic

- *Tinea corporis:* annular lesions with peripheral scale (KOH test and culture are positive), groins most frequently affected ("jock itch")

- *Psoriasis:* scaly rash over the knees, elbows, back, hairline, and scalp; usually nonpruritic; positive Auspitz and Koebner phenomena; histology

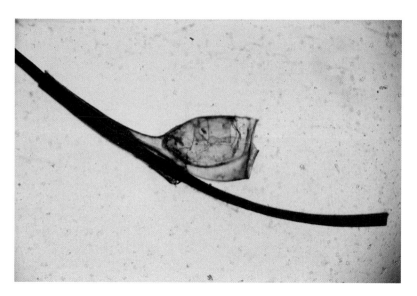

Figure 12.12. A nit attached to the hair shaft.

Treatment

Permethrin (1%) cream applied to affected area and washed off after 10 minutes

Or

Pyrethrins and *piperonyl butoxide* applied to the affected area and washed off after 10 minutes

Or

Lindane 1% shampoo applied for 4 minutes and then thoroughly washed off. (Not recommended for pregnant or lactating women.)

Patients should be reevaluated after a week if symptoms persist. Retreatment is recommended if lice or eggs are found at that time.

Note: In hairy individuals, more widespread application of pediculocide (chiefly to the thighs, chest, and axillary regions) should be considered. At the conclusion of therapy, infested individuals should wear clean underclothes and night clothes.

Clothing and bed linen which may have been contaminated by the patient within the past 2 days should be washed and dried by machine (hot cycle) or dry cleaned.

Special Considerations

Pediculosis of the eyelashes should be managed by the application of occlusive ophthalmic ointment or petrolatum to the eyelid margins twice daily for 8–10 days to smother lice and nits followed by combing with a fine-tooth comb. *Lindane and other pediculocides should not be applied to the eyes.*

Posttreatment Management

Itching often persists for a short time after the lice have been eradicated. Reassurance of patients is very helpful in controlling this problem. Occasionally, oral antipruritics or antihistamines along with topical steroids can be recommended. No resistance of pubic lice to pediculocides has been recorded.[40] If treatment fails, it is usually a result of poor patient compliance or reexposure to an untreated sex partner or another form of reinfestation.

Management of Sex Partners

Sex partners should be treated simultaneously to prevent reinfestation.

Control and Prevention

Effective, simultaneous treatment of the index case and all sex partners and household members is the best way to control pediculosis pubis. Owing to the concomitance of other STDs, careful screening of patients with pediculosis pubis and their sex partners is essential. As a minimum, gonorrhea and *Chlamydia* cultures as well as syphilis blood test are recommended.

REFERENCES

1. Mellanby K: Biology of the parasite, in Orkin M, Maibach HI, Parish LC, Schwartzman RM (eds), *Scabies and Pediculosis.* Philadelphia, Lippincott, 1977, p. 8.
2. Editorial: Whither scabies? *Br Med J* 1:357, 1976.
3. Orkin M: Resurgence of scabies. *JAMA* 217:593–597, 1971.
4. Orkin M: Today's scabies. *JAMA* 233:882–885, 1975.
5. Orkin M, Maibach HI: Scabies, a current pandemic. *Postgrad Med* 66:52–62, 1979.
6. Orkin M, Maibach HI, Holmes KK, et al. (eds): *Scabies in Sexually Transmitted Diseases.* New York, McGraw-Hill, 1984, p. 517.
7. Alexander AM: Role of race in scabies infestations. *Arch Dermatol* 114:627, 1978.
8. Schroeter A: Scabies—A venereal disease, in Orkin M, Maibach HI, Parish LC, Schwartzman RM (eds), *Scabies and Pediculosis.* Philadelphia, Lippincott, 1977, p. 56.
9. Lerche WN, Currier RW, Juranek DD, et al.: Atypical crusted "Norwegian" scabies: Report of nosocomial transmission in a community hospital and approach to control. *Cutis* 31:637–684, 1983.
10. Juranek D, Schultz MG: Epidemiologic investigations of scabies in the U.S., in Orkin M, Maibach HI, Parish LC, Schwartzman RM (eds), *Scabies and Pediculosis.* Philadelphia, Lippincott, 1977, p. 64.
11. Epstein ES, Orkin M: Scabies: Clinical aspects, in Orkin M, Maibach HI, Parish LC, Schwartzman RM (eds), *Scabies and Pediculosis.* Philadelphia, Lippincott, 1977, p. 17.
12. Berge T, Krook G: Persistent nodule in scabies. *Acta Derm Venereol* (Stockh) 47:20–24, 1976.
13. Fischer BF, Warner LC: Cutaneous manifestations of the acquired immunodeficiency syndrome. Update. *Int J Dermatol* 26:615–630, 1987.

14. Espay PD, Jolly HW: Norwegian scabies. *Arch Dermatol* 112;193–196, 1976.

15. Orkin M, Maibach HI: Current views of scabies and pediculosis pubis. *Cutis* 33:85–116, 1984.

16. McMillan TL: Unusual features of scabies associated with topical fluorinated steroids. *Br J Dermatol* 87:496–494, 1972.

17. Hurwitz S: Scabies in babies. *Am J Dis Child* 126:226–228, 1973.

18. Schwartzman RM: Scabies in animals, in Orkin M, Maibach HI, Parish LC, Schwartzman RM (eds), *Scabies and Pediculosis*. Philadelphia, Lippincott, 1977, p. 96.

19. Muller GH: Laboratory diagnosis of scabies, in Orkin M, Maibach HI, Parish LC, Schwartzman RM (eds), *Scabies and Pediculosis*. Philadelphia, Lippincott, 1977, p. 99.

20. Haufe U, Meyer D, Hafe F: Katzenscabies beim Menschen hervorgerufen durch eine an Sarcoptesräude und inchophytie enkrankhte Katze. *Dermatol Wochenschr* 152:977–980, 1966.

21. Chakrabarti A: Human notoedric scabies from contact with cats infested with *Notoedres cati*. *Int J Dermatol* 25:646–648, 1986.

22. Muller G, Jackobs PH, Moore NE: Scraping for human scabies. *Arch Dermatol* 107:70, 1973.

23. Lomholt G: Demonstration of sarcoptes scabiei. *Arch Dermatol* 114:1096, 1978.

24. Martin WE, Wheeler CE Jr: Diagnosis of human scabies by epidermal shave biopsy. *J Am Acad Dermatol* 1:335–337, 1979.

25. Woodley D, Savrot JH: The burrow ink test and the scabies mite. *J Am Acad Dermatol* 4:715–722, 1981.

26. Witkowski JA, Parish LC: Scabies: Subungual area harbor mites. *JAMA* 252:318–319, 1984.

27. Nielsen AO, Secher L, Seier K: Gonorrhoea in patients with scabies. *Br J Vener Dis* 52:394–395, 1976.

28. Beek CH, Mellanby K, Simon RD (eds): Scabies, in *Handbook of Tropical Dermatology and Medical Mycology*. Amsterdam, Elsevier, 1953, p. 875.

29. Nonreported sexually transmissible disease—United States. *MMWR* 28:61–63, 1979.

30. Felman YM, Nikitas JA: Pediculosis pubis. *Cutis* 25:482–559, 1980.

31. Fisher I, Morton RS: Phthirius pubis infestation. *Br J Vener Dis* 46:326–329, 1970.

32. Chapel TA, Katta T, Kuszmar T, et al.: Pediculosis pubis in a clinic for treatment of STD's. *Sex Transm Dis* 6:257–260, 1979.

33. Bushvine JR: Pediculosis: Biology of the parasite, in Orkin M, Maibach HI, Parish LC, Schwartzman RM (eds), *Scabies and Pediculosis*. Philadelphia, Lippincott, 1977, p. 143.

34. Ackerman AB: Crabs—The resurgence of *Phthirius pubis*. *N Engl J Med* 278:950–951, 1968.

35. Alexander J: Scabies and pediculosis. *Practitioner* 200:632–644, 1968.

36. Kraus SJ, Glassman LH: The crab louse: Review of physiology and study of anatomy as seen by the scanning electron microscope. *J Am Vener Dis Assoc* 2:12–18, 1976.

37. Billstein S: Human lice, in Holmes KK, Mardh P-A, Sparling PF, Wiesner PJ (eds), *Sexually Transmitted Diseases*. New York, McGraw-Hill, 1984, p. 513.

38. Miller RAW: Maculae ceruleae. *Cutis* 25:383–384, 1986.

39. Elgart ML, Higdon RS: Pediculosis pubis of the scalp. *Arch Dermatol* 107:916–917, 1973.

40. Schoof HF: The occurrence and distribution of resistance in lice, in *The Control of Lice and Louse-borne Diseases*. Washington DC, 1973, PAHO Scientific Publ. No. 263, p. 223.

13

SEXUALLY TRANSMITTED DISEASES COMMON AMONG HOMOSEXUAL MEN

ENTERIC INFECTONS

Various protozoan, bacterial, viral, and metazoal enteric infections may be transmitted by oral-anal sexual activity (Table 13-1). They are particularly common among homosexual men, but they may occur in heterosexuals practicing orogenital and oral-anal sex.

PROTOZOAN INFECTIONS

Amebiasis

Amebiasis is an infection caused by *Entamoeba histolytica,* a large-bowel parasite of worldwide distribution that is usually associated with poor sanitation and tropical climate and that occurs in travelers returning from tropical areas. Rare urban outbreaks are reported when drinking water is contaminated with raw sewage. During the last decade, a frequent occurrence of amebiasis among homosexual men has been reported.[1-4] The prevalence of sexually acquired amebiasis is not known, but studies of symptomatic gay men showed an 11–27 percent incidence.[5-7]

Infection with *E. histolytica* is acquired mainly by ingestion of the cysts, and oral-anal sexual practices seem to play the major role in the transmission of the

TABLE 13.1. Sexually Transmitted Enteric Infections

Protozoan	Bacterial	Viral	Metazoal
Amebiasis	Shigellosis	Hepatitis A	Enterobiasis
Giardiasis	*Campylobacter enteritis*		Other helminths?
Cryptosporidiosis	Salmonellosis		
Isosporiasis			
Balantidiasis			

disease among homosexuals. Direct infection through the anus is possible (via a shared contaminated enema or via fecally soiled genitalia in group sex situations), but this is probably not the common mode of transmission.

Clinical Manifestations

Following an incubation period of at least 1 week, patients with symptomatic amebiasis present with symptoms ranging from mild diarrhea to severe dysentery; however, fulminant diarrheal disease is rarely encountered in homosexuals. More often the disease is either asymptomatic or with minimal symptoms.[8] Patients with amebiasis usually complain of a change in bowel habits and stool consistency, with both diarrhea and constipation reported. Symptoms vary from increased flatulence, bloating, abdominal cramps, and semiformed stools to the passing of loose or liquid stool, usually several times a day in severe cases. Some patients experience rectal pain, mucus or blood in the stool, and rarely systemic symptoms of fever, prostration, and marked weight loss.

Sigmoidoscopic examination generally reveals normal-appearing rectal mucosa or nonspecific changes, but in about one quarter of patients shallow ulcers with raised and undermined edges can be seen.

Major but rare complications of amebic infection include liver abscess[9], pulmonary abscess, meningitis, peritonitis, and appendicitis.

Genital lesions caused by *E. histolytica* are rare, but they have been decribed on the penis of uncircumcised men[10,11] and on the cervix, vagina, and clitoris in women.[12] Amebiasis of the cervix is characterized by the presence of dark vaginal discharge and ulcerations found on the cervix.[13]

The diagnosis of intestinal amebiasis is made by identifying the trophozoites or cysts in stool specimens (with multiple samples often necessary) or on rectal biopsy. *E. histolytica* can also be cultured from clinical specimen. Various media are in use.

In patients with active intestinal or extraintestinal infection, serologic tests including indirect hemagglutination test (IHA) and precipitation tests may be helpful in establishing the diagnosis, but they are rarely positive in asymptomatic cyst carriers and may remain positive long after the infection has been eradicated. However they are helpful in differentiating inflammatory bowel diseases from amebic colitis. Lately ELISA technic has been employed in detection of amebic infection, however its clinical usefulness has not been established as yet.

Differential Diagnosis

- Other *enteric infections* that occur among homosexual men: stool examination for cysts or trophozoites or bacterial culture should reveal the causative agent.
- Persistent diarrhea in *AIDS:* positive HIV test; other symptoms and signs of AIDS.
- *Irritable bowel syndrome* (funtional disorder): negative stool examination for amebae.
- *Ulcerative colitis, granulomatous colitis, psuedomembranous colitis;* Negative stool examination for amebae; radiologic evidence.
- Gonococcal or chlamydial *proctitis:* positive cultures for *Neisseria gonorrhoeae* or *Chlamydia trachomatis.*
- *LGV:* positive culture for *C. trachomatis,* positive CFT.
- *Primary syphilis:* primary chancre; positive dark-field examination; positive serology.
- *Genital herpes:* vesicle or erosions; positive Tzanck test culture, or other tests.

Treatment

> *Metronidazole,* 750 mg by mouth 3 times daily for 5–10 days
> *Plus*
> *Iodoquinol* (diiodohydroxyquinoline), 650 mg by mouth 3 times daily for 20 days
> (*Diloxanide furoate,* 500 mg by mouth 3 times daily for 10 days, is also effective but is available from the Centers for Disease Control (CDC) only for asymptomatic cyst passers.)

A second choice regimen is *metronidazole* alone, as above, followed by one of the lumenal amebicides if clinical cure is not achieved. The regimen of third choice is *Paromomycin,* 25–30 mg/kg/day in 3 divided doses with meals for 7 days. This drug is used alone. Although it is primarily a lumenal amebicide, it has been noted to exert a superficial tissue effect.

For asymptomatic homosexual male amebic cyst passers, treatment may not be required, or they may be treated with one of the aforementioned regimens. For patients with recurrent or persistent disease, erythromycin, tetracycline, or chloroquine in combination with any of the above drugs except paromomycin should be considered.

Severe colitis or extraintestinal amebiasis should prompt appropriate medical consultation and referral.

Dientamoeba fragilis is another intestinal ameba virulent to humans. Whether infections caused by this protozoan are more frequent in the homosexual community needs to be proved. However, the parasite lives in the cecum and may also be found in the large intestine. Oral-anal sex can with certainty be the route of infection among persons practicing this form of sex. *Dientamoeba fragilis* is asymptomatic in most individuals but may also produce anal pruritus and gastrointestinal symptoms such as nausea, vomiting, and diarrhea. Thus, infection caused by *D. fragilis* should be included in the differential diagnosis of enteric infections in homosexual men. Treatment is as for *E. histolytica*.[14,15]

Giardiasis

Similar to amebiasis, giardiasis is now recognized as a sexually transmitted enteric infection among homosexual men.[6,16-19] The disease is caused by a pear-shaped motile protozoan *Giardia lamblia* that lives in the human duodenum and jejunum. It is estimated the *G. lamblia* is the most common enteric protozoan pathogen isolated within the United States today. The trophozoite is normally attached to the small-bowel epithelial wall where it feeds. The cyst is the infective stage and is transmitted by the fecal-oral route.

Giardiasis is endemic in many countries where sanitary conditions are inadequate. It is usually found in family clusters, among children living in institutions, and among children and adults living in communal groups.[20] The mode of transmission in these settings is probably from contaminated hand to mouth. The disease has been also found in people following exposure to the waters of lakes and mountain streams infected by wild animal reservoirs.[21] Several outbreaks of giardiasis have been reported to be due to inadequate water filtration facilities.[22,23]

Sexually transmitted giardiasis is slightly less frequent than amebiasis,[6,24] and both diseases share the same sexual epidemiologic risk. Simultaneous infections with *G. lamblia* and *E. histolytica* are not uncommon.[6,17]

The major mode of sexual transmissions is via oral-anal sex (primarily anilingus) or fellatio following anal intercourse. Unlike in amebiasis, host factors play an important role. Susceptibility to *G. lambilia* is increased in persons with gastric achlorhydria and hypogammaglobulinemia. Moreover, deficiency of IgA in the intestinal lumen is associated with increased severity of symptoms.

Clinical Manifestations

The incubation period of giardiasis ranges from 1 to 8 weeks (average about 2 weeks). Infectivity, however, precedes the onset of symptoms by several days. Patients may be asymptomatic or may experience upper gastrointestinal symptoms which include epigastric distress, nausea, vomiting, crampy abdominal pains, and foul sulfuric eructation. The typical history for giardiasis is abrupt onset of watery, foul-smelling diarrhea without mucus or blood in the stool. Bloating, flatulence, anorexia, and fatigue may be also present. The disease is usually self-limited, lasting several days to several weeks. In chronic giardiasis, patients experience recurrence of low-grade symptoms separated by periods of normalcy.

Diagnosis

The diagnosis of giardiasis is dependent upon finding the cysts or trophozoites in stool. Since cyst excretion is intermittent, a single stool examination may be inadequate. In patients with repeated negative stool examination but clinically suspected cases, either duodenal aspirate, jejunal biopsy, or a string (Enterotest,

Hedeco, Palo Alto, CA) passed into the duodenum may be necessary to confirm the diagnosis.

It has been suggested that, in some instances, treatment may be given on the basis of presumptive findings without confirmation of the diagnosis by demonstration of pathogen. In recent years several serologic tests have been developed including indirect fluorescent antibody test (IFA), immuno-diffusion test and enzyme-linked immunosorbent (ELISA) assey. All of them can be very useful in detecting *Giardia lamblia* but have not been routinely used as yet.

Differential Diagnosis

Differential diagnosis includes many of the conditions listed under the differential diagnosis of amebiasis. In the case of chronic giardiasis with weight loss and signs of malabsorption, the other causes of malabsorption should be considered: *celiac sprue* (gluten enteropathy), which usually begins in childhood, or *tropical sprue,* which can be confirmed by the fact of recent travel to tropical countries.

Treatment

The drug of choice for symptomatic and asymptomatic infection is *quinacrine,* 100 mg by mouth 3 times daily for 7 days. An alternative regimen is *metronidazole,* 250 mg by mouth 3 times daily for 7 days. In the case of coexistent symptomatic amebiasis and giardiasis, metronidazole in the higher dose may be preferred.

Initial treatment of asymptomatic carriers is indicated. Retreatment for recurrences, either from relapse or reinfection, should depend on individual and epidemiologic circumstances.

Cryptosporidiosis

Cryptosporidium has been regarded for a long time as a opportunistic microorganism, whereas now it is recognized as an important gastrointestinal pathogen causing enteric infections worldwide. *Cryptosporidium* is acquired mainly by ingestion of its oocysts from contaminated water or food products. Similar to other protozoan intestinal pathogens, it can be probably acquired by oral-anal sex.

Clinical manifestations depend a great deal on the immunologic status of the host. In normal patients infection with *Cryptosporidium* results in watery diarrhea with abdominal discomfort and at times nausea and anorexia, whereas in immunocompromised patients, e.g., with AIDS, the disease is more severe. Frequently, the latter develop severe watery diarrhea with subsequent loss of fluids and electrolytes. Severe abdominal cramps and fever are not uncommon. The diagnosis of cryptosporidosis depends upon finding the oocysts in stool. No effective treatment is available as yet. In immunologically healthy persons the disease last for 1−3 weeks followed by full recovery. Immunocompromised patients may require oral or intravenous hydration to replace the loss of fluids.

Isosporiasis

Isospora is another coccidian protozoan capable of infecting the gastrointestinal tract in animals and humans. Three species were found in humans: *Isospora belli, I. hominis,* and *I. natalensis.* In most instances the disease is acquired by ingestion of oocysts with contaminated water or food. It can be also transmitted through oral-anal sex, particularly in homosexual men.[25]

In immunologically healthy persons, isosporiasis is usually asymptomatic and self-limited, whereas in immunocompromised patients it may produce abdominal pain, watery diarrhea, steatorrhea, fever, and weight loss. Diagnosis is established by finding oocysts or sporocysts in the feces. Treatment includes oral administration of trimethoprim-sulfametoxazole, 160/800 mg B.I.D. for 10 days.[26]

Balantidiasis

Balantidum coli is the only ciliate protozoan pathogenic for humans. The infection is usually acquired by ingestion of cysts in contaminated water or food, but oral-anal sex should be also considered as a means of infection, especially in homosexual men. Similar to other protozoan enteric infections, clinical manifestations depend on the immunologic status of the host. In persons with an intact immune system, *Balantidium coli* may reside in the bowel without producing any symptoms. In other individuals, it may cause chronic diarrhea alternating with constipation and intestinal ulcerations similar to those caused by amebiasis, complicated by perforations and peritonitis.[27] In immuncompromised patients fulminant dysentery may occur with watery stools (occasionally with blood) with subsequent loss of fluids and weight.

Diagnosis depends on demonstration of *B. coli* (trophozoites) or cysts in stool specimens or in scrapings of rectal lesions. Treatment is as for amebiasis.

BACTERIAL INFECTIONS

Shigellosis

Shigellosis is an enteric infection caused by the bacteria of the genus *Shigella.* In the United States, mainly two *Shigella* spp. account for most infections: *Shigella sonnei* and *Shigella flexneri.* Shigellosis is commonly recognized in outbreaks, usually in places where crowding and substandard sanitary conditions occur. The disease is frequently recognized in prisons, refugee camps, and among persons in mental institutions as well as in travelers in endemic areas.

Transmission of the disease is person-to-person (humans are the principal vector). Among homosexual men, shigellosis is frequently acquired by oral-anal or oral-genital contact.[28] *Shigella* are highly infectious and are considered the most common cause of bacterial dysentery seen in homosexually active men[29]: they were found in 3% of intestinal infections in homosexual men.[19] In the mid-1970s in Seattle, 30% of all cases of shigellosis occurred in homosexual men, and at about the same time in New York Metropolitan Hospital, gay men comprised almost half of the cases of shigellosis among adult men.[28,30]

Clinical Manifestations

The clinical presentation of shigellosis may vary from a mild afebrile diarrheal illness to a systemic, life-threatening infection. It also may be entirely asymptomatic. It usually begins abruptly, following a 36-hour to 3-day incubation period, with high fever, chills, abdominal cramps, and watery diarrhea. In mild cases, it resolves completely but may also develop into dysentery with severe cramps and proctitis accompanied by tenesmus and bloody mucoid rectal discharge. Some patients may complain of myalgias involving the lower back and thighs. Sigmoidoscopic examination may reveal hyperemic friable mucosa and occasionally multiple small, shallow ulcers with a mucopurulent exudate.

Untreated shigellosis is self-limited, with symptoms resolving over approximately 1 week. The main complications include dehydration and electrolyte imbalance.

Diagnosis

The diagnosis of shigellosis is made by the presence of a positive stool culture. A rectal swab should be rapidly inoculated into the appropriate media and transported to the laboratory without delay to prevent loss of viability of the *Shigella*. A gram-stained smear of a rectal swab in shigellosis usually reveals polymorphonuclear leukocytes, erythrocytes, and macrophages, elements which are not generally present in toxin-induced diarrhea.

Treatment

Treatment consists of correcting fluid and electrolyte losses and administration of specific antimicrobials. The recommended treatment in the United States includes

Trimethoprim-sulfamethoxazole, 160/800 mg by mouth twice daily for 7 days
Or
Ampicillin, 500 mg by mouth 4 times daily for 7 days

Since resistance of *Shigella* spp. to several antimocrobials has been observed, the choice of antibiotic should be based on the sensitivity pattern of the isolate. This is particularly important in case of treatment failures or recurrences.

Campylobacter Enteritis

Campylobacter jejuni is a pathogen causing enteritis in humans. It has been suggested that this microorganism is a more frequent cause of bacterial diarrhea than *Shigella* or *Salmonella*.[31] Transmission of the disease in homosexual men is via the fecal-oral route. In this population, *Campylobacter* may produce colitis as well as proctitis.[19]

Campylobacter enteritis presents with a sudden onset of fever, chills, and abdominal cramps followed by diarrhea. Infection may also cause symptoms of proctitis, with anorectal pain, tenesmus, and mucopurulent or bloody discharge. Bloody diarrhea is present in about half of the cases.

Diagnosis

The diagnosis is based upon recovery of *Campylobacter jejuni* from stool specimens.

Treatment

Although campylobacter enteritis is a self-limited infection, administration of *erythromycin*, 0.5 g by mouth 4 times daily for 7 days, may shorten the clinical course of the disease. Other antibiotics to which *Campylobacter jejuni* is sensitive include: clindamycin or chloramphenicol and gentamycin.

Salmonella Enteritis

Salmonella has been mentioned as a sexually transmitted pathogen causing enteric infection. The fecal to oral route may be the mode of infection among homosexual men. The disease begins within 2 days following infection with fever, chills, nausea, vomiting, and abdominal pain and diarrhea. The range of symptoms is from asymptomatic cases to severe dysentery.

Diagnosis is confirmed by growing the microorganism on appropriate culture.

Treatment is primarily supporting, and no antibiotic is required for uncomplicated symptomatic infections caused by nontyphoidal *Salmonella* species.

VIRAL INFECTIONS

Hepatitis A

Hepatitis A is an enteric infection caused by a small RNA picornavirus classified as enterovirus type 27.[32] The disease is worldwide in distribution, and the frequency of exposure to the virus is related to levels of personal hygiene in the given country.[33] It is estimated that more than half of Americans over 50 years of age have evidence of previous hepatitis A infection, and the prevalence of antibody markers is higher among lower socioeconomic groups and among foreign-born U.S. citizens.[34]

Hepatitis A often occurs in clusters, and the local outbreaks are usually traceable to contaminated water or food. However, transmission by other sources is also possible, since the outbreak frequently occurs among members of a family or within institutions (mental, day care, and military).[35-37]

Similar to other enteric infections, hepatitis A may be sexually transmitted. Several studies have shown a significantly higher incidence of hepatitis A virus infections in homosexuals than in heterosexuals.[38-40] Spread of hepatitis A virus between individuals is primarily via fecal-oral transmissions; the risk of parenteral transmission is extremely low, since viremia is brief and there is no blood-borne carrier state. The frequent practice of anilingus and fellatio among homosexually active men make this population more vulnerable to this infection than other groups. Other risk factors associated with sexually transmitted hepatitis A include duration of homosexuality, number of lifetime sex partners, and frequency of oral-anal exposure.[38,40,41]

Clinical Features

Most cases of hepatitis A are subclinical, and only a small proportion of persons (probably less than 10 percent) who have antibodies recall a compatible illness. The incubation period ranges from 15 to 50 days, with a mean of 33 days. Transient viremia is present during the late incubation period and acute phases. Characteristically, the disease begins with a sudden onset although there may be a prodromal period with flu like symptom, including low-grade fever, malaise, myalgias, nausea, and vomiting. Anorexia is prominent, and patients lose their taste for food. Some of them may develop diarrhea, arthralgias, and skin rashes. Dark urine and light-colored stools generally precede the development of jaundice. When jaundice appears, hepatomegaly and tenderness to palpation in the right upper quadrant of the abdomen may be detected. Serum aminotransferase enzymes (SGOT and SGPT) are significantly elevated. Serum immunoglobulin levels are usually normal, except IgM level, which may be doubled during the course of the disease. Bilirubin level is variably elevated, with a direct-indirect ratio of 1:1. Jaundice usually lasts for 1–2 weeks, and aminotransferase levels return to normal within 5–6 weeks. Most patients recover clinically within a few weeks.

Patients become contagious in the second half of the incubation period, and the fecal shedding of the hepatitis A virus persists up to about 10 days after the onset of jaundice. There is no prolonged carrier stage reported so far, and it seems that one infection produced solid immunity, so reinfection is not considered possible.

Fulminant hepatitis.   Fulminant hepatitis is a rare complication which proceeds to liver necrosis which may be fatal and hepatitis A account for less than 10 percent of this complication. It is characterized by a rapidly rising bilirubin level, severe hypoalbuminemia, and prolonged prothrombin time, which may result in a hemorrhagic diathesis. Liver atrophy may occur (acute yellow atrophy) which progresses to encephalopathy and coma. The reasons why certain individuals develop fulminant hepatitis are unknown, and it is believed that certain defects in the immune system may play an important role in the pathology of this complication. Fulminant hepatitis is more common following hepatitis B virus infection.

Diagnosis

Hepatitis A is usually diagnosed clinically and can be confirmed by detecting specific IgM antihepatitis A antibodies.

For differential diagnosis see Table 13-2.

Treatment

Treatment of hepatitis A is supportive. The patient may be treated on an outpatient basis with rest, adequate nutrition, and avoidance of alcohol and potentially hepatoxic drugs. Frequent small feedings are recommended as is a diet low in fat and high in carbohydrates.

Homosexual men should be advised to refrain from any sexual activities until the acute symptomatic phase has passed.

Prophylaxis

Preexposure or postexposure (within 2 weeks of appearance of symptoms in the index case) administration of immune serum globulin (ISG) intramuscularly is effective in about 80–90 percent of cases.[42,43] The recommended dose for adults is 0.02–0.05 ml/kg of body weight.

METAZOAL INFECTIONS

Enterobiasis

Enterobiasis is a common infection in children caused by *Enterobius vermicularis* (pinworm), an intestinal pathogen. Whereas in children the disease is transmitted by the hand-oral route, the oral-anal route may be the mode of transmission among sexually active gay men. Intense rectal itching is the most common symptom associated with enterobiasis. In a gay man presenting with anal pruritus enterobiasis should be considered in differential diagnosis.

Diagnosis is made by demonstration of worms or their eggs with the cellophane tape impressions from the perianal folds.

Treatment requires administration of *mebendazole* (available under the tradename Vermox), 100 mg (1 tablet) by mouth in a single dose which can be repeated after 2–3 weeks, or *pyrantel pamoate* (available under the tradename Combantrin), 11 mg/kg (maximum 0.1 g) by mouth in a single dose which can be repeated after 2–3 weeks.

Enterobius vermicularis is not the only metazoan which can be transmitted through oral-anal sex; the same practices may facilitate the spread of other helminths.[44]

HEPATITIS B

Hepatitis B is a sexually transmitted disease caused by DNA hepatitis B virus (HBV), also called "Dane particle" after its discoverer. Typically, the virus does not affect organs other than the liver. The disease can be transmitted through both heterosexual and homosexual intercourse but is more prevalent among homosexuals. Synonyms for hepatitis B are serum hepatitis, posttransfusion hepatitis, inoculation hepatitis, and homologous serum hepatitis.

Epidemiology

Hepatitis B occurs worldwide. According to the CDC, about 200,000 new cases occur annually in the United States, and there are more than half a million carriers of the virus.[45] The prevalence of hepatitis B antibodies among the U.S. population is higher among Blacks and persons of oriental ancestry and increases with age and lower socioeconomic status. The disease is more frequent among spouses and household members of carriers of the virus and among health care workers, including nurses, laboratory technicians, and physicians, with surgeons and dentists being a group at special risk.[46-48] Sexually transmitted hepatitis B is more prevalent among homosexuals and prostitutes.

The precise mechanism of hepatitis B infection is not clear: however, viral antigens have been identified in a number of body fluids, including serum, menstrual blood, urine, semen, vaginal fluid, breast milk, and tears. The parenteral transmission occurs by transfusion, vaccination, hemodialysis, needles shared among drug abusers, accidental needle sticks, acupuncture, ear-piercing, tatooing, and dental procedures. Since the early 1970s, several authors have suggested sexual transmission of the disease.[49-52] Confirmation of this hypothesis was accomplished by a series of studies which demonstrated that the prevalence of hepatitis B antigen and its antibody among sexually transmitted disease (STD) clinic patients was much higher than among control groups.[40,53,54] These and other studies have also revealed that the majority of patients with positive tests were homosexual men.[40,49,52-56] Further evidence for sexual transmission of hepatitis B was provided by investigation conducted among prostitutes, which revealed a higher prevalence of hepatitis B antigen[57] and antihepatitis B virus antibodies among them than in control groups.[57,58]

Two large studies conducted a few years ago under the auspices of the CDC shed more light on the sexual transmission of hepatitis B among homosexual men.[59,60] The results indicated that two variables were most significantly related to hepatitis B infection: duration of homosexual activity and the number of nonsteady partners. Another important finding related to homosexual practices was that the orogenital sexual activity, whether passive or active, and regardless of whether ejaculation or swallowing of semen took place, was not associated with an increased risk for infection. The three most important factors were (1) passive anogenital intercourse, (2) active oral-anal sex, and (3) rectal douching.[60] All of these practices involve contact with the rectal mucosa, suggesting that the trauma to rectal mucosa which may occur during intercourse provides both the source of infection as well as a portal of entry for hepatitis B virus. Other investigators noted the presence of hepatitis B surface antigen in lesions of the rectal mucosa in a majority of homosexual men with a positive recent history of receptive anal intercourse.[61] They suggested that these asymptomatic punctate bleeding sites may provide portals for the parenteral infection of hepatitis B virus into the receptive partner and also provide infectious serum that could infect the inserting partner through a microscopic penile lesion or the urethra.

Clinical Features

The clinical spectrum of hepatitis B ranges from inapparent disease to fulminant hepatitis resulting in death. The age of the patients, their general health, the presence of underlying liver diseases, or alterations in patient immunologic status (altered T-cell functions) may influence the course of the disease.[62]

Following the incubation period, which ranges from 30 to 180 days (average is 90 days), there is usually a prodromal phase with constitutional symptoms and signs. Unlike hepatitis A, prodromal symptoms are vague and insidious and include fever, anorexia, nausea, malaise, and fatigue lasting from several days to several weeks. Ten to 20 percent of patients develop a transient serum sickness–like reaction caused by the appearance of anti–hepatitis B virus antibodies and the formation of immune complexes occurring during the preicteric phase; lasting 7–12 days, and usually resolving with the onset of jaundice. The rash is typically urticarial, with pruritic hives appearing in a peripheral distribution. Macular or maculopapular lesions can occur as well as irregular patches of erythema. A migratory and nondeforming arthritis occurs, but arthralgias without arthritis are probably more common. As these symptoms abate, jaundice appears, making the clinical diagnosis apparent. The clinical features of hepatitis B are similar to those of hepatitis A, except that hepatitis B appears to be a more serious disease, has a more prolonged course, and is more likely to progress to a chronic disease. The mechanism of recovery from the disease is unknown, but recovery is almost always accompanied by complete resistance to reinfection. Chronic hepatitis occurs in 10–15 percent of patients, and the factors associated with chronicity are long incubation period, mild infection, nonparenteral acquisition of infection, immunosuppression, and genetic predisposition.

Chronic hepatitis is diagnosed when hepatic inflammation lasts more than 6 months. There are two types of chronic hepatitis: chronic persistent and chronic active hepatitis, both HBsAg positive.

Chronic Persistent Hepatitis

Most homosexual men, chronic carriers of HBsAg, have chronic persistent hepatitis (CPH).[63] Patients with this form of chronic hepatitis are usually asymptomatic but may have mild liver enzyme abnormalities that continue for years. Minimal hepatomegaly is common, and splenomegaly may be present. Liver biopsy shows spotty panlobular inflammation characterized by periportal mononuclear cell infiltrates. CPH is almost always a self-limited disease, with good prognosis for recovery. Liver fibrosis is not seen.

Chronic Active Hepatitis

About 5 percent of patients with acute hepatitis B infection develop chronic active hepatitis (CAH).[64] The most common symptoms are anorexia, weakness, and vague abdominal symptoms. Occasionally, serum-sickness–like syndrome has been observed with urticarial and macular skin lesions. In severe cases, spider angioma may be also present. Clinical signs include hepatomegaly, splenomegaly, and abdominal tenderness. Serum transaminases may be persistently elevated, and serum bilirubin and alkaline phosphatase levels may be increased. Jaundice is not uncommon. Liver biopsy shows cell necrosis with lobular regeneration and fibrosis. In severe cases, cirrhosis and liver failure may occur. This predisposes the infected person to liver cancer.[65,66] For information on fulminant hepatitis see p. 285.

Serologic Diagnosis

The diagnosis of hepatitis B can be established by the presence of HBsAg in serum. The detection of IgM anti-HBcAg and elevation of serum transaminase confirms the acute infection. HBs antigen can be detected with several methods, including radioimmunoassay and enzyme-linked immunosorbent assay and IgM anti-HBcAg is best detected by antibody capture immunoassay. HBsAg is present in the serum 30–50 days after exposure and 1–3 weeks prior to the onset of jaundice. HBsAg may disappear with the onset of jaundice, or it may presist for several weeks. Anti-HBsAg appears during convalesence and 1–3 months after HBsAg has cleared. The peak usually occurs about 6 months after exposure and then gradually decreases. Anti-HBcAg appears during the clinical phase of the disease, peaking at the beginning of recovery and then subsiding faster than anti-HBs. The finding of HBsAg with or without anti-HBc denotes active illness, whereas the presence of anti-HBc alone is suggestive of an early period of convalescence. The presence of anti-HBc and anti-HBs confirms recent infection, whereas the finding of anti-HBs alone implies more remote disease and full recovery. Unlike hepatitis A, a prolonged carrier state for hepatitis B exists, occurring in 6 and 10 percent of patients, with perhaps a greater prevalence among homosexual men.

Differential Diagnosis

- *Hepatitis A:* See Table 13-2.

- *Alcoholic liver disease:* history of prolonged (usually more than 10 years) alcohol intake; WBC count elevated with a left shift, low albumin level, and prolonged prothrombin time; SGOT levels elevated out of proportion to the SGPT level (which is usually normal or even low); negative tests for hepatitis B antigens and antibodies. If the clinical, biochemical, and serological picture is unclear, liver biopsy may be helpful.

- *Cholestatic liver disease:* history of gall bladder or liver problems; prominent symptoms and signs of cholestasis (jaundice, light-colored stools, itching); modest abnormalities in aminotransferase level but significant elevation in alkaline phosphatase levels; leukocytosis with a left shift; negative tests for HBAg and antibodies.

- *Drug-related acute hepatitis:* history of recent intake of drugs or anaesthesia; negative test for HBAg and/or antibodies. Many drugs may induce hepatic injury; the most common causes of drug-related hepatitis in the United States are aspirin, acetaminophen, isoniazid, rifampin, alpha methyldopa, and halothane. Liver biopsy may be necessary.

- *Hepatitis due to other infectious agents:* Elevations in serum enzyme levels and liver disfunction can occur in many infectious diseases due to viruses, bacteria, mycobacteria, ricketsia, and fungi. They can be distinguished by other symptoms and signs and the presence of a positive specific serologic test or demonstration of the microorganisms by a variety of laboratory methods.

TABLE 13.2. Epidemiological and Clinical Features of Viral Hepatitis

	Hepatitis A	*Hepatitis B*	*Non A and Non B*
Incubation period	15–50 days (mean = 30)	30–180 days (mean = 90)	15–150 days (mean = 50)
Sexual transmission	In homosexuals (fecal to oral route)	In homosexuals and spouses (contact with semen and menstrual blood; rectal and penile microtraumas	Probable but not documented
Parenteral transmission	Rare	Common	Common
Onset	Sudden	Insidious	Insidious
Severity	Mild	Mild to severe	Mild to severe
Skin and joint symptoms	Rarely occur	Occur in about 20% of cases	Rarely occur
Fever	Frequently occurs	May occur	May occur
Nausea and vomiting	Frequently occur	May occur	May occur
Prognosis	Benign	More severe in older age	Better than in hepatitis B
Chronic hepatitis	No	May occur	Occur
Fulminant hepatitis	Very rare	May occur	May occur
Duration	1–3 weeks	1–2 months	1–2 months
Mortality	<0.5%	2%	Low

Treatment and Prevention

There is no specific treatment for hepatitis B other than supportive (see treatment of hepatitis A). The effect of interferon and viral DNA inhibitors in some forms of hepatitis B are being investigated, and so far prevention seems to be the best management. Passive immunization with hyperimmune hepatitis B immunoglobulin (HBIG) and active immunization with hepatitis B vaccine (HB vaccine) are presently available. According to CDC recommendations,[67] HBIG should be given to susceptible individuals (no antibodies to HBsAg or HBcAg) who have had sexual contact with an HBsAg-positive person within 14 days of the last sexual contact.

HB vaccine is recommended for sexual and household contacts of hepatitis B carriers, homosexual males and health care workers with exposure to blood or blood products. It should be also considered for promiscuous heterosexuals, men and women (including prostitutes), inmates of correctional facilities and travelers to hepatitis B endemic areas.

Several studies have demonstrated that simultaneous HBIG administration does not interfere with the immune response to HB vaccine and that a combination of HB vaccine and HBIG results in immediate and sustained high levels of antibodies to hepatitis B.[68,69]

For needle-stick, ocular, or mucous-membrane exposure to blood containing HBsAg, a single dose of HBIG (0.06 ml/kg body weight or 5.0 ml for adults) should be administered shortly after exposure (preferably within 24–48 hours). HB vaccine, 20 μg/1.0 ml should be given intramuscularly at a separate site simultaneously with HBIG and then repeated 1 and 6 months later. HB vaccine combined with HBIG appears to be effective in preventing hepatitis B infection in infants of HBsAg-positive mothers.[69-72]

Hepatitis B in Neonates

Perinatal hepatitis B virus infections are well documented.[69,71,73-76] While transplacental infections have been reported, most infections occur during parturition or shortly thereafter. Intrafamilial spread and transmission by transfusion of contaminated blood have been also reported.

The frequency of transmission from asymptomatic mothers, carriers of HBsAg, is relatively low in western countries,[74,77] while in Asia where the carrier stage is more common, 30–40 percent of chronic carriers transmit hepatitis B virus to their newborn infants.[75,78] The risk of transmission is higher when women develop acute hepatitis B during the third trimester of pregnancy. Approximately 75 percent of babies born to these mothers become HBsAg-positive in the first 2 months postpartum.[73-75]

Several investigators reported the importance of HBeAg for vertical transmission of the disease. HBeAg-positive mothers have high levels of virus and are more likely to transmit it to their offspring.[69,79,80] The majority of infants born to HBeAg-positive mothers become infected with hepatitis B virus during the first year of life and become chronic HBsAg carriers.

The course of perinatal hepatitis B infection varies. Clinical illness is relatively infrequent, and only about 10 percent of newborns become icteric at 3–4 months of age. Most infants have no signs of acute infection but may demonstrate mildly elevated liver enzyme levels, which generally resolve. A few infants develop chronic persistent, chronic active, or fulminant hepatitis.

Diagnosis

Diagnosis of hepatitis B in a newborn is made by demonstration of HBsAg in the blood. Liver biopsy may show unresolved hepatitis.

Prevention

Children born to women who developed acute hepatitis B during pregnancy or who are HBeAg-positive at term should be given a single 0.5 ml dose of HBIG the day of birth that is repeated at 3 months and at 6 months. Recent studies, however, suggest that combined prophylaxis with HGIB and hepatitis B vaccine is most effective.[69-72]

Non-A/Non-B Hepatitis

An acute viral hepatitis syndrome in which evidence of hepatitis A and hepatitis B cannot be found is defined as non-A/non-B hepatitis. Non-A/non-B hepatitis is probably caused by at least two different viruses with different modes of spread.[81] The first type, which seems to be the most common type of non-A/non-B hepatitis, is epidemologically similar to hepatitis B and accounts for more than 70 percent of posttransfusion hepatitis in North America and Europe.[82] The disease is a form of what used to be called "post-transfusion hepatitis", (NANB-P) and parenteral transmission seems to be the principal mode of infection. The second type, called enterically transmitted non-A/non-B (NANB-E) hepatitis, is transmitted by the fecal-oral route and has caused large outbreaks in Southern Asia,[83,84] Africa,[85] the Soviet Union,[86] and recently, Mexico.[87] Although person-to-person transmission may take place, sexual transmission, which is most likely in homosexuals conducting oral-anal sex, has not been reported as yet. As with other outbreaks of enteric infection, contaminated water seems to be the source of infection.[87]

The incubation period of hepatitis non-A/non-B ranges from 15 to 150 days and averages 50 days. The clinical severity seems to be between that of hepatitis A and hepatitis B, and the patients are at least as prone to develop chronic hepatitis as patients with type B virus infections.[88]

Diagnosis

Diagnosis of non-A/non-B hepatitis requires serologic testing that excludes hepatitis A and B. Diagnosis of NANB-E can be confirmed by immune electron microscopy (IEM) identification of 23−34 nm viruslike particles in stools of acutely ill patients. Other causes of acute hepatitis should be also excluded (Epstein-Barr virus [EBV], cytomegalovirus, drugs, alcohol, cholestatitic liver disease (see page 289).

Treatment

Similar to hepatitis A and B, there is no specific treatment for non-A/non-B hepatitis. Supportive therapy consists of a high-protein high-carbohydrate diet and avoidance of alcohol and hepatotoxic drugs. Compulsory bed rest is not required, but adequate rest is recommended. Whether immunoserum globulin (ISG) is effective in prevention of non-A/non-B hepatitis is not clear. Since a chronic carrier stage is probable, patients should be instructed about such a possibility.

Hepatitis D

Hepatitis D is caused by the hepatitis virus (HDV) which is a dependent RNA form that requires a simultaneous presence of hepatitis B virus (HBV) for its survival. Thus, HDV infects only individuals who are either HBV carriers (superinfection) or infection may occur simultaneously with hepatitis B virus (coinfection) in an individual who was previously susceptible to hepatitis B virus.

Clinically, hepatitis D virus infection is a more severe and aggressive disease than hepatitis B alone with more patients developing fulminant disease or chronic liver disease or dying as a result of liver damage. The diagnosis is dependent upon demonstration of anti-HD antibodies in serum.

Transmission of HDV is associated with intravenous drug abuse and receipt of contaminated blood or blood products. The question whether hepatitis D virus can be sexually transmitted remains to be answered. However, a recent survey revealed that in Los Angeles and San Francisco HBsAg positive homosexual men have a high prevalence (9 to 15 percent) of anti-HD antibodies. This finding was correlated with sexual promiscuity as well as intravenous drug use.[89]

There is no specific means for prevention of hepatitis D although immunization with hepatitis B vaccine (see p. 290) provides protection by preventing the necessary helper virus infection.

CYTOMEGALOVIRUS INFECTION

Cytomegalovirus (CMV) belongs to the herpes virus group, which also includes herpes simplex virus, varicella-zoster virus, and Epstein-Barr virus. It is morphologically indistinguishable from the remaining members of the group and like them possesses the ability to remain latent or persistent in the host following infection. CMV is distributed worldwide, and most people become infected during the course of their lifetime. In developing countries, the prevalence of antibodies to CMV approaches 100 percent already in early childhood, while in the United States and other industrialized countries, the rate of childhood infection is lower and appears to be associated with increased age. A rise in the prevalence of antibodies to CMV was observed in patients between 15 and 35 years of age,[90-92] and it has been suggested that sexual transmission is to be blamed for at least a portion of this acquisition of CMV by this group of people.[93-95] The infection with CMV may be congenital, acquired at the time of delivery, or acquired later in life. Some people may acquire the virus as a result of blood transfusions or transplantation of organs or bone marrow. Sexual intercourse is only one of many and probably not the main route of infection in heterosexual population, however, there is increasing evidence that the sexual transmission may play an important role in the spreading of CMV.[91,93,96]

The virus has been recovered from many body sites, including the cervix, oropharynx, and urinary tract and was detected in oral, urogenital, and other secretions such as saliva, urine, feces, spermatic fluid, cervical secretions, and breast milk as well as in blood lymphocytes.[97-99]

CMV infection may occur with other sexually transmitted diseases[95,96], was found among the sex partners of infected persons[100] and has been linked to homosexuality.[94,101-104] It has been noted that the sex partners of women with CMV infection are more likely to be positive or shed virus than the partners of uninfected women and that infected sex partners frequently share the same CMV strains, as determined by DNA restriction-enzyme typing.[100] There is also data which suggest that the prevalence of CMV infection is much higher among homosexual men than their heterosexual counterparts.[94,103,104] The prevalence of CMV antibodies measured among homosexual and heterosexual men, patients of one of San Francisco's VD clinics, and among male volunteer blood donors used as a control group was 93.5, 54.3, and 42.7 percent respectively. In the same study, urinary excretion of CMV was observed in 14 of 190 homosexual patients but not in heterosexual men. What is even more interesting is that all patients with viuria were younger than 30 years of age.[94] Homosexual men who excrete CMV frequently have a lower mean ratio of T-helper to T-suppressor cells than control groups.[105-107] Based on this observation, it was suggested that CMV may act as a cofactor in the pathogenesis of AIDS.[108,109] These and other data clearly suggest that sexual contact may be an important mode of acquisition of CMV among adults and that homosexual men are exposed to CMV at an earlier age[94,104] and may be at greater risk for CMV infection than heterosexual men. Whether the latter should be attributed to the greater sexual promiscuity observed among gay men[102,110] or certain sexual behavior[101,110] or to other factors remains to be determined.

Clinical Manifestations

Congenital Infection

The clinical spectrum of intrauterine infection is quite broad and varies from inapparent or asymptomatic (95 percent) infections to a fulminant disease ranging from isolated organ involvement to the multiorgan system dysfunction which may result although rarely, in death.[99,111] The major feature of CMV infection includes hepatomegaly, splenomegaly, jaundice, petechiae, or purpuric exanthem, microcephaly and motor disabilities, chorioretinitis, cerebral calcifications, and thrombocytopenia. Other manifestations include low birth weight, failure to thrive, mental retardation, and deafness. The prognosis for subsequent development for babies in whom disease is clinically apparent at birth is rather poor, since many of them suffer from severe mental retardation. The prognosis for asymptomatic infants is much better; however, hearing loss and subnormal intelligence was noted among these children.[112,113]

Perinatal and Postnatal Infection

The newborn may become infected during the passage through the infected birth canal or the virus may be transmitted through breast milk. The vast majority of infants will remain asymptomatic, and those who are symptomatic may present with pneumonitis, lymphadenopathy, hepatosplenomegaly, and skin rash. The majority of symptomatic disease occurs within the first 3 months of life. These children do not appear at risk for neurologic or mental sequelae.[114]

Infection in Adults

The overwhelming majority of infections with CMV in adults are asymptomatic. In apparent cases the disease is similar and clinically almost indistinguishable from infectious mononucleosis. However, severe tonsillopharyngitis, cervical lymphadenopathy, severe hepatosplenomegaly, and jaundice are rare or absent in CMV infection. The most striking clinical feature can be the abrupt onset of a spiking fever which may persist for 2–3 weeks or longer.[111] Other features include headache, back and/or abdominal pain, morbilliform rash or purpura, conjunctivitis, lymphadenopathy, acute polyneuritis, and rarely hepatitis and splenomegaly. Other rare complications such as pneumonitis, pericarditis, myocarditis, and hemolytic anemia may also occur.[99] Typical hematologic abnormalities include leukocytosis (with relative and absolute lymphocytosis), atypical lymphocytes, and nondiagnostic heterophilic titers. Adult patients usually improve within a couple of weeks; however, some patients may suffer from recurrent fevers, headache and backache, malaise, and lymphocytosis for a period of several months.

In general, CMV infection in adults is mild and frequently overlooked and underdiagnosed. However, in immunosuppressed patients, e.g., transplant recipients or patients with AIDS or other immunopathies, the course of the disease can be more dramatic and occasionally fatal.

Diagnosis

The best and definite method for diagnosis of CMV infection is isolation of the virus in tissue culture. CMV is identified by development of typical cytopathic effect which occurs only in cultures of human diploid fibroblasts. Although culture appears to be the most reliable method of diagnosis of CMV infection, it is of little clinical value since the isolation of the virus often requires several weeks. Alternatively, demonstration of large basophilic intranuclear inclusions in biopsy specimens or in epithelial cells obtained from centrifuged urine may aid in the diagnosis. However, this method is insensitive when compared with tissue culture.

Various serologic techniques have been employed to establish a diagnosis of CMV infection. Complement fixation test is most practical and has been most widely used. (A four fold or greater rise in antibody titer or seroconversion is suggestive for an acute infection). Other serologic techniques are also available.

Treatment and Prevention

Despite a number of trials with various antiviral agents, including cytosine arabinoside, adenine arabinoside, idoxuridine, acyclovir, ganciclovir, interferons, and transfer factor, the results are rather disappointing.[115-120] At least two experimental vaccines also have been studied.[121-123] Unfortunately, despite initial development of cellular and humoral immunity, their recipients were unable to maintain complement-fixing antibodies several years after immunization.

REFERENCES

1. Most H: Manhattan: "A tropical isle." *Am J Trop Med* 17:333–354, 1968.
2. Schmerin MJ, Gelston A, Jones TC: Amebiasis: An increasing problem among homosexuals in New York City. *JAMA* 238:1386–1387, 1977.
3. Pearce RB: Intestinal protozoal infections and AIDS. *Lancet* 2:51, 1983.
4. Markell EK, Havens RF, Kuritsubo RA, et al.: Intestinal protozoa in homosexual men of the San Francisco Bay area: Prevalence and correlates of infection. *Am J Trop Med Hyg* 33:239–245, 1984.
5. Sargeaunt PG, Oates JK, MacLennan I, et al.: *Entamoeba histolytica* in male homosexuals. *Br J Vener Dis* 59:193–195, 1983.
6. William DC, Shookhoff HB, Felman YM, et al.: High rates of enteric protozoal infections in selected homosexual men attending a venerial disease clinic. *Sex Transm Dis* 5:155–157, 1973.
7. Keystone JS, Keystone DL, Proctor EM: Intestinal parasitic infections in homosexual men: Prevalence, symptoms and factors in transmission. *Can Med Assoc J* 123:512–514, 1980.

8. William DC: Enteric diseases. *Cutis* 27:278–285, 1981.

9. Adams EB, MacLeod IN: Invasis amebiasis II: Amebic liver abscess and its complications. *Medicine* 56:325–334, 1977.

10. Purpon I, Jimenez D, Engelking RL: Amebiasis of the penis. *J Urol* 98:372–374, 1967.

11. Thomas JA, Anthony AJ: Amoebiasis of the penis. *Br J Urol* 48:269–273, 1976.

12. Majmudar B, Chaiken ML, Lee KU: Amoebiasis of clitoris mimicking carcinoma. *JAMA* 236:1145–1146, 1975.

13. Cohen C: Three cases of amoebiasis of the cervix uteri. *Br J Obstet Gynecol* 80:476–478, 1973.

14. Spencer KJ, Chapin MR, Carcia LS: *Dientamoeba fragilis.* A gastrointestinal protozoan infection in adults. *Am J Gastroenterol* 77:565–569, 1982.

15. Shein R, Gelb A: Colitis due to *Dieantamoeba fragilis. Am J Gastroenterol* 78:634–636, 1983.

16. Meyers JD, Kuharic HA, Holmes KK: *Giardia lamblia* infection in homosexual men. *Br J Vener Dis* 53:54–55, 1977.

17. Mildvan D, Gelb AM, William D: Venereal transmission of enteric pathogens in male homosexuals: Two case reports. *JAMA* 238:1387–1389, 1977.

18. Schmerin MJ, Jones TC, Klein H: Giardiasis: Association with homosexuality. *Ann Intern Med* 88:801–803, 1978.

19. Quinn TC, Stamm WE, Goodell SE, et al.: The polymicrobial origin on intestinal infection in homosexual men. *N Engl J Med* 309:576–582, 1983.

20. Millet VE, Spencer MJ, Chapin MR, et al.: Intestinal protozoan infection in a semicommunal group. *Am J Trop Med Hyg* 32:54–60, 1983.

21. Stevens DP: Giardiasis: Host-pathogen biology. *Rev Infect Dis* 4:851–858, 1982.

22. Maguire JH: Giardiasis: An update. *Infect Dis Pract* 1:1–5, 1978.

23. Brady PG, Wolfe JC: Waterborne giardiasis. *Ann Intern Med* 81:498–499, 1974.

24. Kean BH, William DC, Lumanais SK: Epidemic of amebiasis and giardiasis in biased population. *Br J Vener Dis* 55:375–378, 1979.

25. Forthal DN, Guest SS: *Isospora belli* enteritis in three homosexual men. *Am J Trop Med Hyg* 33:1060–1064, 1984.

26. Westerman EL, Christensen RP: Chronic *Isospora belli* infection treated with cotrimoxazole. *Ann Intern Med* 91:413–414, 1979.

27. Knight R: Giardiasis, isosporiasis and balantidiasis. *Clin Gastroenterol* 7:31–47, 1978.

28. Bader M, Pedersen AHB, Williams R, et al.: Venereal transmission of shigellosis in Seattle King County. *Sex Transm Dis* 4:89–91, 1977.

29. William DC: Shigellosis, in Ostrow DG, Sandholzer TA, Felman YM (eds), *Sexually Transmitted Diseases in Homosexual Men: Diagnosis, Treatment, Research.* New York, Plenum Medical Book Company, 1983, p. 103.

30. Drusin LM, Genvert G, Topf-Olstein B, et al.: Shigellosis, another sexually transmitted disease? *Br J Vener Dis* 52:348–350, 1976.

31. Blaser MJ, Reller LB: Campylobactor enteritis. *N Engl J Med* 305:1444–1452, 1981.

32. Melnick JS: Classification of hepatitis A virus as enterovirus type 72 and hepatitis B virus as hepadnavirus type 1. *Intervirology* 18:105–106, 1982.

33. Szmuness W, Dienstag JL, Purcell RH, et al.: The prevalence of antibody to hepatitis A antigen in various parts of the world: A pilot study. *Am J Epidemiol* 106:392–398, 1977.

34. Szmuness W, Dienstag JL, Purcell RH, et al.: Distribution of antibody to hepatitis A antigen in urban adult population. *N Engl J Med* 295:755–759, 1976.

35. Hooper RR, Juels CW, Routenberg JA, et al.: An outbreak of type A viral hepatitis at the Naval Training Center, San Diego (epidemiologic evaluation). *Am J Epidemiol* 105:148–155, 1977.

36. Benenson MW, Takafuju ET, Bancroft WH, et al.: A military community outbreak of hepatitis type A related to transmission in a child care facility. *Am J Epidemiol* 112:471–481, 1980.

37. Hadler SC, Webster HM, Erben JJ, et al.: Hepatitis A in day-care centers: A community-wide assessment. *N Engl J Med* 302:1222–1227, 1980.

38. Corey L, Holmes KK: Sexual transmission of hepatitis A in homosexual men. *N Engl J Med* 302:435–438, 1980.

39. Hentzer B, Skinhoj P, Hoybye G, et al.: Viral hepatitis in a venereal clinic population: Relation to certain risk factors. *Scand J Infect Dis* 12:245–249, 1980.

40. McFarlane ES, Embil JA, Manuel FR, et al.: Antibodies to hepatitis A antigen in relation to the number of lifetime sexual partners in patients attending an STD clinic. *Br J Vener Dis* 57:58–61, 1981.

41. Kryger P, Pedersen NS, Mathiesen L, et al.: Increased risk of infection with hepatitis A and B viruses in men with a history of syphilis: Relation to sexual contacts. *J Infect Dis* 145:23–26, 1982.

42. Landrigan PJ, Huber DH, Murphy GD, et al.: The protective efficacy of immune serum globulin in hepatitis A: A statistical approach. *JAMA* 223:74–75, 1973.

43. Seeff LB, Hoofnagle JH: Immunoprophylaxis of viral hepatitis. *Gastroenterology* 77:161–182, 1979.

44. Phillips SC, Mildvan D, William DC, et al.: Sexual transmission of enteric protozoa and helminths in a venereal-disease-clinic population. *N Engl J Med* 305:603–606, 1981.

45. Centers for Disease Control: Inactivated hepatitis B virus vaccine: Recommendations of the Immunization Practices Advisory Committee. *Ann Intern Med* 97:379–383, 1982.

46. Szmuness W, Prince AM, Grady GF, et al.: Hepatitis B infection—A point prevalence study in 15 US hemodialysis centers. *JAMA* 227:901–906, 1974.

47. Denes AE, Smith JL, Maynard JE, et al.: Hepatitis infections in physicians—Results of a national survey. *JAMA* 239:210–212, 1978.

48. Segal HE, Llevewellyn CH, Irwin G, et al.: Hepatitis B antigen and antibody in the US Army. Prevalence in health care personnel. *Am J Public Health* 66:667–671, 1976.

49. Fulford KWM, Dane DS, Catteral RD, et al.: Australia antigen and antibody among patients attending a clinic for sexually transmitted diseases. *Lancet* 1:1470–1473, 1973.

50. Heathcote J, Sherlock S: Spread of acute type B hepatitis in London. *Lancet* 1:1468–1470, 1973.

51. Fass RJ: Sexual transmission of viral hepatitis? *JAMA* 230:861–862, 1974.

52. Szmuness W, Much MI, Prince AM, et al.: On the role of sexual behavior in the spread of hepatitis B infection. *Ann Intern Med* 83:489–495, 1975.

53. Jeffries DJ, James WH, Heffries FJG, et al.: Australia (hepatitis associated) antigen in patients attending a venereal disease clinic. *Br Med J* 2:455–456, 1973.

54. Dietzman DE, Harnisch JP, Ray CG, et al.: Hepatitis B surface antigen (BHsAg) and antibody to HBsAg. Prevalence in homosexual and heterosexual men. *JAMA* 238:2625–2626, 1977.

55. Lim KS, Taam-Wong V, Fulford KWM, et al.: Role of sexual and non-sexual practices in the transmission of hepatitis B. *Br J Vener Dis* 53:190–192, 1977.

56. Hoybye G, Skinhoj P, Hentzer B, et al.: An epidemic of acute viral hepatitis in male homosexuals. Etiology and clinical characteristics. *Scand J Infect Dis* 12:241–244, 1980.

57. Papaevangelou G, Trichopoulos D, Kremastinou T, et al.: Prevalence of hepatitis B antigen and antibodies in prostitutes. *Br Med J* 2:256–258, 1974.

58. Frosner GG, Buchholz HM, Gerth HJ: Prevalence of hepatitis B antibody in prostitutes. *Am J Epidemiol* 102:241–250, 1975.

59. Schreeder MT, Thompson SE, Hadler SC, et al.: Epidemiology of hepatitis B infection in gay men. *J Homosex* 5:307–310, 1980.

60. Schreeder MT, Thompson SE, Hadler SC, et al.: Hepatitis B in homosexual men. Prevalence of infection and factors related to transmission. *J Infect Dis* 146:7–14, 1982.

61. Reiner NE, Judson FN, Bond WW, et al.: Asymptomatic rectal mucosal lesions and hepatitis B surface antigen at sites of sexual contact in homosexual men with persistent hepatitis B virus infection: Evidence for de facto perenteral transmission. *Ann Int Med* 96:170–173, 1982.

62. Anderson MG, Eddleston AL, Murray-Lyon IM: Altered natural history of hepatitis B in homosexual males—A reflection of altered immune responsiveness? *J Med Virol* 17:167–173, 1985.

63. Skinhoj P, Hoybye G, Hentzer B, et al.: Chronic hepatitis B in male homosexuals. *J Clin Pathol* 32:783–785, 1979.

64. Redeker AG: Viral hepatitis: Clinical aspects. *Am J Med Sci* 270:9–16, 1975.

65. Kubo Y, Okuda K, Shimokawa Y, et al.: Hepatitis B surface antigenemia in patients with hepatocellular carcinoma in relation to clinical course and alpha-fetoprotein. *Gastroenterology* 72:1212–1216, 1977.

66. Trichopoulos D, Gerety RJ, Sparros L, et al.: Hepatitis B and primary hepatocellular carcinoma in a European population. *Lancet* 2:1217–1219, 1978.

67. Postexposure prophylaxis of hepatitis B. *MMWR* 33:285–290, 1984.

68. Szmuness W, Stevens CD, Eleszko WR, et al.: Passive-active immunization against hepatitis B: Immunogenicity studies in adult Americans. *Lancet* 1:575–577, 1981.

69. Chung WK, Yoo JY, Sun HS, et al.: Prevention of perinatal transmission of hepatitis B virus: A comparison between the efficacy of passive and passive-active immunization in Korea. *J Infect Dis* 151:280–286, 1985.

70. Beasley RP, Hwang L-Y, Lee G, et al.: Chen C-L: Prevention of perinatally transmitted hepatitis B virus infection with hepatitis B immune globulin and hepatitis B vaccine. *Lancet* 2:1022–1102, 1983.

71. Hair PV, Weisman JY, Tong MJ, et al.: Efficacy of hepatitis B immune globulin in prevention of perinatal transmission of hepatitis B virus. *Gastroenterology* 87:293–298, 1984.

72. Kanai K, Takehiro A, Noto H, et al.: Prevention of perinatal transmission of hepatitis B virus (HBV) to children of e-antigen-positive HBV carrier mothers by hepatitis B immune globulin and HBV vaccine. *J Infect Dis* 151:287–290, 1985.

73. Schweitzer IL, Dumm AEG, Peters RL, et al.: Viral hepatitis B in neonates and infants. *Am J Med* 55:762–771, 1973.

74. Schweitzer IL, Mosley JW, Ashcavai M, et al.: Factors influencing neonatal infection by hepatitis B virus. *Gastroenterology* 65:277–283, 1973.

75. Stevens CE, Beasley RP, Tsui J, et al.: Vertical transmission of hepatitis B antigen in Taiwan. *N Engl J Med* 292:771–774, 1975.

76. Gerety RJ, Schweitzer IL: Viral hepatitis type B during pregnancy, the neonatal period and infancy. *J Pediatr* 90:368–374, 1977.

77. Skinhoj P, Sardermann H, Cohen J: Hepatitis associated antigen (HAA) in pregnant women and their newborn infants.. *Am J Dis Child* 123:380–381, 1972.

78. Derso A, Boxall EH, Tarlow MJ, et al.: Transmission of HBsAg from mother to infant in four ethnic groups. *Br Med J* 1:949–952, 1978.

79. Lee AKY, Ip HMH, Wong VCW: Mechanism of maternal-fetal transmission of hepatitis B virus. *J Infect Dis* 138:668–671, 1978.

80. Stevens CE, Neurath RA, Beasley RP, et al.: HBeAg and anti-HBe detection by radio-immunoassay: Correlation with vertical transmission of hepatitis B virus in Taiwan. *J Med Virol* 3:237–241, 1979.

81. Mosley JW, Redeker AG, Feinstone SM, et al.: Multiple hepatitis viruses in multiple attacks of acute viral hepatitis. *N Engl J Med* 296:75–78, 1977.

82. Prince AM, Brotman B, Grady GF, et al.: Long incubation post-transfusion hepatitis without serological evidence of exposure to hepatitis B virus. *Lancet* 2:241–246, 1974.

83. Khuroo MS, Study of an epidemic of non-A, non-B hepatitis: Possibility of another human hepatitis virus distinct from post-transfusion non-A, non-B type. *Am J Med* 68:818–824, 1980.

84. Tandon BN, Joshi YK, Jain SK, et al.: An epidemic of non-A non-B hepatitis in North India. *Indian J Med Res* 75:739–744, 1982.

85. Enterically transmitted non-A non-B hepatitis—East Africa. *MMWR* 36:241–244, 1987.

86. Balayan MS, Andjaparidze AG, Savinskaja SS: Evidence for a virus in non-A non-B hepatitis, transmitted via the fecal-oral route. *Intervirology* 20:23–31, 1983.

87. Enterically transmitted non-A non-B hepatitis—Mexico. *MMWR* 36:597–602, 1987.

88. Iwarson S, Lindberg J, Lundin P: Progression of hepatitis non-A, non-B to chronic active hepatitis: A histological follow up of two cases. *J Clin Pathol* 32:351–355, 1979.

89. Solomon RE, Kaslow RA, Phair JP, et al.: Human immunodeficiency virus and hepatitis delta virus in homosexual men. A study of four cohorts. *Ann Intern Med* 108:51–54, 1988.

90. Wentworth BB, Alexander ER: Seroepidemiology of infections due to members of the herpesvirus group. *Am J Epidemiol* 94:496–507, 1971.

91. Lang DJ, Kummer JF, Hartley DP: Cytomegalovirus in semen: Persistence and demonstration in extracellular fluids. *N Engl J Med* 291:121–123, 1974.

92. Davis LE, Steward JA, Garvin S: Cytomegalovirus infection: A serologic comparison of nuns and women from a veneral disease clinic. *Am J Epidemiol* 102:327–330, 1975.

93. Chretien JH, McGinniss CG, Muller A: A venereal cause of cytomegalovirus mononucleosis. *JAMA* 238:1644–1645, 1977.

94. Drew WL, Mintz L, Miner RC, et al.: Prevalence of cytomegalovirus infection in homosexual men. *J Infect Dis* 143:188–192, 1981.

95. Chandler SH, Holmes KK, Wentworth BB, et al.: The epidemiology of cytomegalovirus infection in women attending a sexually transmitted disease clinic. *J Infect Dis* 152:597–605, 1985.

96. Jordan MC, Rousseau WE, Noble GR, et al.: Association of cervical cytomegalovirus with venereal disease. *N Engl J Med* 288:932–934, 1973.

97. Lang DJ, Kummer JF: Cytomegalovirus in semen: Observations in selected populations. *J Infect Dis* 132:472–473, 1975.

98. Montgomery R, Youngblood L, Medearis DN: Recovery of cytomegalovirus from the cervix in pregnancy. *Pediatrics* 49:524–531, 1972.

99. Felman YM, Nikitas JA: Sexually transmitted diseases: Cytomegalovirus infection. *Cutis* 27:562–604, 1981.

100. Handsfield HH, Chandler SH, Caine VA, et al.: Cytomegalovirus infection in sex partners: Evidence for sexual transmission. *J Infect Dis* 151:344–348, 1985.

101. Mintz L, Drew WL, Miner RC, et al.: Cytomegalovirus infections in homosexual men: An epidemiological study. *Ann Intern Med* 99:326–329, 1983.

102. Melbye M, Biggar RJ, Ebbesen P, et al.: Lifestyle and antiviral antibody studies among homosexual men in Denmark. *Acta Pathol Microbiol Immunol Scand (B)* 91:357–364, 1983.

103. Mindel A, Sutherland S: Antibodies of cytomegalovirus in homosexual and heterosexual men attending STD clinic. *Br J Vener Dis* 60:189–192, 1984.

104. Embil JA, Pereira LH, MacNeil JP, et al.: Levels of cytomegalovirus seropositivity in homosexual men. *Sex Transm Dis* 15:85–87, 1988.

105. Biggar RJ, Andersen HK, Ebbesen P, et al,: Seminal fluid excretion of cytomegalovirus related to immunosuppression in homosexual men. *Br Med J* 286:2010–2012, 1983.

106. Greenberg SB, Linder S, Baxter B, et al.: Lymphocyte subset and urinary excretion of cytomegalovirus among homosexual men attending a clinic for sexually transmitted diseases. *J Infect Dis* 150:330–333, 1984.

107. Hirsch MS, Schooley RT, Ho DD, et al.: Possible viral interactions in the acquired immunodeficiency syndrome (AIDS). *Rev Infect Dis* 6:726–731, 1984.

108. Quinnan GV, Siegal JP, Epstein JS, et al.: Mechanism of T-cell functional deficiency in the acquired immunodeficiency syndrome. *Ann Intern Med* 103:710–714, 1985.

109. Gottlieb MS: Immunologic aspects of the acquired immunodeficiency syndrome and male homosexuality. *Med Clin North Am* 70:651–664, 1986.

110. Coutinho RA, Wertheim-van Dillen P, Albrecht-van Lent P, et al.: Infection with cytomegalovirus in homosexual men. *Br J Vener Dis* 60:249–252, 1984.

111. Knox GE: Cytomegalovirus: Import of sexual transmission. *Clin Obstet Gynecol* 26:173–177, 1983.

112. Reynolds DW, Stagno S, Stubbs KG, et al.: Inapparent congenital cytomegalovirus infection with elevated cord IgM levels. *N Engl J Med* 290:291–296, 1974.

113. Hanshaw JB, Scheiner AP, Moxley AW, et al.: School failure and deafness after "silent" congenital cytomegalovirus infection. *N Engl J Med* 295:468–470, 1976.

114. Kumar ML, Nankervis GA, Jacobs IB, et al.: Congenital and postnatally acquired cytomegalovirus infection: Long-term follow up. *J Pediatr* 104:674–679, 1984.

115. Barton BW, Tobin JO: The effect of idoxuridine on the excretion of cytomegalovirus in congenital infection. *Ann NY Acad Sci* 173:90, 1970.

116. McCracken GH, Luby JP: Cytosine arabinoside in the treatment of congenital cytomegalic inclusion disease. *J Pediatr* 80:488–495, 1972.

117. Ch'ien LT, Cannon NJ, Whitley RJ, et al.: Effect of adenine-arabinoside on cytomegalovirus infections. *J Infect Dis* 130:32–39, 1974.

118. Emodi G, O'Reilly R, Muller A, et al.: Effect of human exogenous leukocyte interferon in cytomegalovirus infections. *J Infect Dis* 133:A199–204, 1976.

119. Thomas LT, Hawkins GT, Soothill JF, et al.: Transfer-factor treatment in congenital cytomegalovirus infection. *Lancet* 2:1056–1057, 1977.

120. Chachoua A, Dieterich D, Krasinski K, et al.: 9-(1,3-Dihydroxy-2-propoxymethyl) guanine (Ganciclovir) in the treatment of cytomegalovirus gastrointestinal disease with the acquired immunodeficiency syndrome. *Ann Intern Med* 107:133–137, 1987.

121. Elek SD, Stern H: Development of a vaccine against mental retardation caused by cytomegalovirus infection in utero. *Lancet* 1:1–5, 1974.

122. Plotkin SA, Furukawa T, Zygraich N, et al.: Candidate cytomegalovirus strain for human vaccination. *Infect Immun* 12:521–527, 1975.

123. Plotkin SA, Farguar J, Hornberger E: Clinical trials with Towne 125 strains of human cytomegalovirus. *J Infect Dis* 134:470–475, 1976.

14

ACQUIRED IMMUNODEFICIENCY SYNDROME

The acquired immunodeficiency syndrome (AIDS) is a disease of the human immune system caused by the human immunodeficiency virus type 1 (HIV-1) formerly called HTLV-III or LAV. The infection results in a wide array of clinical manifestations such as opportunistic infections, neoplasia, and neurologic and psychiatric disorders. The syndrome is also characterized by certain hematologic and autoimmune abnormalities. Unusual skin manifestations are common.

EPIDEMIOLOGY

Although cases of the disease compatible with the present definition of AIDS were seen in the late 1970s, the first cases of AIDS in the United States were reported in mid-1981.[1] Since then, the number of reported AIDS cases has rapidly increased, exceeding 100,000 cases by the middle of 1989, of which 58,000 have died so far. The Centers for Disease Control projects a cumulative total of 270,000 cases by the end of 1991. It is estimated that presently in the United States there are 1–2 million people infected with HIV. Many of them are unaware of this.

AIDS is not confined to the United States: the syndrome has been reported from approximately 90 countries. It is estimated that several million people worldwide have been infected with the HIV so far,[2,3] and as many as 10–30 percent of them may develop AIDS within the next 5–10 years.[4-6] Especially high rates have been reported from central Africa, Haiti, and Brazil. In the United States, New York, New Jersey, Florida, California, and Texas account for approximately 85 percent of all cases. In the United States, 73 percent of AIDS cases have occurred in homosexual or bisexual men (of whom 8 percent have also been intravenous drug users), 17 percent in intravenous drug users, 2 percent in recipients of contaminated blood or blood products, 2 percent among heterosexual contacts of a per-

TABLE 14.1.   Risk Groups in the United States and Europe

Homosexual or bisexual men
Intravenous drug users
Recipients of contaminated blood
Sex partners of the risk group members
Hemophiliacs
Children born to HIV-positive mothers

son in a high risk group, 1 percent in hemophiliacs, and 5 percent in others (Table 14.1).

Epidemiologic characteristics of AIDS vary in different continents and countries. In Europe, for example, similar to United States, homosexual and bisexual men account for about 80 percent of cases, but intravenous drug users comprise only 5 percent, hemophiliacs 4 percent, and blood transfusion recipients 2 percent; in 7 percent no risk factor could be identified. A small percentage (2 percent) of cases have occurred in persons immigrating to Europe either from central Africa or the Caribbean.[7] In Africa, the male-to-female ratio of AIDS cases is almost 1:1, with heterosexual transmission being the dominant factor. In contrast to American and European AIDS patients, Africans with AIDS rarely report a history of homosexual activity or use of intravenous drugs. Prostitution, contacts with prostitutes, multiple sex partners, and the presence of other sexually transmitted diseases are important risk factors in this part of the world.[8-11]

Modes of Transmission

Despite numerous sources from which HIV has been isolated (Table 14.2), there are only three really important routes of transmission: sexual transmission, transmission through blood (transfusion of blood or blood products, contaminated needles, and other drug paraphernalia), and perinatal transmission (Table 14.3).[12]

Sexual Transmission

HIV can be transmitted by both homosexual and heterosexual intercourse. Most cases of AIDS in the United States and in European countries have occurred among homosexual or bisexual men, and male-to-male activity appears to be the primary mode of transmission in these countries. Receptive anal intercourse and multiple sex partners have been implicated as major behavioral risk factors.[13,14]

TABLE 14.2.   Sources of HIV Isolates

Mononuclear cells	Cerebrospinal fluid
Plasma	Placenta tissue
Semen	Lymph-node
Saliva	Brain
Urine	Bone marrow
Tears	Cervical/vaginal secretions
Breast milk	

TABLE 14.3. Methods of Transmission of HIV

Bidirectional sexual transmission
   Homosexual: male to male
   Heterosexual: male to female
                female to male
Transmission by blood
   Transfusion of blood and blood products
   Sharing blood-contaminated drug paraphernalia
   Injection with unsterilized needles
   Needle stick, open wound, and mucous-membrane exposure
Perinatal
   Transplacental transmission
   Peripartum infection
   Breast feeding?

Transmission of the virus through receptive anal intercourse has been explained by the observation that semen contains lymphocytes, including T-helper lymphocytes, which bear a receptor for HIV and harbor the virus in an infected person. During anal intercourse, which is frequently traumatic to the receptive partner, contaminated semen is deposited in the lower intestinal tract, to enter the bloodstream of the receptive partner.[15]

HIV can be transmitted through heterosexual activity as well,[16] and anal intercourse is not required for transmission between heterosexuals,[11,17-19] although it may increase the risk. Various studies have pointed to efficient male-to-female transmission of HIV,[20-22] and approximately 30–50 percent of women with AIDS in the United States have become infected this way.[17] Data from Africa, where the male-to-female ratio is 1:1 and where 27–88 percent of female prostitutes have antibodies to HIV, speak in favor of heterosexual transmission of HIV.[8] HIV has been isolated not only from the semen of infected men but also in menstrual blood and cervical secretions.[23,24] These facts can make it easier to understand female-to-male transmission of the AIDS virus. In the United States, heterosexual transmission is currently of less quantitative importance; however, the proportion of AIDS cases in this country attributable to heterosexual transmission is increasing faster than in any other risk groups.[25]

Although sexual intercourse seems to be the most important route of infection, the HIV virus may infect human genitalia by other means. Accidental inoculation which occurred upon artificial insemination[26] suggests that sexual intercourse with associated microtrauma may not be necessary for the virus to enter the human body.

Transmission by Blood

Transfusion of blood and blood products. Many hemophiliacs and other blood recipients become infected with HIV after transfusion of contaminated blood or blood products.[27-31] Data obtained through January 1987 show that 2 percent of adults and 12 percent of children with AIDS in the United States become infected in this manner.[12] It is estimated that approximately 12,000 persons in the United States were infected with HIV through transfusion, including 70–80 percent of hemophiliacs before screening of donated blood began.[32] Data from Europe and Africa also indicated a relatively high proportion of HIV positivity rates among blood transfusion recipients.[33,34]

Whole blood, blood cellular components, plasma, and clotting factors were found to have transmitted HIV, while other products such as immunoglobulin, albumin, and plasma protein fraction have not been implicated.[35] Since April 1985, all blood donated in the United States is screened for antibody to HIV, and repeatedly positive blood is discarded. Members of high-risk groups have been asked not to donate blood, so that today the risk of acquiring HIV associated with transfusion of blood or blood products in the United States is extremely low. In less-developed countries where the infrastructure and resources for screening donated blood are limited, chances for acquiring HIV via blood transfusion remain real.

Transmission by sharing needles or other contaminated drug paraphernalia.   In the United States and other developed countries, intravenous drug users comprise a significant proportion of AIDS victims,[7,36-39] the virus being transmitted via contaminated unsterilized needles, syringes, or other paraphernalia.[38,40,41] The habit of sharing needles and other equipment in the group is common. The quantity of virus transmitted in this manner is considerably greater than that which can be transmitted by a simple needle stick; it is also important that this is a repetitive process, thus increasing the chances of acquiring infection. In other countries, it is probable that HIV transmission may be attributable also to medical and paramedical instruments such as skin-piercing devices, tattooing or acupuncture needles, instruments used for circumcision or other rituals, and the reuse of inadequately sterilized needles.[8,42,43]

Transmission by parenteral inoculation.   Although occupational infection through needle stick as well as transmission across mucous membranes and inflamed skin have been reported,[44-46] the risk of acquiring AIDS in this manner is very low.

Inoculum size plays an important role in determining the risk and, although the exact amount of blood involved in a needle stick accident is unknown, experimental data indicate that the mean volume of blood inoculated during needle stick injuries is very small (1.4 µl).[47] Even though the risk of acquiring AIDS by parenteral exposure is very low, it is very important to adhere to established precautions for hospital and laboratory staff in order to avoid nosocomial infection.

Perinatal Transmission

In the United States, about 80% of children with AIDS are known to have a parent who has AIDS or is at risk for the disease.[12] Most pediatric AIDS cases have been reported in New York, New Jersey, and Florida. The incidence of the disease among Hispanic and black children is 9 and 15 times higher than in white children.[48]

Precise data on the routes of perinatal transmission of HIV are lacking, but three ways of virus transmission are possible:

1. Transmission in utero, with HIV infecting the fetus through the maternal circulation[49,50]

2. During labor by inoculation or ingestion of blood or other fluids
3. After birth by breast feeding[51]

The rate of perinatal transmission has not been precisely established as yet, but it is probably much less than 100 percent. Infected as well as uninfected infants have been born to HIV-positive mothers who had previously borne an infected baby.[52] Friedland and Klein suggest that the rate of perinatal transmission of AIDS is probably between 40 and 50 percent.[12]

ETIOLOGY

AIDS is caused by the human immunodeficiency virus type 1 (HIV-1), a retrovirus which belongs to subfamily Lentivirinae.[2,3] This is the third known human T-lymphotropic virus. It was originally designated by some investigators as HTLV-III and by others as lymphadenopathy-associated virus (LAV)[53] or AIDS-associated retrovirus (ARV).[54]

The origin of the virus is not entirely understood, but mounting evidence suggests that HIV mutated from a primate retrovirus and invaded the human host, probably in Africa. Recently, another retrovirus related to HIV-1 was isolated from an AIDS patients in West Africa[55] with similar ultrastructural and biological properties. An analysis of the nucleotide sequence shows that it is evolutionarily distant from the previously known HIV, and most patients infected with this newly discovered HIV do not have detectable titres of antibodies against HIV-1. The new HIV was designated as HIV type 2 and appears to be closely related to the simian immunodeficiency viruses (SIV), which can cause an AIDS-like disease in monkeys.[56]

As with other retroviruses, HIV has RNA as its genetic material, and the special enzyme reverse transcriptase converts viral RNA into DNA. When the virus infects the host cell, the following sequence of events occurs:

1. Virus penetrates the host cell, where it sheds its protein coat, exposing the RNA core.
2. Viral RNA is converted into proviral DNA.
3. Proviral DNA travels to the cell nucleus, where it is integrated into the host cell genome.
4. The cell, after being immunologically activated, induces production of viral particles leading to their release and cell death.

The HIV particularly infects T4 (helper/inducer) lymphocytes and other cells bearing CD4 molecule in their outer protein-like monocytes and macrophages. It appears that CD4-carrying monocytes and macrophages are among the first targets of infection by the HIV and that many T helper lymphocytes may become infected in the lymph node during contact with macrophages. It has been also shown that HIV can infect B cells that are infected with Epstein-Barr virus, the dermal Langerhans cells and neuronal cells.[57-60]

As mentioned above, reproduction of the virus within the T helper lymphocytes and other cells with CD4 cell surface antigen leads to their death, and in this manner gradual depletion of the T helper cell population results. Since T helper lymphocytes lie at the very center of the immune system network, their destruction results in a breakdown of all responses that depend on these cells.

The immunodeficiency of AIDS is manifested as a loss of delayed-type cutaneous hypersensitivity reaction, excessive immunoglobulin production by B cells, and a loss of (in vitro) cytotoxic T-cell responses just to mention the most important phenomena.

As a result of T helper lymphocyte destruction, AIDS patients are unable to mount an adequate cellular or humoral response to infection caused by such agents as *Pneumocystis carini*, *Mycobacterium avium*, or *Candida albicans;* are more prone to develop certain forms of neoplasms; and because of the loss of immunoregulation, may suffer from autoimmune disorders (thrombocytopenia, neutropenia, etc.).

In addition to its effects on the immune system, there is a growing recognition that HIV can cause serious neurologic disorders. Several mechanisms have been proposed to explain neurological manifestation observed in HIV-infected individuals including the infection by HIV of brain macrophages, endothelial cells and glial cells. The chief pathologies observed in the brain were abnormal proliferation of the glial cells surrounding the neurons and lesions resulting from loss of white matter.[61] A high percentage of HIV-infected patients manifest a wide range of symptoms and signs, but the pathogenesis of these neurologic as well as psychotic disorders is unknown.

CLINICAL FEATURES

Incubation

The incubation period of AIDS varies, depending on the mode of its transmission as well as other less well understood factors. Infants born to mothers with HIV infection usually develop symptoms and signs in less than 6 months. The incubation period in recipients of infected blood may be prolonged—greater than 6 years—and the incubation period for sexually acquired AIDS may range from 3 to 10 years or more.

Acute HIV Syndrome

Most patients infected with HIV are asymptomatic during the first period of the disease. Some (10–20 percent) develop a clinical syndrome characteristic for acute viral infection.[62,63] That includes a "mononucleosislike" illness with fever, generalized lymphadenopathy, headache, sore throat, myalgias, arthralgias, and fatigue. On occasion, headache and meningoencephalitic symptoms may dominate. Some patients develop transient macular, maculopapular, urticarial or vesicular rash usually confined to the trunk (Figure 14.1). Laboratory abnormalities may include leukopenia, lymphopenia and thrombocytopenia. There is also relative monocytosis and an elevated sedimentation rate. The T4/T8 ratio may be inverted. This acute syndrome is self-limited and usually subsides within 2–4 weeks, although

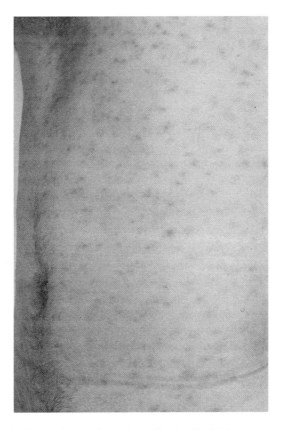

Figure 14.1. Transient maculopapular rash on the trunk which may occur in the acute HIV syndrome.

chronic lymphadenopathy may persist. Such symptoms are of course highly nonspecific and can be seen in a variety of common viral infections. Seroconversion follows the acute HIV syndrome usually in 1 to 10 weeks.

The natural course of HIV infection is not clearly defined. The time from infection to the development of AIDS is highly variable, with a mean time of 7 to 9 years. There have also been reports that transient infection with AIDS virus may occur.[67] The remaining patients may develop a spectrum of symptoms and signs ranging from benign, generalized chronic lymphadenopathy to severe, life-threatening opportunistic infections or neoplasms. This spectrum has been arbitrarily subdivided into several clinical categories, which are schematically depicted in Figure 14.2.

Generalized Persistent Lymphadenopathy

Generalized persistent lymphadenopathy (GPL) may appear in HIV-infected persons during an acute HIV syndrome, can be a separate feature of HIV infection, or may be a cardinal clinical finding in AIDS-related complex.[5] To meet the diagnostic criteria, the lymph nodes should be larger than 1.5 cm and located in two or

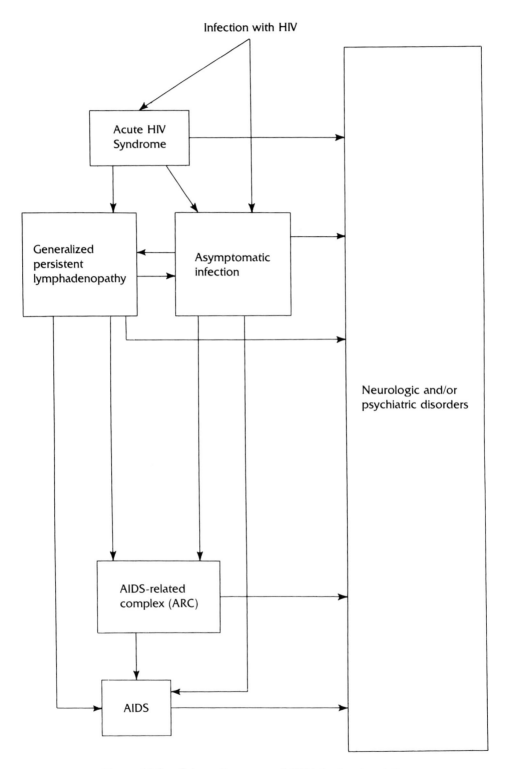

Figure 14.2. Schematic course of HIV infection in adults.

more extrainguinal areas. Other causes of lymphadenopathy or lymphangitis such as infections or neoplastic diseases should be excluded. The lymph nodes vary in size and may occasionally cause discomfort to the patient but are rarely so large as to result in obstructing symptoms. If biopsied, histopathology reveals pronounced nonspecific follicular hyperplasia with prominent capillary endothelial cell proliferation and an abundance of B lymphocytes. Occasionally HIV particles may be observed within follicular dendritic cells.

AIDS-Related Complex

AIDS-Related Complex (ARC) is a collection of clinical signs and laboratory abnormalities that have been found in HIV-infected patients but which do not meet the AIDS diagnostic criteria (see the appendixes). The complex has not been identified in a uniformly accepted fashion, and there are many classification systems which attempt to categorize the spectrum of HIV infections.[68-71] Besides GPL, patients with ARC may develop oral candidiasis, multidermatomal herpes zoster, or hairy leukoplakia. Other frequently encountered symptoms include persistent diarrhea, long-lasting fever, night sweats, fatigue and weight loss.

Minor Opportunistic Infections

Oral candidiasis (thrush) and herpes zoster are considered the "minor" opportunistic infections which often occur in patients with ARC.[72-74] These infections are common in the general population; their occurrence may not be related to HIV infection or may be the first signs of depression of the cellular immune system and may show ominous signs of progression from ARC to AIDS.[8] Appearance of oral candidiasis or herpes zoster in a person in one of the risk groups should alert the physician to testing for HIV antibodies and evaluation of the T4/T8 ratio.

Diarrhea and Other Manifestations

Persistent or intermittent diarrhea is frequently seen in ARC patients. The role of HIV itself as a cause of gastrointestinal disorder is unclear.[75] Necessary laboratory evaluation should be undertaken to find the causes of enteropathy, including bowel opportunistic infections common among patients with full blown disease. Patients with ARC also exhibit prolonged constitutional symptoms such as unexplained fever (over 100° F) lasting longer than 3 months, fatigue, frequent night sweats, and loss of weight. These are also very nonspecific symptoms and can be classified as ARC only with other clinical and laboratory abnormalities.

Laboratory Abnormalities in ARC

Laboratory abnormalities seen in ARC just to mention only some of them include hematological manifestations, such as leukopenia (nearly always lymphopenia and frequently granulocytopenia), trombocytopenia, and anemia. The number of T4 (helper) lymphocytes is usually below 400/mm,[3] and the T4 (helper) to T8 (suppressor) ratio is less than 1.0. The bone marrow often shows a mild dysplastic picture and cytopenias. Patients with ARC may display elevated serum globulins (with circulating immune complexes), elevated levels of acid-labile interferon, beta-2 microglobulin, and alpha-thymosin.[76] Patients with ARC may have intact cutaneous hypersensitivity, but many of them display different degrees of anergy. The immunologic abnormalities differ in degree and frequency and increase as the disease progresses.[77]

AIDS

AIDS is the final stage of HIV infection. It is characterized by progressive deficiency in the immune system and is manifested by the presence of severe opportunistic infections, unusual neoplasms (Kaposi's sarcoma and high-grade lymphomas), neurologic disorders, or wasting syndrome.

Opportunistic Infections

As a result of profound immunosuppression, patients infected with HIV are predisposed to multiple opportunistic infections (Table 14.4). In patients with AIDS, such opportunistic infections are often severe, persistent, and may relapse despite appropriate therapy. Moreover, several opportunistic infections may occur simultaneously, which significantly complicates treatment. Kaposi's sarcoma and central nervous system lymphoma were included as two neoplasms, along with certain opportunistic infections, that form the original criteria for diagnosis of AIDS prior to discovery of HIV as the etiologic agent. A variety of malignancies have been associated with AIDS (Table 14.5). It is possible that occurrence of certain malig-

TABLE 14.4. Microorganisms Associated with Opportunistic Infections in Patients with AIDS

Viruses	*Fungi*
Herpes simplex (types 1 and 2)	Candida
Cytomegalovirus	Cryptococcus
Varicella-zoster virus	Histoplasma
Epstein-Barr virus	Coccidioides
Adenoviruses	(and probably others)
Enteroviruses	*Protozoa*
Human papillomavirus	Pneumocystis carini
(and probably others)	Toxoplasma gondii
Bacteria	Cryptosporidia
Mycobacterium avium-intracellulare	Isospora belli
Mycobacterium tuberculosis	(and probably others)
Salmonella sp.	
Shigella sp.	
Legionella sp.	
Nocardia sp.	
Listeria monocytogenes	
Streptococcus pneumoniae	
Haemophilus influenzae	
Staphylococcus aureus	
(and others)	

TABLE 14.5. Malignancies Associated with AIDS

Kaposi's sarcoma
Burkitt's lymphoma
Non-Hodgkin's lymphomas
Hodgkin's disease
Chronic lymphocytic leukemia
Hepatocellular carcinoma
Adenosquamous carcinoma of the lung
Carcinoma of the oropharynx
Squamous cell carcinoma (?)
Melanoma malignum (?)

nancies in AIDS patients is similarly the result of prior exposure to certain micro-organisms thought to be involved in their pathogenesis (e.g., cytomegalovirus, Epstein-Barr virus, HTLV-I, and HTLV-II). Differences in the frequency of Kaposi's sarcoma among AIDS risk groups (primarily homosexuals and, rarely, in other risk groups) may suggest a higher prevalence of unknown infectious agents among homosexual men.

The detailed clinical description of clinical manifestations of full-blown AIDS goes far beyond the scope of this book, and only the clinical moieties which are of importance to dermatologists and venereologists will be discussed.

Kaposi's Sarcoma

The etiology of Kaposi's sarcoma (KS) has not been definitely determined as yet. However, recently Kaposi's sarcoma cells have been shown to secrete basement membrane-specific macromolecules, which confirms the theory that Kaposi's sarcoma cells are derived from the endothelium of the blood microvasculature.[78] Neoangiogenesis and spindle-cell formation is induced by newly discovered Kaposi's sarcoma growth factor (KSGF), a substance which is released after infection with HIV (R. Gallo, International Conference on AIDS, Stockholm, 1988).

Kaposi's sarcoma was previously considered to be a rare malignant neoplasm usually seen in elderly men of Jewish, Mediterranean, or Eastern European descent or in young men from subsaharan Africa. It also has been seen in patients with terminal cancer, patients receiving immunosuppressive medication, patients with inherited immune disorders,[79] and now AIDS patients.[80-82]

There are several epidemiologic and clinical differences between the classical or European form of KS, the African form, and that seen in AIDS patients (Table 14.6).

In classic Kaposi's sarcoma, the lesions begin symmetrically on the lower extremities, and they may spread to involve large areas. The lesions are red-blue to brown violaceous macules and papules which progress to plaques or nodules which may ulcerate.[83] Petechiae and ecchymoses may be present, and they are usually associated with hemosiderin pigmentation (Figure 14.3). Venous stasis and lymphedema have been observed.[84] The course of the disease is indolent, with rare

TABLE 14.6. Various Types of Kaposi's Sarcoma

	Classic	*African*	*AIDS*
Age	Elderly	Children and young adults	Mean age: 35
Sex	Male	Male and female	Predominantly male
Ethnic background	Jewish, Mediterranean, East European	Sub-Saharan tribes	Diverse
Distribution	Lower extremities	No specific location (3 variants)	Head, neck, trunk (tendency for regions of cutaneous cleavage)
Lymph node lesions	Infrequent	Frequent	Frequent
Prevalence	0.02% of all malignancies	9% of all malignancies	Epidemic proportions
Prognosis	Rarely causing death	Fatal	Rapidly fatal
Response to treatment	Good	Fair; relapses occur	Poor; some response to chemotherapy, but relapses are common

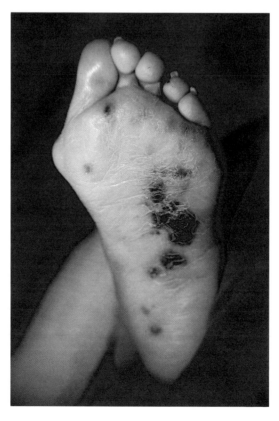

Figure 14.3. Classical variant (non-AIDS) of Kaposi's sarcoma: ecchymoses, petechiae, and hemosiderin hyperpigmentation on the sole of 80-year-old white female.

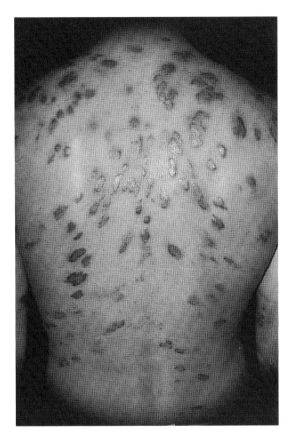

Figure 14.4. Kaposi's sarcoma on the trunk associated with AIDS. Many of the oval or elongated plaques are parallel to the skin tension lines.

involvement of lymph nodes and visceral organs.[85,86] Patients commonly die of other diseases.

The African form of disease is more disseminated anatomically and was described in three variants: (1) nodular, usually confined to extremities; (2) locally aggressive, characterized by florid, exophytic growth or deeply infiltrating underlying structures, including bones and localized primarily on extremities, and (3) lymphadenopathic, with skin lesions often absent. The disease is frequently fatal, with a worse prognosis among patients with locally aggressive and lymphadenopathic types.

AIDS-associated KS is similar to the African variety. However, it appears to be even more aggressive and more difficult to treat. Typically, lesions seen in HIV-infected patients are moderately infiltrated, oval or elongated, poorly demarcated pink to purple plaques parallel to the skin tension lines (Figures 14.4 and 14.5). In contrast to the classical KS, the lesions in AIDS patients tend to be smaller and located on the upper trunk, neck, and head,[82] and from the onset they are widespread and multifocal. The Kaposi's sarcoma lesions are polymorphous, varying from a solitary red or bluish macule to large red-brownish papules to smooth,

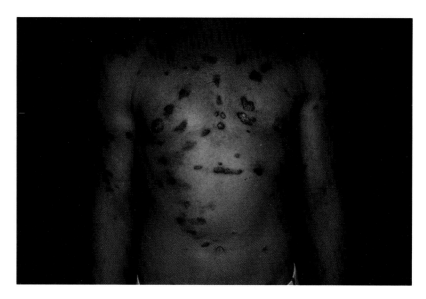

Figure 14.5. Pink, oval, and elongated plaques, parallel to the skin tension lines, on the upper trunk in patients with AIDS-associated Kaposi's sarcoma.

raised, widespread violaceous tumors. Practically any newly detected macule, papule, plaque, or nodule seen in an individual at risk for harboring HIV should be considered as being Kaposi's sarcoma, and a biopsy should be done.[87] Frequent involvement of the mucous membranes (30 percent),[87] lymph nodes, and/or gastrointestinal tract are characteristics of KS in AIDS patients. Oral lesions present as prominent violaceous plaques or tumors, and this manifestation may suggest the possible involvement of the gastrointestinal tract.[66]

The gastrointestinal tract is the most common extracutaneous site; however, lesions in the lung, liver, pancreas, testis, and larynx have been also reported.[88,89] These patients may manifest systemic complaints of fever, malaise, anorexia, diarrhea, and weight loss. The disease often pursues a fatal course. When the gastrointestinal tract or other viscera become involved, mortality may reach 80% over 2 years.[90]

Histopathology. Histologically, the typical lesion of Kaposi's sarcoma is a proliferation of mixed cellularity with irregular vascular slits embedded in spindle-shaped endothelial cells. Collagen bundles; an inflammatory infiltrate composed of lymphocytes, histiocytes, and plasma cells; as well as erythrocytes may be seen between the fascicles of spindle cells. Early lesions may be nonspecific and resemble granulation tissue.[84] Biopsies of lymph nodes show replacement of the normal architecture with irregular vascular spaces, fascicles of spindle cells, extravasated red blood cells, and plasma cells. In some homosexual patients with unexplained lymphadenopathy and the absence of skin lesions, lymph node biopsies have revealed, in addition to hypervascular follicular hyperplasia, small foci of Kaposi's sarcoma.

There is a suggestion that clinically discernible Kaposi's sarcoma lesions in

AIDS patients represent an "iceberg-tip" phenomenon. Atypical vascular proliferations were seen in the clinically uninvolved skin of AIDS patients and was defined as "pre-Kaposi's sarcoma."[91]

Differential diagnosis. The variety of clinical presentations of Kaposi's sarcoma gives an extensive differential diagnosis. Biopsy is necessary to confirm diagnosis and histology to differentiate lesions from stasis dermatitis, pyogenic granulomas, capillary hemangiomas, angiosarcomas, etc. True KS should also be distinguished from pseudo-Kaposi's sarcoma, which are a benign reactive blood vessel proliferation. One of them is acroangiodermatitis of Mali, characterized by purple vascular lesions on the dorsal surface of the forefoot in patients with chronic venous insufficiency; the other is the so-called "Stewart-Bluefarb syndrome," which occurs when Kaposi-like vessel proliferations are seen on the lower extremities of young persons in association with arteriovenous shunts.[92]

Treatment. Treatment of Kaposi's sarcoma in patients with AIDS is hampered by the fact that administration of cytostatic drugs may further compromise the severely damaged immune systems and worsen prognosis.

Radiation therapy is useful for superficial lesions, but chemotherapy is necessary in those cases with widespread disease. The *Vinca* alkaloids (vinblastine and vincristine) and the new podophyllotoxin etoposide have been tested extensively[93,94] as well as combination therapy using adriamycin, bleomycin, vinblastine, vincristine, and/or dacarbazine.[84] Interferons appear to hold some promise, with a 30–40 percent response to parenteral administration of alpha interferon.[95,96] However, it has not yet been shown conclusively whether that treatment of Kaposi's sarcoma increases patients' survival. Among AIDS patients with KS, the opportunistic infections rather than KS are the predominant cause of death.[97]

Lymphomas and Carcinomas

Other malignancies that have been reported in patients with AIDS[98-101] include several types of lymphomas.[98,99,102] The most common forms of AIDS-associated lymphomatous malignancies appear to be the high-grade lymphomas, including small noncleaved lymphomas (Burkitt or Burkitt-like) and B-cell immunoblastic sarcoma.[103] Other types of low-grade lymphomas, such as plasmacytoid lymphocytic lymphoma, have also been reported. Characteristically, the lymphomas in AIDS patients have multiple sites of extranodal disease, including the bone marrow and central nervous system. Other organs involved are the rectum and anus, heart, liver, kidney, small bowel, stomach, lung, and bladder. Levine et al. suggest that widely disseminated lymphoma may be a distinctive feature of the AIDS-related lymphomas.[104] Involvement of skin and subcutaneous tissue is rare. Hodgkin's disease is uncommon and does not involve the skin.[84] Skin tumor nodules containing both Kaposi's sarcoma and undifferentiated lymphoma have been also described.[99]

Basal and squamous cell carcinomas as well as malignant melanomas have been reported in association with AIDS.[101,105-108] The occurrence of these neoplasms in men with AIDS may be coincidental but is similar to the incidence of mucocutaneous squamous cell carcinomas in renal transplant recipients and other

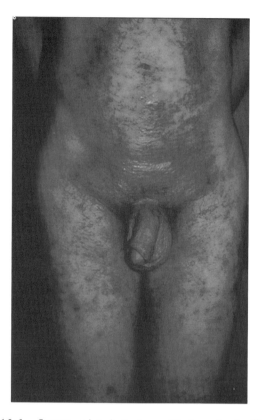

Figure 14.6.   Severe seborrheic dermatitis in patient with AIDS.

immunosuppressed patients.[109,110] This may be due to long-lasting infection with potentially oncogenic viruses proliferating in the absence of host immune surveillance.[103] Reports of an association between anorectal dysplasia, human papillomavirus, and HIV infection in homosexual men as well as the finding of the Epstein-Barr virus genome in certain lymphomas may well illustrate this theory.[111,112]

Cutaneous Manifestations of HIV Infection
(Table 14-7)

Seborrheic Dermatitis. Seborrheic dermatitis is a common, chronic, papulosquamous eruption frequently affecting patients infected with AIDS virus. Its prevalence ranges from 24 percent in ARC patients up to 83 percent in AIDS patients.[113,114] The disease in this population is often more explosive and inflammatory than in otherwise healthy patients[113,115] and may involve areas such as the trunk and extremities which are not typically involved in seborrheic dermatitis (Figure 14.6).[107] It has been suggested that *Pityrosporum ovale* is important in the etiology of seborrheic dermatitis, and the increased susceptibility to fungal infection is presumably partially accountable for the increased frequency and severity of this skin condition in HIV-infected patients. It has also been demonstrated that the severity of seborrheic dermatitis in HIV-infected persons may have prognostic sig-

TABLE 14.7. Skin Manifestations Associated with HIV Infection

Infections	*Protozoan Infections*
Viral	Amoebiasis cutis
Herpes zoster	Pneumocytosis cutis
Herpes simplex	*Mixed Infections (bacterial, viral, fungal)*
Warts and other lesions caused	*Neoplasms*
by human papillomavirus	Lymphoma
Molluscum contagiosum	Squamous cell carcinoma
Oral hairy leukoplakia	Kaposi's sarcoma
Acute HIV exanthema (?)	Basal cell carcinoma
Cytomegalovirus exanthema	Melanoma
Epstein-Barr virus exanthema	*Miscellaneous*
Bacterial	Seborrheic dermatitis
Mycobacterial infections	Papular eruptions
Staphylococcal and other	Acneiform folliculitis
bacterial skin infections;	Eosinophilic pustular folliculitis
e.g., folliculitis, ulcers	Granuloma annulare
carbuncles, ecthymata,	Xeroderma
cellulitis, impetigo, abscesses	Atopic dermatitis
Fungal	Yellow nail syndrome
Candidiasis	Telangiectasiae
Angular cheilitis	Nutritional deficiency
Dermatophytosis	Norwegian scabies
Histoplasmosis cutis	Adverse drug eruptions
Cryptococcosis cutis	Aphthous ulcerations
Sporotrichosis	Gingivitis
Scopulariopsis	Gum recession
Tinea versicolor	

nificance[114] and that this kind of dermatitis may be the initial manifestation of AIDS[115,116] or precede the onset of other symptoms of AIDS by up to 2 years.[113] Based on the finding that seborrheic dermatitis associated with AIDS shows a distinctive histologic pattern,[117] it has been suggested that the disease seen in HIV-infected patients may be a distinct clinical entity of unknown cause, bearing no relation to the seborrheic dermatitis of the banal type.[84] Some authors believe that many cases of seborrheic dermatitis found in AIDS patients if examined by KOH or by culture may turn out to be tinea[118] and recommend performing these tests in all such patients with seborrheic dermatitis–like lesions.[66]

The appearance of seborrheic dermatitis in HIV-infected patients may vary from mild to severe. Patients with HIV infection present with moderate to severe scaling of the scalp and eyebrows with a scaling erythema in the aural, perinasal, and infraorbital areas. A butterfly pattern on the face is a striking finding.[113] The lesion may also appear in the axillae and groin and on the chest and genitals. They may vary from a dry, flaky desquamation to greasy, yellowish red patches with indistinct borders. The disease is usually more severe than in otherwise healthy persons.

Seborrheic dermatitis can be treated in the usual manner with tar-containing

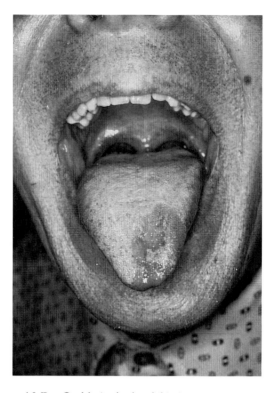

Figure 14.7. Oral hairy leukoplakia in patient with AIDS.

shampoos, and low-to-high potency corticosteroid lotions, or creams. Many patients with AIDS-associated seborrheic dermatitis responded to ketoconazole in tablets or 2 percent cream.[119,120]

Oral Hairy Leukoplakia. Oral hairy leukoplakia (Figure 14.7) appears to be a separate clinical entity first described in AIDS patients by Greenspan et al.[121] The sign has been identified almost exclusively in male homosexuals with HIV infection.[121-123]

The lesions of oral hairy leukoplakia occur principally on the lateral borders of the tongue. They are usually solitary, although bilateral lesions have been seen as well. Clinically, oral hairy leukoplakia appears as a slightly raised, poorly demarcated plaque which shows a corrugated or ''hairy'' surface. The size of the lesions ranges from a few millimeters to 3 cm. The condition is usually asymptomatic but occasionally may be painful. Some lesions were reported to come and go as a consequence of stress,[122] but complete, spontaneous regression has never been reported.

Histologically the lesion closely resembles that of a warty or papillomavirus-induced condylomatous lesion. It is characterized by acanthosis, parakeratosis, and keratin projections on the surface so fine that, macroscopically, they resemble hair.[121] In addition, large pale-staining cells with pyknotic nuclei are seen in the upper stratum malpighii, which appear similar to the koilocytes described in cervi-

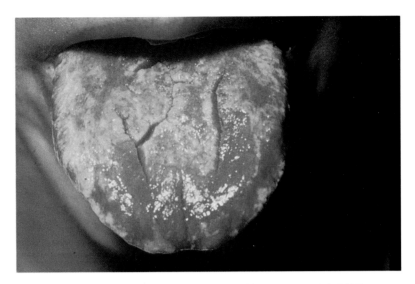

Figure 14.8. Oral candidiasis (thrush) in patient with AIDS.

cal condylomata.[122] Two viruses have been identified in oral hairy leukoplakia lesions: a human papillomavirus (HPV) and Epstein-Barr virus (EBV). The lesions appear to be the product of the symbiotic action of those two viruses. EBV was found to replicate within the cells of the lesions.[124] Differential diagnosis includes leukoplakia, characterized by epithelial hyperplasia or atypia, oral candidiasis, geographic tongue, white sponge nevus, and oral lichen planus. In conclusion, oral hairy leukoplakia is the first example of leukoplakia caused by a virus or viruses, and because of its close association with HIV infection, it may serve as an important marker for AIDS.

Candidiasis. Oral candidiasis (Figure 14.8) (thrush) and angular cheilitis (perléche) are frequent opportunistic infections in ARC and AIDS patients.[115] These are very rare in a previously healthy person who has not received antibiotic or immunosuppressive therapy. When seen in an otherwise healthy individual who belongs to one of the risk groups for AIDS may be the harbinger of HIV infection.[125] Examination of the mouth may reveal only small grayish white patches on the tongue or buccal mucosa, or on occasion, the entire mucous membrane of the oral cavity may be affected with erythema and cheesy white or dirty gray exudate. The presence of *Candida* can be confirmed by microscopic examination of a KOH preparation, by gram-stain, or by culture.

In severely immunocompromised patients, infection may progress to involve the esophagus and small and large intestines. The most common symptoms of *Candida* esophagitis are dysphagia and odynophagia. Patients frequently complain of food sticking when swallowed followed by substernal burning sensations. Liver and brain abscesses due to *Candida* infection were described in AIDS patients.[126] Oral lesions, including angular cheilitis, can be treated with nystatin (mouthwash or tablets). Refractory cases respond better to ketoconazole (200 mg tablets once daily). Candidiasis of the GI tract or of other internal organs should be treated either with oral ketoconazole or parenterally administered amphotericin B.

Candidal intertrigo of inguinal and anal regions may run a severe course in HIV-infected patients. The lesion tends to spread to the adjacent skin, perineum, and beyond the gluteal fold. Large parts of the skin may be affected with widespread satellite lesions. In women *Candida* can be the cause of severe intractable vaginitis, and in children with AIDS it can cause a particularly extensive diaper rash.[107] Nail dystrophies due to *Candida* infection involving both hands and feet have been reported, and these lesions appeared to corelate with severe T-cell depletion and were refractory to topical and systemic antifungal treatment.[107]

Fungal Infection Associated with HIV Infection. Disseminated cryptococcosis with skin lesions has been reported in homosexual men with AIDS.[127-129] Although this opportunistic infection primarily affects the central nervous system and lungs, *Cryptococcus neoformans* was also found in skin lesions.[130] Cutaneous cryptococcosis may present as papules and pustules, cellulitis, vegetating plaques, or subcutaneous abscesses or ulcerations. There are reports of two AIDS patients, one of whom developed facial papules resembling molluscum contagiosum[128] and the other lesions resembling herpes simplex.[127] In both instances, *Cryptococcus neoformans* was found to be the cause of disease. Histologic study and culture of skin specimens along with appropriate studies of CSF, serum, or sputum are essential for diagnosis. Treatment with amphotericin B may reduce the mortality rate.

Disseminated histoplasmosis is another fungal opportunistic infection that has been reported in patients with AIDS but is probably rare. The cutaneous manifestations of histoplasmosis may be very nonspecific. In AIDS patients it has been described as (1) a widespread, erythematous, maculopapular eruption, with slight scaling, on the trunk and extremities;[131] (2) as papular lesions on the arms, forearms, dorsa of the hands, palms, and feet with several papules having central keratinous plugs;[132] and (3) as folliculitis, pustules, papulonecrotic lesions surrounded by red halos, and perianal ulcers.[133] The diagnosis of cutaneous histoplasmosis should be verified by direct microscopy and/or by culture. The disease is more likely to occur where *Histoplasma capsulatum* is endemic, e.g., eastern and central parts of the United States.

Systemic sporotrichosis and patchy alopecia caused by scopulariopsosis have been described in patients with HIV infection.[107] In contrast to typical cutaneous sporotrichosis when exposure to soil or plants is a common history, the portal of entry for AIDS patients is presumably the lungs with subsequent hematogenous spread. In both instances fungi can be demonstrated by cultures.[108]

Superficial fungal infections have been frequently observed in AIDS patients.[84,115] An extensive infection with *Trichophyton rubrum* can be an important sign of the immunosuppression which occurs in HIV-positive patients.[107,134] *Trichophyton rubrum* was found to be the cause of keratoderma-blennorhagica–like lesions on the palms and soles of AIDS patients as well as plamoplantar keratoderma with and without simultaneous nail involvement.[107] Superficial fungal infection in AIDS may also present as extensive tinea pedis, tinea cruris, or tinea versicolor. Tinea faciale resembling erythema multiforme and tinea of the neck which presented as flat-topped papules have also been reported.[135]

Herpes Zoster. Localized herpes zoster is a disorder of older persons (mean age in excess of 60 years) and is thought to arise as a result of deficient T-cell or killer cell

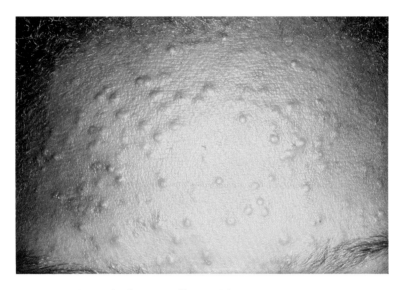

Figure 14.9. Varicella in adult patient with AIDS.

activity associated with aging. The appearance of herpes zoster in an otherwise healthy young homosexual man may be suggestive of immunologic compromise similar to that occurring in elderly persons with shingles which can ultimately evolve into AIDS.[136,137] Localized herpes zoster has been reported in patients after AIDS has been diagnosed.[115] Disseminated zoster in AIDS patients has been also reported.[107,138]

Varicella in adults with AIDS or in young children exposed to HIV may run a very severe course with extensive cutaneous and internal manifestations (Figure 14.9).[107,139] The disease can be life threatening, and intravenous acyclovir and intravenous gammaglobulin may be required.[107,108]

Herpes Simplex. An increased incidence of herpes simplex infections has been reported in AIDS patients (Figure 14.10).[140-143] The disease may run an unusually severe and prolonged course.[135,140,143] Many patients have atypical and often chronic oral or genital lesions. Atypical distribution is also not uncommon.[135,141] Patients with recurrent infection suffer from pronounced attacks and usually have prolonged healing time with persistent shedding of virus. The lesions are wider spread, and ulceration may be deeper and larger.[87] Severe nonhealing ulcerative lesions of herpes simplex involving the perianal region are a frequent type of herpes infection in homosexual men.[140] These patients present with perianal pain associated with exudative ulceration which may persist for months unless aggressively treated. The rectum may also become infected, giving rise to herpetic proctitis.[144] Patients with multiple erosions on the face with biopsy suggestive for herpes,[87] lesions in the nasolabial fold and on the hands, fingers, and legs also have been described.[135,141] Herpetic esophagitis and involvement of tracheobronchial mucosa have been reported.[145] The disease usually responds promptly to a 7–10-day course of intravenous acyclovir which reduces the shedding of the virus and accelerates epithelization of the ulcers. Continuous administration of oral acyclovir may prevent recurrences.[87]

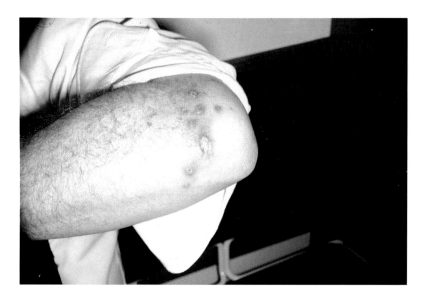

Figure 14.10. Vesicular, pustular, and erosive lesions caused by herpes simplex virus in patient with AIDS.

Molluscum Contagiosum. Molluscum contagiosum is commonly seen in young children and can be seen in adolescents, especially in the genital region, where it is probably transmitted by sexual contact.[146,147] In patients with AIDS, mollusca frequently appear as facial papules (Figure 14.11) which, over a period of time, disseminate, increasing not only in number but also in size.[87,148] The individual lesions appear as round, shiny, pearly umbilicated papules or nodules located all over the body. Typically, infection consists of fewer than 20 lesions that resolve

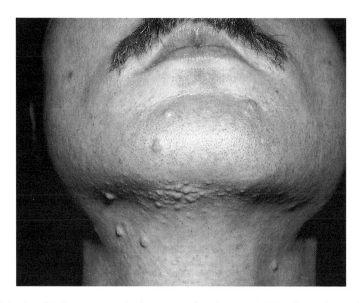

Figure 14.11. Molluscum contagiosum on the face and chin of a patient with AIDS.

spontaneously in less than 12 months. In patients with AIDS, the lesions are more numerous (can be more than 100) and more persistent.[149,150] The pox virus (an etiologic agent of molluscum contagiosum) is believed to be controlled not only by T helper lymphocytes but also by Langerhans cells, both of which have been shown to be decreased in number in AIDS.[58] This may in part explain the frequent appearance of molluscum contagiosum in AIDS patients, the widespread lesions, and the more persistent course and recurrences after the usual treatment.[107] Several hundred molluscum lesions have been reported in one AIDS patient.[151] In an aim to prevent recurrences, surgical excision or cryotherapy is recommended.[107]

Acute Exanthema. Transient macular, papular, and urticarial lesions have been reported to accompany the acute HIV infection and seroconversion.[107] The appearance of skin lesion is preceded by about a 1-week period of influenzalike symptoms, including malaise, fever, myalgia, arthralgia, encephalopathy, lymphadenopathy, sore throat, and diarrhea.[62,65,139] European authors reported syphilitic roseolalike eruption predominantly located on the trunk with few elements on the face and neck and no lesions on the peripheral part of the extremities.[66] The macular lesions were without any scaling, which was an important feature allowing the differentiation of the eruption from pityriasis rosea.[66] During the acute stage, patients with exanthema frequently demonstrate blood abnormalities similar to those seen in more advanced stages of HIV infection, such as leukopenia, thrombocytopenia, and decreased T-cell helper to suppressor ratio.[108] The HIV test is usually negative at this stage, and seroconversion occurs within less than a 5-week period.[64] Biopsy specimens from macular lesions are nonspecific, showing pericapillary lymphocyte infiltration in the upper dermis, plasma cells, and histiocytes.[66]

Not only histology but the whole syndrome is very nonspecific. The pathomechanism of it is unknown, and several viral exanthemas (EBV, CMV, hepatitis B virus) should be included in the differential diagnosis. Perhaps the recently found antigenemia and the presence of circulating antigens during the course of this self-limited illness may help to understand the nature of the acute illness associated with HIV infection.[152] Regardless of the unclear origin of so-called acute HIV exanthema, its appearance in a patient of one of the risk groups may be significant and should alert the physician to prompt necessary evaluation. Early recognition of this syndrome may permit one to introduce appropriate epidemiologic and therapeutic approaches.

Other Viral-induced Skin Lesions. Besides its presence in hairy leukoplakia, human papillomavirus has been found in association with anorectal epithelial dysplasia in patients with HIV infection.[111] By analogy to the relation between HPV-associated cervical intraepithelial neoplasia in women, dysplasia in the anorectal epithelium of homosexual men may be the marker for future anorectal carcinoma. The association of anorectal dysplasia and HIV infection has been found and may suggest that HIV infection may be a cofactor in anorectal dysplasia or that transmission of both HPV and HIV infections depends on common risk factors. Further studies, however, are needed to elucidate this finding. Besides its association with precancerous lesions, HPV can produce large, perianal condylomata acuminata, particularly in homosexual men.[107] Also, common warts have been found frequently in HIV-infected individuals. They did not cause any significant clinical problems except that they frequently recurred.[107]

Cytomegalovirus appears to be the cause of pruritic rash in AIDS patients. Inclusions typical for cytomegalovirus were found in biopsies from pruritic macules on the lower portions of the legs and on the feet of patients with AIDS.[135]

Mycobacterial and Bacterial Skin Infection. *Mycobacterium avium-intracellulare* infection has been surprisingly common in AIDS patients.[153,154] It is generally, but not always, a late complication of AIDS. Rarely, the infection can present skin manifestations. A reported case had ill-defined macular discolored lesions on the forearms thought to be Kaposi's sarcoma. Histology revealed acid-fast organisms within histiocytes, which is a typical finding in infection with *Mycobacterium avium-intracellulare.*[135] Infections caused by another mycobacterium, *Mycobacterium tuberculosis,* frequently occur in AIDS patients, presumably as a reactivation of primary infection. Tuberculosis is increasing in incidence, especially in areas with a high prevalence of HIV infection. The disease in patients with AIDS is often extrapulmonary, runs a severe course, and is difficult to treat. Scrofuloderma in association with AIDS has been reported.[135,155] Because of the interaction between tuberculosis and HIV infection, the CDC recommends that people with tuberculosis who have risk factors for AIDS be tested for antibody to HIV. Similarly HIV-positive persons should be evaluated for infection with *Mycobacterium tuberculosis* in an aim to start a prophylactic treatment if evidence for infection exists. Additionally, HIV testing should be considered in patients with "severe or unusual manifestations of tuberculosis."[156,157]

Multiple abscesses, furunculosis, cellulitis, severe widespread forms of folliculitis, and extensive impetigo have been reported in association with AIDS,[107,115,139] with staphylococci, and streptococci the most frequently cultured organisms. *Staphylococcus aureus* was found in ecthymatous lesions and pyomyositis in homosexuals infected with HIV.[107] There was also a report of staphylococcal scalded skin syndrome in a homosexual with ARC secondary to *S. aureus* septicemia.[158] *Hemophilus influenzae* was cultured from severe cellulitis, and another patient developed an abscess caused by *Rhodococcus equi.*[107] Skin lesions caused by *Pseudomonas* and *Actinomyces israeli* were also reported.[107] Just recently I have consulted a patient with AIDS who presented with subcutaneous abscesses and superficial oozing ulcerations which grew *Nocardia asteroides* Figure 14.12.

Protozoan Skin Infections. *Pneumocystis carinii* pneumonia has been the hallmark of the opportunistic infections affecting AIDS patients. Recently, a first report of biopsy-proved *Pneumocystis carini*-produced skin lesions has been published.[159] It presented as bilateral polypoid mass in the external auditory canals of an AIDS patient with a history of progressive hearing loss. Treatment with intravenous trimethoprim and oral trimethoprim-sulfamethoxazole resulted in marked reduction of the size of the lesions.

A case of a homosexual man with disseminated infection caused by *Acanthamoeba castellani* with skin lesion was reported. The lesion noted at autopsy appeared as a papule on the thigh. Biopsy revealed amebic trophozoites within the inflammatory infiltrate.[135]

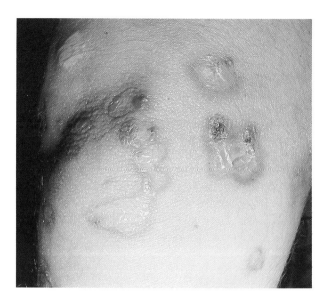

Figure 14.12. Oozing ulcerations and subcutaneous abscesses caused by *Nocardia asteroides* in HIV infected patient.

Mixed Infections. Skin lesions in which mixed viral, bacterial, and/or fungal pathogens were found have been described in AIDS patients.[108,160] Mixed infections may produce in immunocompromised patients unusual skin lesions never previously seen. Few AIDS patients with keratotic, vegetating plaques were described. Skin biopsies showed cytopathic changes typical for herpes or papillomavirus infections as well as fungal elements. It has been suggested that these lesions might be considered as the cutaneous equivalent of oral hairy leukoplakia.[160]

Miscellaneous Skin Diseases

PAPULAR ERUPTION. A clinically characteristic yet histologically nonspecific papular eruption has been reported in several patients with AIDS.[161] The lesions presented as noncoalescing 2–5-mm skin-colored papules located on the head, neck, upper trunk, and extremities. In many instances, the lesions were persistent for more than 9 months, but the number of papules varied with time. The eruption was often but not always pruritic. Histology was nonspecific, with a chronic, perivascular infiltrate of mononuclear cells. The presence of a similar papular eruption in AIDS patients was confirmed by other authors.[87] The cause is unknown. A similar papular eruption was reported in hepatitis B carriers[162] and Gianotti-Crosti syndrome.[107]

ACNEIFORM FOLLICULITIS. HIV-positive patients often complain of a recurrence of their teen-age acne, and indeed several authors reported widespread acneiform folliculitis in ARC and AIDS patients.[66,84,87,134] The folliculitis is usually widespread, involving the face, neck, back, chest, upper arms, thighs, and axillary and perianal areas. *Staphylococcus aureus* occasionally is grown, but the lesions are often sterile. Biopsy shows a severe mixed perifollicular infiltrate with polymorphonuclear cells, lymphocytes, plasma cells, and granulomatous inflammation.[134]

A rare form of eosinophilic pustular folliculitis reminiscent of the eruption reported from Japan by Ise and Ofuji has been described in patients with ARC and AIDS.[87,163] Since, in some biopsy specimens, *Demodex folliculorum* was found, it has been suggested that this kind of folliculitis may result from aberrant immunologic reaction to *Demodex folliculorum* and dermatophytes.[163]

YELLOW NAIL SYNDROME. The yellow nail syndrome, formerly associated with chronic respiratory infections, has been described in patients with AIDS.[164] However, all four patients out of eight reported by the authors suffered from *Pneumocystis carini* pneumonia. The nail changes included yellow discoloration of the distal part of the nails, transverse and/or longitudinal riding, onycholysis, loss or decrease of lunula, and opaqueness. Despite its association with several diseases, the cause of yellow nail syndrome has never been fully explained.

XERODERMA. Dry skin similar to that observed in other conditions associated with immunodeficiency (Hodgkin's lymphoma, sarcoidosis, lepromatous leprosy) or malabsorption syndrome can occasionally be seen in AIDS patients.[115] Acquired ichthyosis and asteatotic eczema of the lower legs have also been reported.[115]

ATOPIC DERMATITIS. Atopic dermatitis is particularly common in children with pediatric AIDS. As many as 50 percent of them may have lesions compatible with atopic skin.[165] However, this condition has been also described in adults with AIDS who have never had atopic dermatitis in childhood.[108] These findings along with the frequent occurrence of atopic dermatitis in Brutons hypo–gamma-globulinemia, ataxia-telangiectasia, and Wiskott-Aldrich syndrome provide additional support for the hypothesis that certain immunodysfunctions lie at the basis of the pathogenesis of this disease.

TELANGIECTASIA. Telangiectases of unusual distribution (across the chest and on the neck, as well as on the palms, fingers, and ears) were reported in HIV-positive patients. Biopsy showed dilated blood vessels and small-cell perivascular infiltrates.[87]

NUTRITIONAL DEFICIENCY–LIKE CHANGES. This kind of lesion has been seen in children with AIDS.[135] Verrucous, hyperpigmented lesions on the legs and follicular petechial eruption, also on the legs, along with bleeding of the gums have been reported. In the first case, skin biopsy revealed changes compatible with pellagra, zinc deficiency, or acquired acrodermatitis enteropathica.[135]

ORAL CAVITY DISORDERS. Besides oral candidiasis, angular cheilitis and oral hairy leukoplakia, patients infected with HIV may demonstrate various disorders in the oral cavity.[100] For example gingivitis is very common in patients with ARC and AIDS and many of them suffer from gum recession. Some of them develop dental abscesses and tooth extractions are frequently required. The oral cavity can be the site where warts appear in great numbers and in a minority of patients with AIDS and ARC aphtous ulcerations, severe at time, may be seen.[166]

OTHER SKIN DISEASES ASSOCIATED WITH HIV INFECTION. A number of other skin symptoms have been noted in association with AIDS or ARC. These include granuloma annulare and granuloma annulare–like eruption,[167,168] hyperalgesic pseudothrombophlebitis, thrombocytopenic purpura, erythema elevatum diutinum, pityriasis rosea, vasculitis, cutis marmorata, drug eruptions, aphthosis, psoriasis, Reiter's syndrome, and chronic photosensitivity.[87,107,108,169,170] It is possible that these and other aforementioned skin conditions have no causal relationship with HIV infection. However, when a patient at high risk for AIDS presents with any of the cutaneous manifestations discussed, the physician should be alert to the possibility of HIV infection and undertake all necessary procedures, including tests for HIV, biopsy, culture, and acid-fast and fungal staining to confirm or rule out this diagnosis.

Sexually Transmitted Diseases and HIV Infection

Promiscuous individuals are the prime risk category not only for HIV infection but also for other sexually transmitted diseases. It has been mentioned before that diseases such as genital herpes, molluscum contagiosum, genital warts, or scabies (Figure 14.13) may run unusually severe courses in HIV-infected individuals. Because of the impaired immune system, skin lesions in these diseases are usually larger, more widespread, and deeper than in individuals with an intact immunity. Similarly, other sexually transmitted diseases may also run an altered course. It has been noted that in HIV positive individuals infections caused by *Chlamydia*

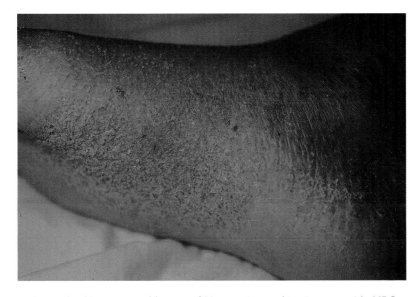

Figure 14.13. Unusual lesion of Norwegian scabies in man with AIDS.

trachomatis can be more severe,[84] and patients with secondary syphilis develop granulomatous skin lesions normally not seen during this stage of disease.[171] Abundant treponemes were seen in the biopsies of skin lesions in men with syphilis and simultaneous HIV infection.[172] There is also a report of a patient with AIDS (Kaposi's sarcoma) who developed typical lesions of syphilis (proven by demonstration of spirochetes in biopsy specimens) but with negative serologic tests.[173] HIV can be the cause of neurologic relapse of previously adequately treated syphilis or may significantly alter the course of neurosyphilis.[174,175] It has been also suggested that patients infected with HIV who require simultaneous treatment for syphilis should be treated as for neurosyphilis since their impaired immune system may be unable to cope with treponemal infection in the same manner as in individuals with intact immunity.

Physicians working with homosexual patients with AIDS or ARC should bear in mind that their patients may have, for example, chronic diarrhea not necessarily due to HIV infection but may suffer from enteric infections which are more prevalent among gay men than in the normal population. Generalized lymphadenopathy, which appears to be a common sign of HIV infection, may be also seen in early symptomatic syphilis, and inguinal lymphadenopathy may be the sign of primary syphilis, chancroid, LGV, or genital herpes.

Sexually transmitted diseases, especially those which present with genital ulcerations, were found to be the risk factor for AIDS, especially in African patients.

In conclusion, one must remember that gay patients with AIDS can be at risk for other sexually transmitted infections and that gay patients with sexually transmitted disease may be infected with HIV. Both conditions are associated with a particular lifestyle rather than other factors. However, one must also know that the AIDS epidemic which has caused anxiety, social isolation, and abstinence from sex has also resulted in the reduction in the rate of STDs in the population at risk for AIDS.[176,177]

DIAGNOSIS

Diagnosis of HIV infection is based on the presence of symptoms and the signs of diseases predictive of underlying cellular immunodeficiency in the absence of any other causes for susceptibility to that disease and/or positive HIV tests. A strict definition of AIDS was proposed by the Centers for Disease Control in 1982[178] and revised in 1985[179] and 1987 (see the appendix).

Serologic Testing for HIV Infection

After a seronegative period which ranges from 4 to 12 weeks most of the patients infected with HIV will have circulating antibodies which can be detected with a number of tests. Currently the enzyme immunoassay (EIA) is the most commonly used screening test. If performed under optimal laboratory conditions it is highly sensitive (99 percent) and specific (99 percent).[180] EIA detects circulating antibodies to multiple viral agents and its specificity can be increased by repetition of the test on all specimens which were initially positive. Positive EIA results require confirmation with the use of a supplemental test. The most widely used confirmatory test is the Western blot test, but other methods such as radioim-munoprecipitation and immunofluorescence can also be used. All of them detect antibody to individual viral protein and thus are more specific. Confirmatory tests are intended to distinguish the false positive results of EIA from those truly infected. The so-called second and third generation assays have been recently developed. The second generation tests detect antibodies to individual, specific viral proteins and they utilize either recombinant DNA technology or chemically synthesized peptides representing immunodominant regions of the viral proteins. Second generation tests should be more specific that EIA, cheaper and safer in production. They can also be helpful in monitoring the progress of the disease.

The third generation tests detect viral antigens or viral RNA and DNA. Antigen detection may be of value in the early phase of the infection before the antibodies appear in circulation and in patients receiving antiviral treatment informing the therapist about the amount of circulating antigen.

Sensitivity and specificity of currently used serologic methods of detection of HIV infection is very high. However, one must remember that during the first weeks of infection patients may not have detectable antibodies or even antigens. In patients who may have symptoms or signs predictable for early HIV infection (acute mononucleosis-like symptoms, acute aseptic meningitis) the test should be repeated after 6, 9 and 24 weeks because of the possibility of delayed antibody response to HIV.

Guidelines for HIV Testing

There are presently two main goals for testing for HIV infection. The first can be called epidemiologic: picking up the highest number of asymptomatic and usually unaware individuals infected with HIV and in this way slowing down the spread of the virus; the second goal is medical or diagnostic. In the latter category, HIV serologic tests are used in order to confirm or rule out HIV infection in patients with symptoms and signs compatible with clinical features of early HIV infection (Table 14.8). These guidelines are not final nor complete and they certainly will be revised in the future depending on developments in the AIDS epidemic.

TREATMENT

There currently is no available curative therapy for HIV infection and treatment for AIDS patients is basically supportive. It consists of attending to all infections and tumors that can be treated with chemotherapeutics or other means. Zidovudine (ZDV—previously known as azidothymidine [AZT]), which in vitro inhibits replication of HIV, has been shown to reduce the frequency of opportunistic infections and mortality in the later stages of this disease.[181] However, serious adverse reactions, particularly bone marrow suppression, were observed.[182] Additionally, the drug is very expensive and not widely available as yet. According to the results of just completed studies, ZDV appears to be effective in the early stages of the disease and appears to be working in half of the previously administered

TABLE 14.8. Guidelines for HIV Testing*

Medical Indications	Epidemiological Indications
1) Generalized lymphadenopathy	1) Persons at risk for HIV infection:
2) Chronic unexplained fever	a) homosexual men
3) Chronic unexplained diarrhea	b) intravenous drug abusers
4) Unexplained weight loss	c) blood and blood product
5) Tuberculosis	recipients including hemophiliacs
6) Kaposi's sarcoma	d) Sex partners of members of risk
7) Disseminated forms of herpes virus	groups
infections (zoster or simplex)	2) Persons with sexually transmitted
8) Chronic or disseminated candidiasis	diseases
9) Rare, unusual forms of lymphoma	3) Prostitutes (female and male)
10) Premature dementia or unexplained	4) Blood or organ donors
encephalopathy	5) Future mothers with identifiable risk
	for HIV infection (1b,c,d, 2, 3) or who
	have lived in communities of high
	prevalence of infection among
	women
	6) Persons admitted to the hospital (age
	groups deemed to have high
	prevalence of HIV infection)
	7) Persons in correctional institutions

*Based on the Public Health Service guidelines for counseling and testing to prevent HIV infections and AIDS. *MMWR* 36:509–515, 1987.

daily dose. Given to patients with early symptoms of HIV infection, it significantly slows the progression of the disease.

A number of groups are evaluating new drugs or combinations of drugs that can be administered to persons with different stages of HIV infections including asymptomatic infection. Hope lies in a vaccine which will prevent HIV infection in susceptible persons, but it is unlikely it will be available in the near future.

PREVENTION

The topic of preventing AIDS goes far beyond the scope of this book. However, there are a few cardinal features that should be stressed whenever the AIDS issue is discussed. Because neither an effective vaccine nor a cure is currently available the only way to prevent AIDS is to prevent the infection with HIV. This can be achieved by appropriate sex education and counseling advocating safe sex (monogamous relationship, with uninfected partner), using condoms and avoiding contacts with intravenous drug users and other high risk persons. Recent data on the effectiveness of early treatment with ZDV on slowing the progress of HIV infection makes the issue of early detection of HIV infection more important than ever. It emphasizes how critical it is that persons at risk for HIV infection be tested and seek, if positive, prompt medical care. Voluntary and confidential HIV antibody testing is essential in detecting early infections with HIV and prevention of further transmission of the virus.

REFERENCES

1. Pneumocystis pneumonia—Los Angeles. *MMWR* 30:250–252, 1981.

2. Gallo RC, Salahuddin SZ, Popovic M, et al.: Frequent detection and isolation of cytopathic retroviruses (HTLV-III) from patients with AIDS and at risk for AIDS. *Science* 224:500–503, 1984.

3. Coffin J, Hasse A, Levy JA, et al.: Human immunodeficiency virus (letter). *Science* 232:697, 1986.

4. Curran JW: The epidemiology and prevention of the acquired immunodeficiency syndrome. *Ann Intern Med* 103:657–662, 1985.

5. Jaffe HW, Darrow WW, Echenberg DF, et al.: The acquired immunodeficiency syndrome in a cohort of homosexual men. *Ann Intern Med* 103:210–214, 1985.

6. Goedert JJ, Ginzburg HM, Grossman RJ, et al.: Three-year incidence of AIDS in five cohorts of HTLV-III–infected risk group members. *Science* 231:992–995, 1986.

7. Coutinho RA, Bos JM, Ruitenberg EJ: The epidemiology of LAV/HTLV-III infection in Europe, in Staguet M, Hemmer R, Baert T. (eds), *Clinical Aspects of AIDS and AIDS-related Complex.* Oxford University Press, Oxford, 1986, p. 7–13.

8. Quinn TC, Mann JM, Curran JW, et al.: AIDS in Africa: An epidemiologic paradigm. *Science* 234:955–963, 1986.

9. Clumeck N, Van de Perre P, Carael M, et al.: Heterosexual promiscuity among African patients with AIDS. *N Engl J Med* 313:182, 1985.

10. Van de Perre P, Clumeck N, Carael M, et al.: Female prostitutes: A risk group for infection with human T-cell lymphotropic virus type III. *Lancet* 2:524–527, 1985.

11. Kreiss JK, Koech D, Plummer FA, et al.: AIDS virus infection in Nairobi prostitutes: Spread of the epidemic to East Africa. *N Engl J Med* 314:414–418, 1986.

12. Friedland GH, Klein RS: Transmission of the human immunodeficiency virus. *N Engl J Med* 317:1125–1135, 1987.

13. Marmor M, Friedman-Kien AE, Zolla-Pazner S, et al.: Kaposi's sarcoma in homosexual men: A seroepidemiologic case-control study. *Ann Intern Med* 100:809–815, 1984.

14. Blattner WA, Biggar RJ, Weiss SH, et al.: Epidemiology of human T-lymphotropic virus type III and the risk of the acquired immunodeficiency syndrome. *Ann Intern Med* 103:662–664, 1985.

15. Polk BF: Updates on HIV infection: Epidemiologic and clinical aspects. *Md Med J* 36:31–32, 1987.

16. Clumeck N: Heterosexual transmission of AIDS: No time for complacency. *Eur J Clin Microbiol* 5:609–616, 1986.

17. Guinan ME, Hardy A: Epidemiology of AIDS in women in the United States: 1981 through 1986. *JAMA* 257:2039–2042, 1987.

18. Mann JM, Quinn TC, Francis H, et al.: Prevalence of HTLV-III/LAV in household contacts of patients with confirmed AIDS and controls in Kinshasa, Zaire. *JAMA* 256:721–724, 1986.

19. Fischl MA, Dickinson GM, Scott GM, et al.: Evaluation of heterosexual partners, children and household contacts of adults with AIDS. *JAMA* 257:640–644, 1987.

20. Pitchenik AE, Shafron RD, Glasser RM, et al.: The acquired immunodeficiency syndrome in the wife of a hemophiliac. *Ann Intern Med* 100:62–65, 1984.

21. Redfield RR, Markham PD, Salahuddin SZ, et al.: Frequent transmission of HTLV-III among spouses of patients with AIDS-related complex and AIDS. *JAMA* 253:1571–1573, 1985.

22. Harris C, Butkus-Small C, Klein RS, et al.: Immunodeficiency in female sexual partners of men with the acquired immunodeficiency syndrome. *N Engl J Med* 308:1181–1184, 1983.

23. Wofsy CB, Cohen JB, Hauer LB, et al.: Isolation of AIDS-associated retrovirus from genital secretions of women with antibody to the virus. *Lancet* 1:527–529, 1986.

24. Vogt MW, Witt DJ, Craven DE, et al.: Isolation patterns of the human immunodeficiency virus from cervical secretion during the menstrual cycle of women at risk for the acquired immunodeficiency syndrome. *Ann Intern Med* 106:380–382, 1987.

25. Public Health Service plan for prevention and control of AIDS and the AIDS virus. *Public Health Rep* 101:341–348, 1986.

26. Stewart GJ, Cunningham AL, Driscoll GL, et al.: Transmission of human T-cell lymphotropic virus type III (HTLV-III) by artificial insemination by donor, *Lancet* 2:581–584, 1985.

27. Curran JW, Lawrence DN, Jaffe H, et al.: Acquired immunodeficiency syndrome (AIDS) associated with transfusions. *N Engl J Med* 310:69–75, 1984.

28. *Pneumocystis carini* pneumonia among persons with hemophilia, *MMWR* 31:365–368, 1982.

29. Evatt BL, Ramsley RB, Lawrence DN, et al.: The acquired immunodeficiency syndrome in patients with hemophilia. *Ann Intern Med* 100:499–504, 1984.

30. Feorino PM, Jaffe HW, Palmer E, et al.: Transfusion-associated acquired immunodeficiency syndrome: evidence for persistent infection in blood donors, *N Engl J Med* 312:1293–1296, 1985.

31. Allen JR: Epidemiologic considerations in the transmission of LAV/HTLV-III by blood and blood products, in Petricciani JC, Gust ID, Hoppe PA, Krijnen HW (eds), AIDS: *The Safety of Blood and Blood Products.* Chichester, John Wiley & Sons Ltd., WHO, 1987 p. 33–45.

32. Human immunodeficiency virus infection in transfusion recipients and their family members. *MMWR* 36:137–140, 1987.

33. Mariani G, Verani P, DeRossi G, et al.: The spread of the HTLV-III/LAV infection in a population of hemophiliacs treated exclusively with commercial concentrates, in Stagnet M, Hemmer R, Baert (eds), *Clinical Aspects of AIDS and AIDS-related Complex.* Oxford University Press, Oxford 1986, pp. 63–71.

34. Mann JM, Francis H, Quinn TC, et al.: Surveillance for AIDS in Central African City, Kinshasa, Zaire. *JAMA* 255:3255–3259, 1986.

35. Provisional public health service interagency recommendations for screening donated blood and plasma for antibody to the virus causing acquired immunodeficiency syndrome. *MMWR* 34:1–5, 1985.

36. Wendt D, Sadowski L, Markowitz N, et al.: Prevalence of serum antibody to human immunodeficiency virus among hospitalized intravenous drug abusers in a low-risk geographic area. *J Infect Dis* 155:151–152, 1987.

37. Chaisson RE, Moss AR, Onishi R, et al.: Human immunodeficiency virus infection in heterosexual intravenous drug users in San Francisco. *Am J Public Health* 77:169–172, 1987.

38. Ferroni P, Geroldi D, Galli C, et al.: HTLV-III antibody among Italian drug addicts. *Lancet* 2:52–53, 1985.

39. Rodrigo JM, Serra MA, Aguilar E, et al.: HTLV-III antibodies in drug addicts in Spain. *Lancet* 2:156–157, 1985.

40. Friedland GH, Harris C, Butkus-Small C, et al.: Intravenous drug abusers and the

acquired immunodeficiency syndrome (AIDS): Demographic drug use, and needle-sharing patterns. *Arch Intern Med* 145:1413–1417, 1985.

41. Black JL, Polan MP, DeFord HA, et al.: Sharing of needles among users of intravenous drugs. *N Engl J Med* 314:446–447, 1986.

42. Pape JW, Liautaud B, Thomas F, et al.: The acquired immunodeficiency syndrome in Haiti. *Ann Intern Med* 103:674–678, 1985.

43. Mann JM, Francis H, Davachi F, et al.: Human immunodeficiency virus seroprevalence in pediatric patients 2 to 14 years of age at Mama Yemo Hospital, Kinshasa, Zaire. *Pediatrics* 78:673–677, 1986.

44. Anonymous: Needlestick transmission of HTLV-III from a patient infected in Africa. *Lancet* 2:1376–1377, 1984.

45. Oksenhendler E, Harzil M, LeRoux J-M, et al.: HIV infection with seroconversion after a superficial needlestick injury to the finger. *N Engl J Med* 315:582, 1986.

46. CDC Update: Human immunodeficiency virus infections in health-care workers exposed to blood of infected patients. *MMWR* 36:285–289, 1987.

47. Napoli VM, McGowan JE: How much blood is in a needlestick? *J Infect Dis* 155:828, 1987.

48. Acquired immunodeficiency syndrome (AIDS) among blacks and Hispanics-United States. *MMWR* 35:655–666, 1986.

49. Lapointe N, Michand J, Pekovic D, et al.: Transplacental transmission of HTLV-III virus. *N Engl J Med* 312:1325–1326, 1985.

50. Marion RW, Wiznia AA, Hutcheon RG, et al.: Human T-cell lymphotropic virus type III (HTLV-III) embryopathy: A new dysmorphic syndrome associated with intra-uterine HTLV-III infection. *Am J Dis Child* 140:638–640, 1986.

51. Thiry L, Sprecher-Goldberger S, Jonckheer T, et al.: Isolation of AIDS virus from cell-free breast milk of three healthy carriers. *Lancet* 2:891–892, 1985.

52. Scott GB, Fischl MA, Klimas N, et al.: Mothers of infants with the acquired immuno-deficiency syndrome: Evidence for both symptomatic and asymptomatic carriers. *JAMA* 253:363–366, 1985.

53. Barré-Sinoussi F, Chermann JC, Rey F, et al.: Isolation of a T-lymphotropic retrovirus from a patient at risk for acquired immune deficiency syndrome (AIDS). *Science* 220:868–871, 1983.

54. Levy JA, Hoffman AD, Kramer SM, et al.: Isolation of lymphocytopathic retroviruses from San Francisco patients with AIDS. *Science* 225:840–842, 1984.

55. Guyader M, Emerman M, Sonigo P, et al.: Genome organization and transactivation of the human immunodeficiency virus type 2. *Nature* 326:662–669, 1987.

56. Daniel MD, Letvin NL, King NW, et al.: Isolation of T-cell tropic HTLV-III-like retro-virus from macaques. *Science* 228:1199–1204, 1985.

57. Montagnier L, Gruest J, Chamaret S, et al.: Adaptation of lymphadenopathy associated virus (LAV) to replication in EBV transformed B lymphoblastoid cell lines. *Science* 225:63–66, 1984.

58. Belsito DV, Sanchez MR, Baer RL, et al.: Reduced Langerhans cells Ia antigen and ATPase activity in patients with the acquired immunodeficiency syndrome. *N Engl J Med* 310:1279–1282, 1984.

59. Shaw GM, Harper ME, Hahn BH, et al.: HTLV-III infection in brains of children and adults with AIDS encephalopathy. *Science* 227:177–182, 1985.

60. Koenig S, Gendelman HE, Orenstein JM, et al.: Detection of AIDS virus in macro-phages in brain tissue from AIDS patients with encephalopathy. *Science* 233:1089–1093, 1986.

61. Gallo R: The AIDS virus. *Sci Am* 256:47–56, 1987.

62. Cooper DA, Gold J, Maclean P, et al.: Acute AIDS retrovirus infection. *Lancet* 1:537–540, 1985.

63. Ho DD, Sarngadharan MG, Resnick L, et al.: Primary human T-lymphotropic virus type III infection. *Ann Intern Med* 103:880–885, 1985.

64. Lindskov R, Orskov-Lindhardt B, Weissman K, et al.: Acute HTLV-III infection with roseolalike rash. *Lancet* 1:447, 1986.

65. Wantzin GRL, Lindhardt BO, Weismann K, et al.: Acute HTLV-III infection associated with exanthema diagnosed by seroconversion. *Br J Dermatol* 115:601–606, 1986.

66. Sindrup JH, Lisby G, Weismann K, et al.: Skin manifestations in AIDS, HIV infection and AIDS-related complex. *Int J Dermatol* 26:267–272, 1987.

67. Burger H, Weiser B, Robinson WS, et al.: Transient antibody to lymphadenopathy-associated virus/human T-lymphotrophic virus type III and T-lymphocyte abnormalities in the wife of man who developed the acquired immunodeficiency syndrome. *Ann Intern Med* 103:545–547, 1985.

68. Revision of the case definition of acquired immunodeficiency syndrome for national reporting—United States. *MMWR* 34:373–375, 1985.

69. Classification system for human T-lymphotropic virus type III/lymphadenopathy-associated virus infections. *MMWR* 35:334–339, 1986.

70. Redfield RR, Wright DC, Tramont EC: The Walter Reed staging classification for HTLV-III/LAV infection. *N Engl J Med* 314:131–132, 1986.

71. Haverkos HW, Gottlieb MS, Killen JY, et al.: Classification of HTLV III/LAV-related diseases (letter). *J Infect Dis* 152:1095, 1985.

72. Goedert JJ, Sarngadharan MG, Biggar RJ, et al.: Determinants of retrovirus (HTLV-III) antibody and immunodeficiency conditions in homosexual men. *Lancet* 2:711–716, 1984.

73. Cone LA, Schiffman MA: Herpes zoster and the acquired immunodeficiency syndrome. *Ann Intern Med* 100:462, 1984.

74. Groopman JE: Spectrum of HTLV-III infection, in Broeder S (ed), *AIDS: Modern Concepts and Therapeutic Challenges.* New York, Marcel Dekker, 1987, pp. 135–142.

75. Armstrong D, Gold JWM, Dryjanski J, et al.: Treatment of infections in patients with the acquired immunodeficiency syndrome. *Ann Intern Med* 103:738–743, 1985.

76. Ziegler JL: The natural history of AIDS, in Petricciani JC, Gust ID, Hoppe PA, et al. (eds), *AIDS: The Safety of Blood and Blood Products.* Chichester, John Wiley & Sons, 1987, pp. 21–31.

77. Seligmann M, Pinching AJ, Rosen FS, et al.: Immunology of human immunodeficiency virus infection and the acquired immunodeficiency syndrome: An update. *Ann Intern Med* 107:234–242, 1987.

78. Kramer RH, Fuh G-M, Hwamg CBC, et al.: Basement membrane and connective tissue proteins in early lesions of Kaposi's sarcoma associated with AIDS. *J Invest Dermatol* 84:516–520, 1985.

79. Klepp O, Dahl O, Stenning JT: Association of Kaposi's sarcoma with prior immunosuppressive therapy. A 5-year study of Kaposi's sarcoma in Norway. *Cancer* 12:2626–2630, 1978.

80. Kaposi's sarcoma and *Pneumocystis* pneumonia among homosexual men—New York City and California. *MMWR* 30:305–308, 1981.

81. Myskowski PL, Romano JF, Safai B: Kaposi's sarcoma in young homosexual men. *Cutis* 29:31–34, 1982.

82. Urmacher C, Myskowski PL, Ochoa M, et al.: Outbreak of Kaposi's sarcoma in young homosexual men. *Am J Med* 72:569–575, 1982.

83. Martin J: Acquired immunodeficiency syndrome (AIDS) and Kaposi's sarcoma. *Int J Dermatol* 23:483–486, 1984.

84. Rampen FHJ: AIDS and the dermatologist. *Int J Dermatol* 26:1–7, 1987.

85. Finkbeiner WE, Ekbert BM, Groundwater JR, et al.: Kaposi's sarcoma in young homosexual men: A histopathological study with particular reference to lymph node involvement. *Arch Pathol Lab Med* 106:261–264, 1982.

86. Epstein DM, Gefter WB, Conrad K, et al.: Lung disease in homosexual men. *Radiology* 143:7–20, 1982.

87. Warner LC, Fisher BK: Cutaneous manifestation of the acquired immunodeficiency syndrome. *Int J Dermatol* 25:337–350, 1986.

88. Friedman-Kien AE: Disseminated Kaposi's sarcoma syndrome in young homosexual men. *J Am Acad Dermatol* 5:468–471, 1981.

89. Safai B: Kaposi's sarcoma: An overview of classical and epidemic forms, in Broder S (ed), *AIDS: Modern Concepts and Therapeutic Challenges.* New York, Marcel Dekker, 1987, pp. 205–218.

90. Volberding P: Therapy of Kaposi's sarcoma in AIDS. *Semin Oncol* 11:60–67, 1984.

91. Schwartz JL, Muhlbauer JE, Steigbigel RT: Pre-Kaposi's sarcoma. *J Am Acad Dermatol* 11:377–380, 1984.

92. Rudlinger R: Kaposiforme Akroangiodermatiden (Pseudokaposi). *Hautarzt* 36:65–68, 1985.

93. Mintzer DM, Real FX, Jovino L, et al.: Treatment of Kaposi's sarcoma and thrombocytopenia with Vincristine in patients with the acquired immunodeficiency syndrome. *Ann Intern Med* 102:200–202, 1985.

94. Laubenstein LJ, Krigel RL, Odajnyk CM, et al.: Treatment of epidemic Kaposi's sarcoma with Etoposide or a combination of Doxorubicin, Bleomycin, and Vinblastine. *J Clin Oncol* 2:1115–1120, 1984.

95. Groopman JE, Gottlieb MS, Goodman J, et al.: Recombinant alpha-2 interferon therapy for Kaposi's sarcoma associated with the acquired immunodeficiency syndrome. *Ann Intern Med* 100:671–676, 1984.

96. Fauci AS, Masur H, Gelmann EP, et al.: NIH conference: New concepts in Kaposi's sarcoma. The acquired immunodeficiency syndrome: An update. *Ann Intern Med* 102:800–813, 1985.

97. Moskowitz L, Hensley GT, Chan JC, et al.: Immediate causes of death in acquired immunodeficiency syndrome. *Arch Pathol Lab Med* 109:735–738, 1985.

98. Ziegler JL, Drew WL, Miner RC, et al.: Outbreak of Burkitt's-like lymphoma in homosexual men. *Lancet* 2:631–633, 1982.

99. Lind SE, Gross PL, Andiman WA, et al.: Malignant lymphoma presenting as Kaposi's sarcoma in a homosexual man with acquired immunodeficiency syndrome. *Ann Intern Med* 102:338–340, 1985.

100. Levine A, Parkash SG, Meyer PR, et al.: Retrovirus and malignant lymphoma in homosexual men. *JAMA* 254:1921–1925.

101. Conant MA, Volberding P, Fletcher V, et al.: Squamous cell carcinoma in sexual partner of Kaposi's sarcoma patient. *Lancet* 1:286, 1982.

102. Schoeppel SL, Hoppe RT, Dorfman RF, et al.: Hodgkin's disease in homosexual men with generalized lymphadenopathy. *Ann Intern Med* 102:68–70, 1985.

103. Levine AM, Gill PS, Rasheed S: AIDS-related malignant B-cell lymphoms, in Broder S

(ed), *AIDS: Modern Concepts and Therapeutic Challenges*. New York, Mercel Dekker, 1987, pp. 233–244.

104. Levine AM, Gill PS, Meyer PR, et al.: Retrovirus and malignant lymphoma in homosexual men. *JAMA* 254:1921–1925, 1985.

105. Slazinski L, Stall JR, Mathews CR: Basal cell carcinoma in a man with acquired immunodeficiency syndrome. *J Am Acad Dermatol* 11:140–141, 1984.

106. Li FP, Osborn D, Cronin CM: Anorectal squamous carcinoma in two homosexual men. *Lancet* 2:391, 1982.

107. Kaplan MH, Sadick N, McNutt S, et al.: Dermatologic findings and manifestations of acquired immunodeficiency syndrome (AIDS). *J Am Acad Dermatol* 16:485–506, 1987.

108. Fisher BF, Warner LC: Cutaneous manifestations of the acquired immunodeficiency syndrome: Update 1987. *Int J Dermatol* 26:615–630, 1987.

109. Maize JC: Skin cancer in immunosuppressed patients. *JAMA* 237:1857–1858, 1977.

110. Marshall V: Premalignant and malignant skin tumors in immunosuppressed patients. *Transplantation* 17:272–275, 1974.

111. Frazer IH, Medley G, Crapper RM, et al.: Association between anorectal dysplasia, human papillomavirus and human immunodeficiency virus infection in homosexual men. *Lancet* 2:657–660, 1986.

112. Purtillo DT: Immune deficiency predisposing to Epstein-Barr virus-induced lymphoproliferative diseases: The x-linked lymphoproliferative syndrome as a model. *Adv Cancer Res* 34:279–312, 1981.

113. Eisenstat B, Wormser GP: Seborrheic dermatitis and butterfly rash in AIDS. *N Engl J Med* 311:189, 1984.

114. Mathes BM, Douglass MC: Seborrheic dermatitis in patients with acquired immunodeficiency syndrome. *J Am Acad Dermatol* 13:947–951, 1985.

115. Farthing CF, Staughton RCD, Rowland Payne CME: Skin disease in homosexual patients with acquired immune deficiency syndrome (AIDS) and lesser forms of human T-cell leukemia virus (HTLV-III) disease. *Clin Exp Dermatol* 10:3–12, 1985.

116. delaLoma A, Manrique A, Rubio R, et al.: Generalized tuberculosis in a patient with acquired immunodeficiency syndrome. *J Infect* 10:57–59, 1985.

117. Soeprono FF, Schinella RA, Cockerell CJ, et al.: Seborrheic-like dermatitis of acquired immunodeficiency syndrome: A clinicopathologic study. *J Am Acad Dermatol* 14:242–248, 1986.

118. Perniciaro C, Peters MS: Tinea faciale mimicking seborrheic dermatitis in patients with AIDS. *N Engl J Med* 314:315–316, 1986.

119. Ford GP, Farr PM, Ive FA, et al.: The response of seborrhoeic dermatitis to ketoconazole. *Br J Dermatol* 26(Suppl 3):25, 1984.

120. Skinner RB, Zanolli MD, et al.: Seborrheic dermatitis and acquired immunodeficiency syndrome. *J Am Acad Dermatol* 14:147–148, 1986.

121. Greenspan D, Greenspan JS, Conant M, et al.: Oral "hairy" leukoplakia in male homosexuals: Evidence of association with both papillomavirus and herpes group virus. *Lancet* 2:831–834, 1984.

122. Conant MA: Hairy leukoplakia: A new disease of the oral mucosa. *Arch Dermatol* 123:585–587, 1987.

123. Lupton GO, James WD, Redfield RR, et al.: Oral hairy leukoplakia: A distinctive marker of human T-cell lymphotropic virus Type III (HTLV-III) infection. *Arch Dermatol* 123:624–628, 1987.

124. Greenspan JS, Greenspan D, Lennette ET, et al.: Replication of Epstein-Barr virus within the epithelial cells of oral "hairy" leukoplakia, an AIDS-associated lesion. *N Engl J Med* 313:1564–1571, 1985.

125. Klein RS, Harris CA, Small CB, et al.: Oral candidiasis in high risk patients as the initial manifestation of the acquired immunodeficiency syndrome. *N Engl J Med* 311:354–358, 1984.

126. Busch DF: Overview of infectious diseases and other nonmalignant conditions in the acquired immune deficiency syndrome. *Front Radiat Ther Oncol* 19:52–58, 1985.

127. Borton LK, Wintroub BV: Disseminated cryptococcosis presenting as herpetiform lesions in homosexual men with acquired immunodeficiency syndrome. *J Am Acad Dermatol* 10:387–390, 1984.

128. Rico MJ, Penneys NS: Cutaneous cryptococcosis resembling molluscum contagiosum in a patient with AIDS. *Arch Dermatol* 121:901–902, 1985.

129. Kovacs JA, Kovacs AA, Polis M, et al.: Cryptococcosis in the acquired immunodeficiency syndrome. *Ann Intern Med* 103:533–538, 1985.

130. Koger OW, Steck WD, Kantor GR, et al.: Cutaneous manifestations of *Cryptococcus neoformans* infections in two AIDS patients. Paper presented during the 46th annual meeting of American Academy of Dermatology, San Antonio, December 5–10, 1987.

131. Kalter DC, Tschen JA, Klimar M: Maculopapular rash in a patient with acquired immunodeficiency syndrome. *Arch Dermatol* 121:1455–1460, 1985.

132. Mayorla F, Penneys NS: Disseminated histoplasmosis presenting as a transepidermal elimination disorder in an AIDS victim. *J Am Acad Dermatol* 13:842–844, 1985.

133. Hazelhurst JA, Vismer HF: Histoplasmosis presenting with unusual skin lesions in acquired immunodeficiency syndrome (AIDS). *Br J Dermatol* 113:345–348, 1985.

134. Muhlemann MF, Anderson MG, Paradinas FJ, et al.: Early warning skin signs in AIDS and persistent generalized lymphadenopathy. *Br J Dermatol* 114:419–424, 1986.

135. Penneys NS, Hick B: Unusual cutaneous lesions associated with acquired immunodeficiency syndrome. *J Am Acad Dermatol* 13:845–852, 1985.

136. Cone LA, Schiffman MA: Herpes zoster and acquired immunodeficiency syndrome. *Ann Intern Med* 100:462, 1984.

137. Friedland-Kien AE, Lafleur FL, Gendler E, et al.: Herpes zoster: A possible early clinical sign for development of acquired immunodeficiency syndrome in high-risk individuals. *J Am Acad Dermatol* 14:1023–1028, 1986.

138. Quinnan GV, Masur H, Rook AH, et al.: Herpesvirus infections in the acquired immune deficiency syndrome. *JAMA* 252:72–77, 1984.

139. Resnick L, Herbst JS: Dermatological (non-Kaposi's sarcoma) manifestations associated with HTLV-III/LAV infection, in Broder S (ed), *AIDS: Modern Concepts and Therapeutic Challenges*. New York, Marcel Dekker, 1987, pp. 258–302.

140. Siegal FP, Lopez C, Hammer GS, et al.: Severe acquired immunodeficiency in male homosexuals manifested by chronic perianal ulcerative herpes simplex lesions. *N Engl J Med* 305:1439–1444, 1981.

141. Dotz WI, Berman B: Kaposi's sarcoma, chronic ulcerative herpes simplex and acquired immunodeficiency. *Arch Dermatol* 119:93–94, 1983.

142. DeMaubeuge J, Mascart-Lemone F, Clumeck N, et al.: Acquired immunodeficiency manifested as severe genital herpes. *Dermatologica* 168:105–111, 1984.

143. Kalb RE, Grossman ME: Chronic perianal herpes simplex in immunocompromised host. *Am J Med* 80:486–490, 1986.

144. Goodell SE, Quinn TC, Mkrtichian E, et al.: Corey L: Herpes simplex virus proctitis in homosexual men. *N Engl J Med* 308:868–871, 1983.

145. Fauci AS, Macher AM, Longo DL, et al.: NIH Conference. Acquired immunodeficiency syndrome: Epidemiologic, clinical, immunologic and therapeutic consideration. *Ann Intern Med* 100:92–106, 1984.

146. Brown ST, Nalley JF, Kraus SJ: Molluscum contagiosum. *Sex Transm Dis* 8:227–234, 1984.

147. Hook EW, Stamm WE: Sexually transmitted diseases in men. *Med Clin North Am* 67:235–251, 1983.

148. Katzman M, Elmats CA, Lederman MM: Molluscum contagiosum in the acquired immunodeficiency syndrome. *Ann Intern Med* 102:413–414, 1985.

149. Lombardo PC: Molluscum contagiosum and the acquired immunodeficiency syndrome. *Arch Dermatol* 121:834–835, 1985.

150. Sarma DP, Weilbacher TG. Molluscum contagiosum in the acquired immunodeficiency syndrome. *J Am Acad Dermatol* 13:682–683, 1985.

151. Redfield RR, James WD, Wright DC, et al.: Severe molluscum contagiosum infection in a patient with human T-cell lymphotropic (HTLV-III) disease. *J Am Acad Dermatol* 13:821–824, 1985.

152. Kessler HA, Blaauw B, Spear J, et al.: Diagnosis of human immunodeficiency virus infection in seronegative homosexuals presenting with an acute viral syndrome. *JAMA* 258:1196–1199, 1987.

153. Zakowski P, Fligiel S, Berlin OG, et al.: Disseminated *Mycobacterium avium intracellulare* infection in homosexual men dying of acquired immunodeficiency. *JAMA* 248:2980–2982, 1982.

154. Wong B, Edwards FF, Kiehn TE, et al.: Continuous high-grade *Mycobacterium avium intracellulare* bacteremia in patients with acquired immunodeficiency syndrome. *Am J Med* 78:35–40, 1985.

155. Marchiando A: Scrofula followed by AIDS. *Ear Nose Throat J* 63:197–198, 1984.

156. Diagnosis and managements of mycobacterial infection and disease in persons with HTLV-III/LAV infection. *MMWR* 35:448–452, 1986.

157. Sunderam G, McDonald RJ, Maniatis T, et al.: Tuberculosis as a manifestation of the AIDS. *JAMA* 256:362–366, 1986.

158. Richard M, Mathieu-Serra A: Staphylococcal scalded skin syndrome in a homosexual adult. *J Am Acad Dermatol* 15:385–389, 1986.

159. Coulman CU, Greene I, Archibald WR: Cutaneous pneumocystosis. *Ann Intern Med* 106:396–398, 1987.

160. Gretzula JC, Penneys NS: Complex viral and fungal skin lesions of patient with acquired immunodeficiency syndrome. *J Am Acad Dermatol* 16:1151–1154, 1987.

161. James WD, Redfield RR, Lupton GP, et al.: A papular eruption associated with human T-cell lymphotropic virus type III disease. *J Am Acad Dermatol* 13:563–566, 1985.

162. Martinez MI, Sanchez JL, Lopez-Malpica F: Peculiar papular skin lesions occurring in hepatitis B carriers. *J Am Acad Dermatol* 16:31–34, 1987.

163. Soeprono FF, Schinella RA: Eosinophilic pustular folliculitis in patients with acquired immunodeficiency syndrome. *J Am Acad Dermatol* 14:1020–1022, 1986.

164. Chernosky ME, Finley VK: Yellow nail syndrome in patients with acquired immunodeficiency disease: *J Am Acad Dermatol* 13:731–736, 1985.

165. McLeod AW: Dermatologic manifestations of AIDS. *Medicine N America* (2nd series) 32:4448–4454, 1986.

166. Farthing CF, Brown SE, Staughton RCD, et al.: Colour Atlas of AIDS. London, Wolfe Medical Publications, Ltd., 1986, pp. 51–56.

167. Ghadially R, Sibbald RG, Walter JB, et al.: Granuloma annulare in HTLV-III positive patients. Paper presented during the 46th Annual Meeting of the American Academy of Dermatology, San Antonio, December, 5–10, 1987.

168. Chren M-M: Granulomatous skin lesions in patients with human immunodeficiency virus (HIV) infection. Paper presented during the 46th Annual Meeting of the American Academy of Dermatology, San Antonio, December, 5–10, 1987.

169. Nemeth AJ, Taylor JR, Halprin K: Chronic photosensitivity associated with AIDS: Therapy with PUVA. Paper presented during the 46th Annual Meeting of the American Academy of Dermatology, San Antonio, December, 5–10, 1987.

170. Duvic M, Johnson TM, Rapini RP, et al.: Acquired immunodeficiency syndrome-associated psoriasis and Reiter's Syndrome. *Arch Dermatol* 123:1622–1632, 1987.

171. Krueger JG, Scott R, Hambrick GW: Granulomatous secondary syphilis in HIV-I antibody positive man. Paper presented during the 46th Annual Meeting of the American Academy of Dermatology, San Antonio, December, 5–10, 1987.

172. Logan MA, Lupton F: Secondary syphilis in HIV positive white male with abundant treponemes observed on skin biopsy. Paper presented during the 46th Annual Meeting of the American Academy of Dermatology, San Antonio, December, 5–10, 1987.

173. Hicks CB, Benson PM, Lupton GP, et al.: Seronegative secondary syphilis in a patient infected with the human immunodeficiency virus (HIV) with Kaposi sarcoma. *Ann Intern Med* 107:492–495, 1987.

174. Berry CD, Hooten TM, Collier AC, et al.: Neurologic relapse after benzathine penicillin therapy for secondary syphilis in a patient with HIV infection. *N Engl J Med* 316: 1587–1589, 1987.

175. Johns DR, Tierney M, Selsenstein D: Alternation in the natural history of neurosyphilis by concurrent infection with the human immunodeficiency virus. *N Engl J Med* 316:1569–1572, 1987.

176. Weller IVD, Hindley DJ, Adler MW: Gonorrhea in homosexual men and media coverage of the acquired immunodeficiency syndrome in London 1982–3. *Br Med J* 289: 1041, 1984.

177. Poulusen A, Ullman S: AIDS-induced decline of the incidence of syphilis in Denmark. *Acta Derm Venereol (Stockh)* 65:567–569, 1985.

178. Update on acquired immunodeficiency syndrome (AIDS)—United States. *MMWR* 31:507–514, 1982.

179. Revision of the case definition of acquired immunodeficiency for national reporting—United States. *MMWR* 34:373, 1985.

180. Public Health Service guidelines for counseling and antibody testing to prevent HIV infection and AIDS. *MMWR* 36:509–515, 1987.

181. Fischl MA, Richman DD, Grieco MH, et al.: The efficacy of azidothymidine (AZT) in the treatment of patients with AIDS and AIDS-related complex: A double-blind, placebo-controlled trial. *N Engl J Med* 317:185–191, 1987.

182. Fischl MA, Richman DD, Grieco MH, et al.: The toxicity of azidothymidine (AZT) in the treatment of patients with AIDS and AIDS-related complex: A double-blind, placebo-controlled trial. *N Engl J Med* 317:192–197, 1987.

14

APPENDIX I–V*

APPENDIX I: REVISION OF THE CDC SURVEILLANCE CASE DEFINITION FOR ACQUIRED IMMUNODEFICIENCY SYNDROME

Introduction

The following revised case definition for surveillance of acquired immuno-deficiency syndrome (AIDS) was developed by CDC in collaboration with public health and clinical specialists. The Council of State and Territorial Epidemiologists (CSTE) has officially recommended adoption of the revised definition for national reporting of AIDS. The objectives of the revision are a) to track more effectively the severe disabling morbidity associated with infection with human immunodeficiency virus (HIV) (including HIV-1 and HIV-2); b) to simplify reporting of AIDS cases; c) to increase the sensitivity and specificity of the definition through greater diagnostic application of laboratory evidence for HIV infection; and d) to be consistent with current diagnostic practice, which in some cases includes presumptive, i.e., without confirmatory laboratory evidence, diagnosis of AIDS-indicative diseases (e.g., *Pneumocystis carinii* pneumonia, Kaposi's sarcoma).

The definition is organized into three sections that depend on the status of laboratory evidence of HIV infection (e.g., HIV antibody) (Figure 1). The major proposed changes apply to patients with laboratory evidence for HIV infection: a) inclusion of HIV encephalopathy, HIV wasting syndrome, and a broader range of specific AIDS-indicative diseases (Section II.A); b) inclusion of AIDS patients whose indicator diseases are diagnosed presumptively (Section II.B); and c) elimination of exclusions due to other causes of immunodeficiency (Section I.A).

Application of the definition for children differs from that for adults in two

---

*Reprinted from *Mortality and Morbidity Weekly Reports,* 36(1S):35–155, 1987. Reported by Council of State and Territorial Epidemiologists; AIDS Program, Center for Infectious Diseases, CDC.

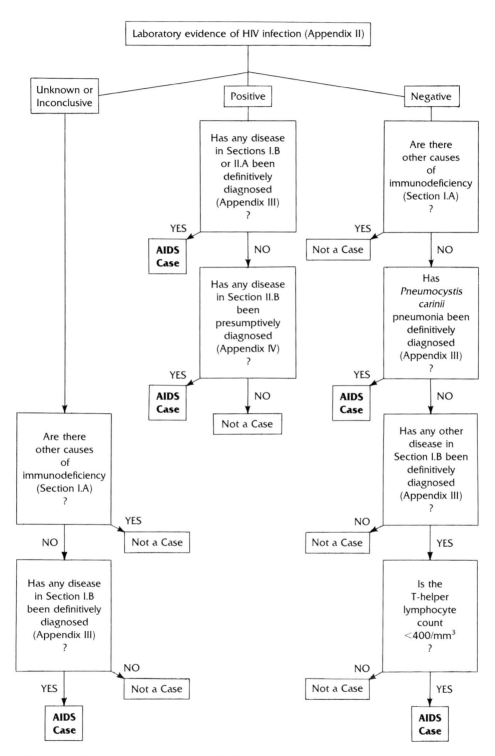

Figure 1. Flow diagram for revised CDC case definition of AIDS, September 1, 1987.

ways. First, multiple or recurrent serious bacterial infections and lymphoid interstitial pneumonia/pulmonary lymphoid hyperplasia are accepted as indicative of AIDS among children but not among adults. Second, for children < 15 months of age whose mothers are thought to have had HIV infection during the child's perinatal period, the laboratory criteria for HIV infection are more stringent, since the presence of HIV antibody in the child is, by itself, insufficient evidence for HIV infection because of the persistence of passively acquired maternal antibodies < 15 months after birth.

The new definition is effective immediately. State and local health departments are requested to apply the new definition henceforth to patients reported to them. The initiation of the actual reporting of cases that meet the new definition is targeted for September 1, 1987, when modified computer software and report forms should be in place to accommodate the changes. CSTE has recommended retrospective application of the revised definition to patients already reported to health departments. The new definition follows:

1987 Revision of Case Definition for AIDS for Surveillance Purposes

For national reporting, a case of AIDS is defined as an illness characterized by one or more of the following "indicator" diseases, depending on the status of laboratory evidence of HIV infection, as shown below.

I. Without Laboratory Evidence Regarding HIV infection

If laboratory tests for HIV were not performed or gave inconclusive results (see appendix II) and the patient had no other cause of immunodeficiency listed in Section I.A below, then any disease listed in Section I.B indicates AIDS if it was diagnosed by a definitive method (*see* Appendix III).

A. Causes of immunodeficiency that disqualify diseases as indicators of AIDS in the absence of laboratory evidence for HIV infection
    1. High-dose or long-term systemic corticosteroid therapy or other immunosuppressive/cytotoxic therapy ≤ 3 months before the onset of the indicator disease
    2. Any of the following diseases diagnosed ≤ 3 months after diagnosis of the indicator disease: Hodgkin's disease, non-Hodgkin's lymphoma (other than primary brain lymphoma), lymphocytic leukemia, multiple myeloma, any other cancer of lymphoreticular or histiocytic tissue, or angioimmunoblastic lymphadenopathy
    3. A genetic (congenital) immunodeficiency syndrome or an acquired immunodeficiency syndrome atypical of HIV infection, such as one involving hypogammaglobulinemia
B. Indicator diseases diagnosed definitively (*see* Appendix III)
    1. Candidiasis of the esophagus, trachea, bronchi, or lungs
    2. Cryptococcosis, extrapulmonary
    3. Cryptosporidiosis with diarrhea persisting > 1 month

4. Cytomegalovirus disease of an organ other than liver, spleen, or lymph nodes in a patient > 1 month of age

5. Herpes simplex virus infection causing a mucocutaneous ulcer that persists longer than 1 month; or bronchitis, pneumonitis, or esophagitis for any duration affecting a patient > 1 month of age

6. Kaposi's sarcoma affecting a patient < 60 years of age

7. Lymphoma of the brain (primary) affecting a patient < 60 years of age

8. Lymphoid interstitial pneumonia and/or pulmonary lymphoid hyperplasia (LIP/PLH complex) affecting a child < 13 years of age

9. *Mycobacterium avium* complex or *M. kansasii* disease, disseminated (at a site other than or in addition to lungs, skin, or cervical or hilar lymph nodes)

10. *Pneumocystis carinii* pneumonia

11. Progressive multifocal leukoencephalopathy

12. Toxoplasmosis of the brain affecting a patient > 1 month of age

II. With Laboratory Evidence for HIV Infection

Regardless of the presence of other causes of immunodeficiency (Section I.A), in the presence of laboratory evidence for HIV infection (*see* Appendix II), any disease listed above (I.B) or below (II.A or II.B) indicates a diagnosis of AIDS.

A. Indicator diseases diagnosed definitively (*see* Appendix III)
1. Bacterial infections, multiple or recurrent (any combination of at least two within a 2-year period), of the following types affecting a child < 13 years of age:

    septicemia, pneumonia, meningitis, bone or joint infection, or abscess of an internal organ or body cavity (excluding otitis media or superficial skin or mucosal abscesses), caused by *Haemophilus, Streptococcus* (including pneumococcus), or other pyogenic bacteria

2. Coccidioidomycosis, disseminated (at a site other than or in addition to lungs or cervical or hilar lymph nodes)

3. HIV encephalopathy (also called "HIV dementia," "AIDS dementia," or "subacute encephalitis due to HIV") (*see* Appendix III for description)

4. Histoplasmosis, disseminated (at a site other than or in addition to lungs or cervical or hilar lymph nodes)

5. Isosporiasis with diarrhea persisting > 1 month

6. Kaposi's sarcoma at any age

7. Lymphoma of the brain (primary) at any age

8. Other non-Hodgkin's lymphoma of B-cell or unknown immunologic phenotype and the following histologic types:
    a. Small noncleaved lymphoma (either Burkitt or non-Burkitt type) (*see* Appendix V for equivalent terms and numeric codes used in the *International Classification of Diseases,* Ninth Revision, Clinical Modification)
    b. Immunoblastic sarcoma (equivalent to any of the following, al-

though not necessarily all in combination: immunoblastic lymphoma, large-cell lymphoma, diffuse histiocytic lymphoma, diffuse undifferentiated lymphoma, or high-grade lymphoma) (*see* Appendix V for equivalent terms and numeric codes used in the *International Classification of Diseases*, Ninth Revision, Clinical Modification) Note: Lymphomas are not included here if they are of T cell immunologic phenotype or their histologic type is not described or is described as "lymphocytic," "lymphoblastic," "small cleaved," or "plasmacytoid lymphocytic"

9. Any mycobacterial disease caused by mycobacteria other than *M. tuberculosis*, disseminated (at a site other than or in addition to lungs, skin, or cervical or hilar lymph nodes)

10. Disease caused by *M tuberculosis*, extrapulmonary (involving at least one site outside the lungs, regardless of whether there is concurrent pulmonary involvement)

11. *Salmonella* (nontyphoid) septicemia, recurrent

12. HIV wasting syndrome (emaciation, "slim disease") (*see* Appendix III for description)

B. Indicator diseases diagnosed presumptively (by a method other than those in Appendix III)
Note: Given the seriousness of diseases indicative of AIDS, it is generally important to diagnose them definitively, especially when therapy that would be used may have serious side effects or when definitive diagnosis is needed for eligibility for antiretroviral therapy. Nonetheless, in some situations, a patient's condition will not permit the performance of definitive tests. In other situations, accepted clinical practice may be to diagnose presumptively based on the presence of characteristic clinical and laboratory abnormalities. Guidelines for presumptive diagnoses are suggested in Appendix IV.

1. Candidiasis of the esophagus

2. Cytomegalovirus retinitis with loss of vision

3. Kaposi's sarcoma

4. Lymphoid interstitial pneumonia and/or pulmonary lymphoid hyperplasia (LIP/PLH complex) affecting a child < 13 years of age

5. Mycobacterial disease (acid-fast bacilli with species not identified by culture), disseminated (involving at least one site other than or in addition to lungs, skin, or cervical or hilar lymph nodes)

6. *Pneumocystis carinii* pneumonia

7. Toxoplasmosis of the brain affecting a patient > 1 month of age

III. With Laboratory Evidence Against HIV Infection

With laboratory test results negative for HIV infection (*see* Appendix II), a diagnosis of AIDS for surveillance purposes is ruled out *unless*

A. All the other causes of immunodeficiency listed above in Section I.A are excluded, *and*

B. The patient has had either
  1. *Pneumocystis carinii* pneumonia diagnosed by a definitive method (*see* Appendix III), *or*
  2. a. Any of the other diseases indicative of AIDS listed above in Section I.B diagnosed by a definitive method (see Appendix II), *and*
      b. A T-helper/inducer (CD4) lymphocyte count $< 400/mm^3$.

Commentary

The surveillance of severe disease associated with HIV infection remains an essential, although not the only, indicator of the course of the HIV epidemic. The number of AIDS cases and the relative distribution of cases by demographic, geographic, and behavioral risk variables are the oldest indices of the epidemic, which began in 1981 and for which data are available retrospectively back to 1978. The original surveillance case definition, based on then-available knowledge, provided useful epidemiologic data on severe HIV disease.[1] To ensure a reasonable predictive value for underlying immunodeficiency caused by what was then an unknown agent, the indicators of AIDS in the old case definition were restricted to particular opportunistic diseases diagnosed by reliable methods in patients without specific known causes of immunodeficiency. After HIV was discovered to be the cause of AIDS, however, and highly sensitive and specific HIV-antibody tests became available, the spectrum of manifestations of HIV infection became better defined, and classification systems for HIV infection were developed.[2–5] It became apparent that some progressive, seriously disabling, and even fatal conditions (e.g., encephalopathy, wasting syndrome) affecting a substantial number of HIV-infected patients were not subject to epidemiologic surveillance, as they were not included in the AIDS case definition. For reporting purposes, the revision adds to the definition most of those severe noninfectious, noncancerous HIV-associated conditions that are categorized in the CDC clinical classification systems for HIV infection among adults and children.[4,5]

Another limitation of the old definition was that AIDS-indicative diseases are diagnosed presumptively (i.e., without confirmation by methods required by the old definition) in 10–15% of patients diagnosed with such diseases; thus, an appreciable proportion of AIDS cases were missed for reporting purposes.[6,7] This proportion may be increasing, which would compromise the old case definition's usefulness as a tool for monitoring trends. The revised case definition permits the reporting of those clinically diagnosed cases as long as there is laboratory evidence of HIV infection.

The effectiveness of the revision will depend on how extensively HIV-antibody tests are used. Approximately one third of AIDS patients in the United States have been from New York City and San Francisco, where, since 1985, $< 7\%$ have been reported with HIV-antibody test results, compared with $> 60\%$ in other areas. The impact on the revision on the reported numbers of AIDS cases will also depend on the proportion of AIDS patients in whom indicator diseases are diagnosed presumptively rather than definitively. The use of presumptive diagnostic criteria varies geographically, being more common in certain rural areas and in urban areas with many indigent AIDS patients.

To avoid confusion about what should be reported to health departments, the term "AIDS" should refer only to conditions meeting the surveillance definition. This definition is intended only to provide consistent statistical data for public health purposes. Clinicians will not rely on this definition alone to diagnose serious disease caused by HIV infection in individual patients because there may be additional information that would lead to a more accurate diagnosis. For example, patients who are not reportable under the definition because they have either a negative HIV-antibody test or, in the presence of HIV antibody, an opportunistic disease not listed in the definition as an indicator of AIDS nonetheless may be diagnosed as having serious HIV disease on consideration of other clinical or laboratory characteristics of HIV infection or a history of exposure to HIV.

Conversely, the AIDS Surveillance definition may rarely misclassify other patients as having serious HIV disease if they have no HIV-antibody test but have an AIDS-indicative disease with a background incidence unrelated to HIV infection, such as cryptococcal meningitis.

The diagnostic criteria accepted by the AIDS surveillance case definition should not be interpreted as the standard of good medical practice. Presumptive diagnoses are accepted in the definition because not to count them would be to ignore substantial morbidity resulting from HIV infection. Likewise, the definition accepts a reactive screening test for HIV antibody without confirmation by a supplemental test because a repeatedly reactive screening test result, in combination with an indicator disease, is highly indicative of true HIV disease. For national surveillance purposes, the tiny proportion of possibly false-positive screening tests in persons with AIDS-indicative diseases is of little consequence. For the individual patient, however, a correct diagnosis is critically important. The use of supplemental tests is, therefore, strongly endorsed. An increase in the diagnostic use of HIV-antibody tests could improve both the quality of medical care and the function of the new case definition as well as assist in providing counseling to prevent transmission of HIV.

REFERENCES

1. World Health Organization: Acquired immunodeficiency syndrome (AIDS): WHO/CDC case definition for AIDS. *WHO Wkly Epidemiol Rec* 61:69–72, 1986.
2. Haverkos HW, Gottlieb MS, Killen JY, et al.: Classification of HTLV-III/LAV-related diseases (letter). *J Infect Dis* 152:1095, 1985.
3. Redfield RR, Wright DC, Tramont EC: The Walter Reed staging classification of HTLV-III infection. *N Engl J Med* 314:131–132, 1986.
4. Classification system for human T-lymphotropic virus type III/lymphadenopathy-associated virus infections. *MMWR* 35:334–339, 1986.
5. Classification system for human immunodeficiency virus (HIV) infection in children under 13 years of age. *MMWR* 36:225–230, 235, 1981.
6. Hardy AM, Starcher ET, Morgan WM, et al.: Review of death certificates to assess completeness of AIDS case reporting. *Pub Hlth Rep* 102:386–391, 1981.
7. Starcher ET, Biel JK, Rivera-Castano R, et al.: The impact of presumptively diagnosed opportunistic infections and cancers on national reporting of AIDS (Abstract). III International Conference on AIDS, Washington, DC, June 1–5, 1987.

APPENDIX II: LABORATORY EVIDENCE FOR OR AGAINST HIV INFECTION

1. For Infection: When a patient has disease consistent with AIDS:
   a. A serum specimen from a patient ≥ 15 months of age, or from a child < 15 months of age whose mother is not thought to have had HIV infection during the child's perinatal period, that is repeatedly reactive for HIV antibody by a screening test (e.g., enzyme-linked immunosorbent assay [ELISA]), as long as subsequent HIV-antibody tests (e.g., Western blot, immunofluorescence assay), if done, are positive; *or*
   b. A serum specimen from a child < 15 months of age, whose mother is thought to have had HIV infection during the child's perinatal period, that is repeatedly reactive for HIV antibody by a screening test (e.g., ELISA), plus increased serum immunoglobulin levels and at least one of the following abnormal immunologic test results; reduced absolute lymphocyte count, depressed CD4 (T-helper) lymphocyte count, or decreased CD4/CD8 (helper/suppressor) ratio, as long as subsequent antibody tests (e.g., Western blot immunofluorescence assay), if done, are positive; *or*
   c. A positive test for HIV serum antigen; *or*
   d. A positive HIV culture confirmed by both reverse transcriptase detection and a specific HIV-antigen test or in situ hybridization using a nucleic acid probe; *or*
   e. A positive result on any other highly specific test for HIV (e.g., nucleic acid probe of peripheral blood lymphocytes).
2. Against Infection: A nonreactive screening test for serum antibody to HIV (e.g., ELISA) without a reactive or positive result on any other test for HIV infection (e.g., antibody, antigen, culture), if done.
3. Inconclusive (Neither For nor Against Infection):
   a. A repeatedly reactive screening test for serum antibody to HIV (e.g., ELISA) followed by a negative or inconclusive supplemental test (e.g., Western blot immunofluorescence assay) without a positive HIV culture or serum antigen test, if done; *or*
   b. A serum specimen from a child < 15 months of age, whose mother is thought to have had HIV infection during the child's perinatal period, that is repeatedly reactive for HIV antibody by a screening test, even if positive by a supplemental test, without additional evidence for immunodeficiency as described above (in 1.b) and without a positive HIV culture or serum antigen test, if done.

APPENDIX III: DEFINITIVE DIAGNOSTIC METHODS FOR DISEASES INDICATIVE OF AIDS

Diseases	Definitive Diagnostic Methods
Cryptosporidiosis Cytomegalovirus Isosporiasis Kaposi's sarcoma Lymphoma Lymphoid pneumonia or hyperplasia *Pneumocystis carinii* pneumonia Progressive multifocal leukoencephalopathy Toxoplasmosis	Microscopy (histology or cytology).
Candidiasis	Gross inspection by endoscopy or autopsy or by microscopy (histology or cytology) on a specimen obtained directly from the tissues affected (including scrapings from the mucosal surface), not from a culture.
Coccidioidomycosis Cryptococcosis Herpes simplex virus Histoplasmosis	Microscopy (histology or cytology), culture, or detection of antigen in a specimen obtained directly from the tissues affected or a fluid from those tissues.
Tuberculosis Other mycobacteriosis Salmonellosis Other bacterial infection	Culture.
HIV encephalopathy* (dementia)	Clinical findings of disabling cognitive and/or motor dysfunction interfering with occupation or activities of daily living, or loss of behavioral developmental milestones affecting a child, progressing over weeks to months, in the absence of a concurrent illness or condition other than HIV infection that could explain the findings. Methods to rule out such concurrent illnesses and conditions must include cerebrospinal fluid examination and either brain imaging (computed tomography or magnetic resonance) or autopsy.
HIV wasting syndrome*	Findings of profound involuntary weight loss > 10% of baseline body weight plus either chronic diarrhea (at least two loose stools per day for ≥ 30 days) or chronic weakness and documented fever (for ≥ 30 days, intermittent or constant) in the absence of a concurrent illness or condition other than HIV infection that could explain the findings (e.g., cancer, tuberculosis, cryptosporidiosis, or other specific enteritis).

*For HIV encephalopathy and HIV wasting syndrome, the methods of diagnosis described here are not truly definitive but are sufficiently rigorous for surveillance purposes.

APPENDIX IV: SUGGESTED GUIDELINES FOR PRESUMPTIVE DIAGNOSIS OF DISEASES INDICATIVE OF AIDS

Diseases	Presumptive Diagnostic Criteria
Candidiasis of esophagus	a. Recent onset of retrosternal pain on swallowing, *and* b. Oral candidiasis diagnosed by the gross appearance of white patches or plaques on an erythematous base or by the microscopic appearance of fungal mycelial filaments in an uncultured specimen scraped from the oral mucosa.
Cytomegalovirus retinitis	A characteristic appearance on serial ophthalmoscopic examinations (e.g., discrete patches of retinal whitening with distinct borders, spreading in a centrifugal manner, following blood vessels, pressing over several months, frequently associated with retinal vasculitis, hemorrhage, and necrosis). Resolution of active disease leaves retinal scarring and atrophy with retinal pigment epithelial mottling.
Mycobacteriosis	Microscopy of a specimen from stool or normally sterile body fluids or tissue from a site other than lungs, skin, or cervical or hilar lymph nodes, showing acid-fast bacilli of a species not identified by culture.
Kaposi's sarcoma	A characteristic gross appearance of an erythematous or violaceous plaque-like lesion on skin or mucous membrane. (Note: Presumptive diagnosis of Kaposi's sarcoma should not be made by clinicians who have seen few cases of it.)
Lymphoid interstitial pneumonia	Bilateral reticulonodular interstitial pulmonary infiltrates present on chest x-ray for $\geq$ 2 months with no pathogen identified and no response to antibiotic treatment.
Pneumocystis *carinii* pneumonia	a. A history of dyspnea on exertion or nonproductive cough of recent onset (within the past 3 months), *and* b. Chest x-ray evidence of diffuse bilateral interstitial infiltrates or gallium scan evidence of diffuse bilateral pulmonary disease, *and* c. Arterial blood gas analysis showing an arterial pO_2 of < 70 mm Hg or a low respiratory diffusing capacity (<80% of predicted values) or an increase in the alveolar-arterial oxygen tension gradient, *and* d. No evidence of a bacterial pneumonia.
Toxoplasmosis of the brain	a. Recent onset of a focal neurologic abnormality consistent with intracranial disease or a reduced level of consciousness, *and* b. Brain imaging evidence of a lesion having a mass effect (on computed tomography or nuclear magnetic resonance) or the radiographic appearance of which is enhanced by injection of contrast medium; *and* c. Serum antibody to toxoplasmosis or successful response to therapy for toxoplasmosis.

APPENDIX V: EQUIVALENT TERMS AND INTERNATIONAL CLASSIFICATION OF DISEASE (ICD) CODES FOR AIDS-INDICATIVE LYMPHOMAS

The following terms and codes describe lymphomas indicative of AIDS in patients with antibody evidence for HIV infection (Section II.A.8 of the AIDS case definition). Many of these terms are obsolete or equivalent to one another. ICD-9-CM (1978)

Codes	Terms
200.0	*Reticulosarcoma* lymphoma (malignant); histiocytic (diffuse) reticulum cell sarcoma; pleomorphic cell type or not otherwise specified
200.2	*Burkitt's tumor or lymphoma* malignant lymphoma, Burkitt's type

ICD-O (Oncologic Histologic Types 1976)

Code	Terms
9600/3	*Malignant lymphoma, undifferentiated cell type* non-Burkitt's or not otherwise specified
9601/3	*Malignant lymphoma, stem cell type* stem cell lymphoma
9612/3	*Malignant lymphoma, immunoblastic type* immunoblastic sarcoma, immunoblastic lymphoma, or immunoblastic lymphosarcoma
9632/3	*Malignant lymphoma, centroblastic type* diffuse or not otherwise specified, or germinoblastic sarcoma; diffuse or not otherwise specified
9633/3	*Malignant lymphoma, follicular center cell, non-cleaved* diffuse or not otherwise specified
9640/3	*Reticulosarcoma, not otherwise specified* malignant lymphoma, histiocytic; diffuse or not otherwise specified reticulum cell sarcoma, not otherwise specified malignant lymphoma, reticulum cell type
9641/3	*Reticulosarcoma, pleomorphic cell type* malignant lymphoma, histiocytic, pleomorphic cell type reticulum cell sarcoma, pleomorphic cell type
9750/3	*Burkitt's lymphoma or Burkitt's tumor* malignant lymphoma, undifferentiated, Burkitt's type malignant lymphoma, lymphoblastic, Burkitt's type

15

SKIN DISEASES COMMONLY AFFECTING THE ANOGENITAL REGION

BACTERIAL, FUNGAL, AND VIRAL INFECTIONS OF THE SKIN

Balanitis—Balanoposthitis

Balanitis is an inflammatory disease of the glans of the penis. In uncircumcised men the inflammatory process frequently involves the inner surface of the overlying prepuce—balanoposthitis.

Balanoposthitis or balanitis can be caused by yeasts or fungi, bacteria, viruses, and/or protozoa.[1-11] Poor hygiene, chemical or mechanical injuries of the glans of the penis or inner surface of the prepuce are factors predisposing to these infections. Some of them can be acquired from sexual partners.[12,13] When the prepuce is difficult to retract or when phimosis is present secretions accumulated under the prepuce are very likely to be secondarily infected causing inflammation of the glans and the prepuce. The symptoms consist of itching and burning. In more severe cases discharge from underneath the prepuce as well as urinary symptoms may be present. The glans or the inner surface of the prepuce is usually erythematous and covered with a maculopapular rash (Figure 15.1). "Cuts" and erosions, often covered with exudate are not uncommon.

Patients with diabetes and those receiving immunosuppressive therapy are at increased risk of candidal balanitis or candidal balanoposthitis. In this form of balanoposthitis small white plaques can be seen or dry glazed erythematous glans or small eroded papules may be present. In severe cases ulcerations with edema

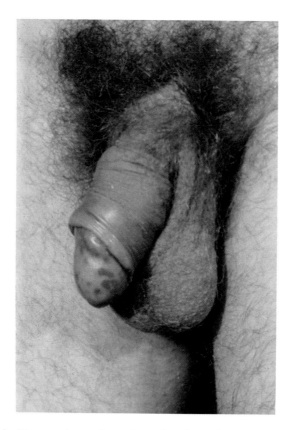

Figure 15.1.   Balanitis: maculopapular rash on the glans of penis caused by mixed bacterial/yeast infection.

may occur. Secondary phimosis is not uncommon. Female sex partners of men with candidal balanitis frequently suffer from vaginal candidiasis.[13]

Diagnosis is based on the clinical picture and can be confirmed by culture growing either *C. albicans* or other pathogenic microorganisms.

The differential diagnosis includes genital herpes, chancroid, primary syphilis (balanitis of Follmann), secondary syphilis, balanitis circinata (Reiter's syndrome), contact dermatitis, dermatitis artefacta, erythema multiforme, Stevens-Johnson syndrome, scabies, erythroplasia of Queyrat, balanitis plasmocellularis of Zoon.

Treatment

In mild cases cleaning the glans of the penis with an emollient nondetergent soap is usually sufficient. More severe cases may require application of frequently changed compresses (every 1 to 2 hours) with saline or 0.25% silver nitrate several times a day. In case of severe inflammation 1% hydrocortisone cream with or without antiseptic twice daily is very helpful. If *Candida albicans* is the cause of disease, clotrimazole or miconazole creams applied twice daily are recommended.[3] If the prepuce cannot be retracted (phimosis) subpreputial irrigation with saline or 0.25% silver nitrate solution at frequent intervals may be very helpful. Recurrent

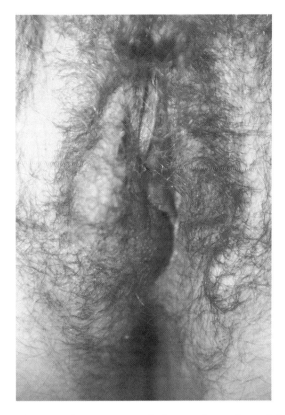

Figure 15.2. Bartholinitis: inflammation and abscess formation of the right Bartholin's gland.

balanitis or balanoposthitis can be prevented by circumcision. Moreover, whenever candidal balanitis becomes unusually recurrent or resistant to treatment, the possibility of underlying systemic diseases such as diabetes mellitus and AIDS should be ruled out and the patient should be asked about concomitant treatment with systemic broad spectrum antibiotics or immunosuppressive drugs.

Bartholinitis

Bartholinitis may result from infections of Bartholin's gland (Figure 15.2) with sexually transmitted microorganisms such as *Neisseria gonorrhoeae, Trichomonas vaginalis*, and *Chlamydia trachomatis* but may also be caused by streptococci, staphylococci, *Escherichia coli*, and others.[14,15] Clinically, bartholinitis varies from slight painless enlargement of the gland to acute infection with formation of an abscess requiring emergency surgery.

In acute bartholinitis the affected labium is swollen and painful and the pus can be expressed through the external opening of the duct, which usually shows an erythematous halo. If abscess formation occurs there may be considerable enlargement of the extremely tender gland accompanied by fever. Following infection, a cyst of Bartholin's gland may form.

Diagnosis: painful swelling or abscess formation on one of the labia majora; pus expressed through the opening of the duct or obtained by aspiration or drainage reveal the causative pathogen.

Differential diagnosis: the most common cause of bartholinitis is gonococcal infection; however, other microorganisms such as *T. vaginalis* and *C. trachomatis* and other typical skin pathogens such as staphylococci or streptococci can be the cause of infection of this gland as well.

Treatment

Systemic antibiotics depend upon the causative agent. If abscess develops aspiration with a wide-bore needle under local anesthesia or incision and drainage may be required. In case of recurring abscesses, excision of the gland under general anesthesia should be considered.

Pyogenic Lesions

Pyodermas of the anogenital region, as in other parts of the body, are commonly caused by streptococci and staphylococci. The region is particularly prone to skin infections because of hairy skin, flexures, a variety of glandular structures, and proximity to the vagina and anus.[16] Pyogenic lesions include folliculitis, furuncles, carbuncles, and cellulitis, including erysipelas, abscesses, and impetigo.

Folliculitis.   Folliculitis (Figure 15.3) is an inflammatory reaction in the hair follicle mainly caused by *Staphylococcus aureus*. It is usually asymptomatic or produces mild discomfort. Clinically, the lesion appears as a pustule, often with central hairs.

Furuncles and carbuncles.   Furuncles (boils) and carbuncles are pus-filled cutaneous nodules usually caused by *S. aureus*, but other bacteria including streptococci also can be the cause. Furuncles usually arise from infected hair follicles. Initially small pustules with an erythematous periphery appear, but after destruction of the follicle wall, infection spreads, causing local pain and even systemic symptoms. As the lesions progress they may burst, discharging a central necrotic plug of pus. A carbuncle is a group of furuncles that have coalesced. Since more skin is involved, there is also more tissue reaction, including erythema, edema, and local tenderness. Fever is not uncommon.

Furuncles should be treated with systemic antibiotics (the antibiotics should be active against beta-lactamase producing *Staphylococci*). Local measures include application of cleansing agents. The area should be kept clean of discharge and any dressing should be changed frequently. Some cases may require small incision and drainage.

Abscess and cellulitis.   Abscess (Figure 15.4) and cellulitis are infections of the skin and subcutaneous tissue caused by pyogenic bacteria. When the lesion is well circumscribed, it is termed an abscess, and when it is diffuse and spreading, the preferred term is cellulitis. The skin shows several signs, which include erythema, swelling, elevated local temperature, and tenderness or pain. When an abscess is formed fluctuation can be felt on palpation. Fever may be present.

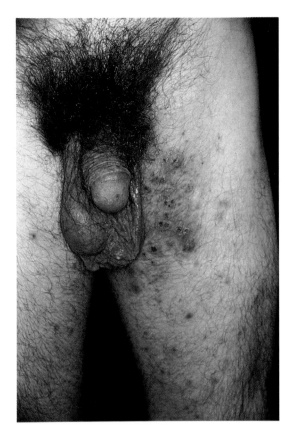

Figure 15.3. Folliculitis on the skin of the thighs and scrotum caused by *Staphylococcus aureus*.

Abscess and cellulitis should be treated with systemic antibiotics. Abscesses may need a surgical incision and drainage.

Impetigo. Impetigo is a rare infection of the skin caused by *S. aureus* and group A streptococci. The early lesions are pustules, which quickly break to form crusts. The hallmark of the disease is a lesion covered with honey-colored crust. The disease occurs in children on the face and hands but rarely may affect the genital region (the skin of the pubis and scrotum or the vulva are most frequently affected).

Impetigo should be treated with systemic and topical antibiotics. Soaks with topical antibiotics and keratolytic agents may help to remove the crusts.

Hidradenitis Suppurativa

Hidradenitis suppurativa (Figure 15.5) is an inflammatory disease of the apocrine sweat glands. The cause is unknown, but the condition results from obstruction of the apocrine ducts followed by their dilatation. Bacterial infection and hormones are believed to play a significant role in the etiology of the disease.[17] It is frequently associated with severe acne and perifolliculitis.

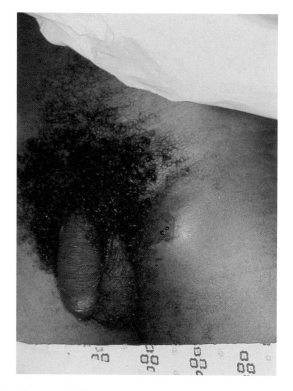

Figure 15.4. Abscess in the groin caused by staphylococci and streptococci.

The apocrine gland areas frequently involved are the axillae, groins, buttocks, and perianal region. Patients usually present with multiple deeply situated inflammatory nodules which are painful and may break down, forming draining abscess, sinuses, and fistulas.[18] Secondary bacterial infection is almost a rule. The disease is chronic and relapses are common. Sequelae such as fibrotic lesions may restrict movement. Due to destruction of the apocrine glands and scarring, the patient may lose the ability to sweat at the affected site.

Diagnosis is based on the clinical picture and typical distribution. Biopsy may be helpful.

Differential diagnosis includes furuncles, carbuncles, abscess, lymphadenitis, cutaneous tuberculosis, actinomycosis, LGV, syphilis, chancroid, and donovanosis.

Treatment

Systemic antibiotics should be administered until inflammation disappears. When induration persists, prednisone 40 to 60 mg daily for 7 to 10 days may be helpful.

Compresses with saline, Burow's solution or 0.5% neomycin may provide relief of discomfort and also disinfect the skin. Large cysts should be incised and drained. Intralesional triamcinolone may result in involution of the nodule or even permanent disappearance of the lesion.[19]

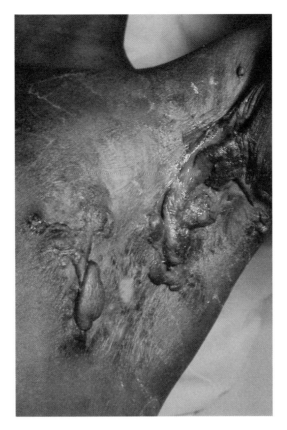

Figure 15.5. Hidradenitis suppurativa: fibrotic lesions, inflammatory nodules, fistulas, and sinuses in the axillae; similar lesion may develop in the groins.

Intertrigo

Intertrigo is an eroded, weeping eruption in areas where two skin surfaces touch (Figure 15.6), It frequently occurs in the anogenital region (groins and between the buttocks) particularly in obese patients. A humid environment, excessive sweating, and vaginal or rectal discharge are important predisposing factors. Regardless of their cause, the lesions are frequently infected by bacteria or fungi, particularly yeast.[20]

The lesions appear as symmetrical, red, macerated half-moon–shaped plaques on both sides of the buttock cleft or on both sides of the groin. In more advanced cases, painful fissures may develop which usually complicate treatment.

In the case of yeast infections, satellite lesions may occur. These are isolated individual lesions which have the same color and appearance as the main lesion and are present around the main area of involvement or on remote parts of the skin. In women candidal intertrigo may accompany vulvovaginitis caused by *C. albicans*.

Diagnosis is based on the presence of macerated, weeping lesions in the body fold of the genital region. Secondary infections can be confirmed by bacteriologic or

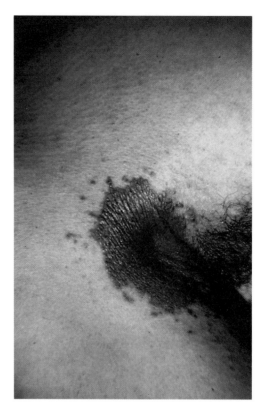

Figure 15.6.   Intertrigo caused by *Candida albicans:* note satellites around the main lesion.

fungal cultures; however, it must be remembered that the presence of *C. albicans* does not necessarily imply its pathogenic role.

Differential diagnosis includes tinea cruris, which is characterized by the presence of active lesions (papules, vesicles) at the margin of skin lesions, erythrasma, and secondary syphilis.

Treatment

Blow-dry the affected area (wear nonocclusive garments). Powders with nystatin may be applied. One-percent hydrocortisone creams with anticandidal agents (vioform, clotrimazole, miconazole) are very helpful. In case of severe maceration, wet compresses with 0.25% silver nitrate or Burow's solution should be applied before other treatment is introduced.

Tinea Cruris

Tinea cruris ("jock itch") (Figure 15.7) is a common itching fungal infection appearing usually in males and often accompanied by tinea pedis ("athletes foot"). The perspiration that occurs with exercise is probably the common predisposing denominator in both diseases.[21,22]

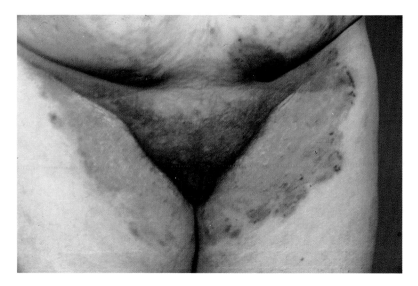

Figure 15.7. Tinea curis caused by *Trichophyton rubrum:* note active lesions on the margin.

The skin lesions are usually bilateral, mildly erythematous scaly patches with slightly raised borders. They have a tendency toward central clearing with active lesions, which include small vesicles and scaling, seen on the margins. Oozing, crusting, and secondary bacterial infections occasionally may be seen. The process spreads by enlargement of the patches and the appearance of satellite lesions that coalesce to form larger plaques. The infection primarily involves the crural folds but frequently extends to the scrotum and thighs. At times, the skin of the penis, the perianal area, and the buttocks may be affected. Infectiousness is minimal even between husband and wife. The diagnosis is made by demonstration of fungal elements in KOH (Figure 15.8) preparation or by culture.[21] Wood's light examination is negative.

Differential diagnosis includes erythrasma, intertrigo (*candidiasis*) and contact dermatitis (deodorants).

Treatment

Apply antifungal creams (clotrimazole, miconazole, econazole) twice daily for at least 10 days. In case of severe inflammation or itching antifungal cream with steroids (Lotrisone® (Schering)) may be preferred. Frequent recurrences can be prevented by use of absorbent powders (Z-Sorb, etc.) which will help to control moisture. Systemic administration of griseofulvin or ketoconazole may also be considered.

Erythrasma

Erythrasma is a chronic superficial skin infection caused by *Corynebacterium minutissimum.*[22] It occurs in the intertriginous areas, most commonly in the groins

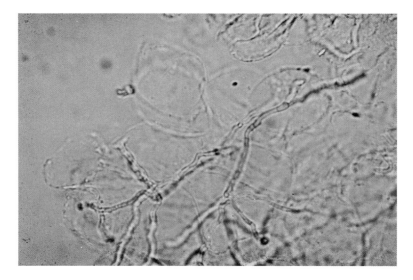

Figure 15.8. KOH preparation demonstrating fungal hyphae.

(Figure 15.9) and axillae. The disease is asymptomatic, although occasionally patients may complain of mild itching. Clinically erythrasma appears as a reddish brown, velvety patch with fine scales. The diagnosis is made with a Wood's light examination, which shows a characteristic coral pink fluorescence [22] (Figure 15.10) and/or gram stain of skin scrapings which may reveal cocciform bacteria. KOH examination is negative.

Differential diagnosis includes tinea cruris and intertrigo.

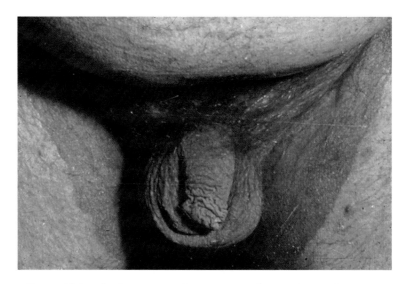

Figure 15.9. Erythrasma: erythematous, scaly eruption in the groin.

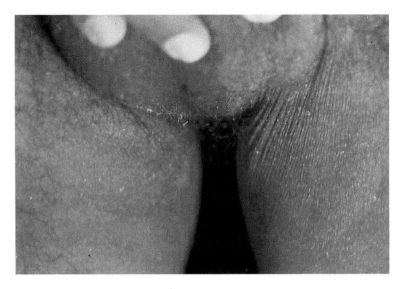

Figure 15.10. Wood's light examination confirms the diagnosis by revealing the coral red fluorescence.

Treatment

Systemic erythromycin 1 g a day for 7 to 10 days and/or topical erythromycin (A/T/S, EryDerm) applied twice daily for 7 to 10 days. Other measures include application of an imidazole like miconazole or clotrimazole creams.

Herpes Zoster (Shingles)

Herpes zoster affects the anogenital region only sporadically. Prodromal symptoms such as local pain and itching precede the appearance of skin lesions. The groups of vesicles or blisters which appear on a red, slightly erythematous base are unilateral and segmentarily arranged (Figure 15.11). The lesions are painful, and postherpetic neuralgia may last for a long time.

Diagnosis: the clinical appearance is usually diagnostic; Tzanck smear, culture, serology, or electron microscopy may aid the diagnosis.

Differential diagnosis includes genital herpes, which does not follow the dermatomal distribution and has a history of recurrences. Tzanck smear and histology can be the same and are of no value in distinguishing between those two diseases; culture and serology may help determine the diagnosis. Other diseases to be distinguished are primary and secondary syphilis, Behçet's syndrome, Stevens-Johnson syndrome, and genital candidiasis.

Treatment

In acute phase, Acyclovir (Zovirax) administered orally 200 mg capsules 5 times daily for 5–10 days should decrease the duration of the disease as well as reduce the pain and inflammation. It has no effect on postherpetic neuralgia. Topically, Burow's solution applied for 20 minutes 3 times a day should help to remove serum and crusts as well as to suppress bacterial growth. In some cases,

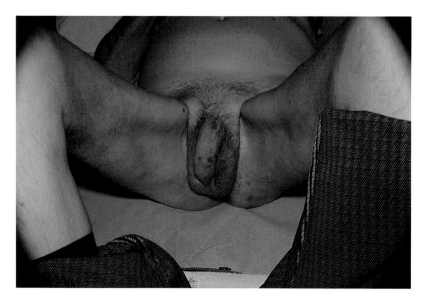

Figure 15.11. Herpes zoster in men with lymphoma: vesicles and pustules on the skin of penis, scotum, and left buttock.

administration of systemic antibiotics, effective against streptococcus and staphylococcus, may be necessary to control infected lesions. Postherpetic neuralgia may be reduced by topically applied capsaicin cream.[23]

BENIGN TUMORS

Angiokeratomas of Fordyce

The angiokeratomas of Fordyce are small red to purple multiple papules with slightly verrucous surfaces which consist of multiple small vessels (Figure 15.12). They may occasionally rupture and bleed when traumatized. The lesions are present mainly in elderly patients and are considered a senile development. They are frequently seen on the scrotum but they may also appear on the penis or vulva.

Diagnosis is usually obvious clinically; biopsy if necessary may confirm diagnosis.

Differential diagnoses include melanoma or melanocytic moles.

Treatment

Treatment is not necessary. If desired a scissor excision, electrodesiccation or laser may be used.

Seborrheic Keratosis

Seborrheic keratoses are common growths that originate in the dermis. They may appear in sun-exposed as well as covered body sites and are generally more

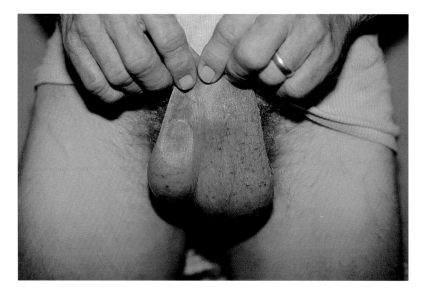

Figure 15.12. Angiokeratoma of Fordyce: redish purple multiple papule on the skin of the scrotum of 66-year-old man.

common with increasing age. Although these tumors tend to occur in other parts of the body, infrequently they may appear in the anogenital region (Figure 15.13). The lesions are sharply circumscribed, stuck to the skin, and vary in size and color. They can also be flat or minimally raised, with a smooth or verrucous brownish surface. The most common lesions, however, are oval or round, flattened domes with granular, irregular surfaces. Seborrheic keratoses are asymptomatic but may itch when manipulated or irritated by clothing or maceration.

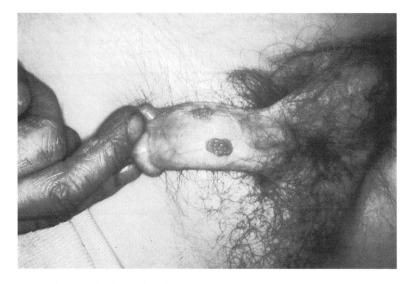

Figure 15.13. Seborrheic ketatosis on the skin of the penis.

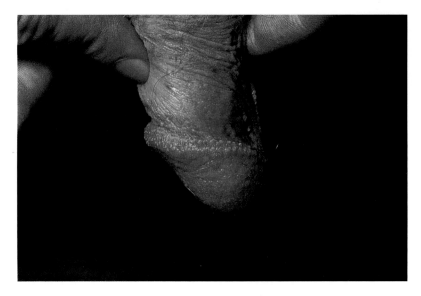

Figure 15.14. Pearly penile papules (papillomatosis coronae penis).

Diagnosis is usually obvious clinically because of the characteristic "stuck on" appearance and brownish granular surface. Biopsy, if necessary, may confirm diagnosis.

Differential diagnosis includes condylomata acuminatum and condylomata lata, pyogenic granuloma, keratoacanthoma, pigmented nevus, besalioma, and squamous cell carcinoma and malignant melanoma.

Treatment

Treatment is not necessary. Flat lesions respond well to cryosurgery. Thick and keratotic lesions often require curettage after initial freezing. Larger seborrheic keratoses can be excised under local anaesthesia.

Pearly Penile Papules

Pearly penile papules (hirsutoid papillomas of the penis, papillomatosis coronae penis) occur in up to 20 percent of the male population. They are congenital abnormalities which histologically resemble fibromas of the oral cavity or fibrous papules of the face (Figure 15.14). The papules are present in one or more rows usually on the corona glandis or more rarely on the coronal sulcus.[24] Occasionally they may also be found along the frenulum or be scattered over the glans of the penis. These hypertropic papillae vary in size from 0.5 to 3–4 mm and are whitish red to whitish yellow in color. Occasionally they may be somewhat brownish and show a filiform configuration.

Diagnosis: the characteristic appearance and location leaves little doubt as to the diagnosis. Biopsy may confirm diagnosis.

Differential diagnosis: these normal excrescences are frequently confused with

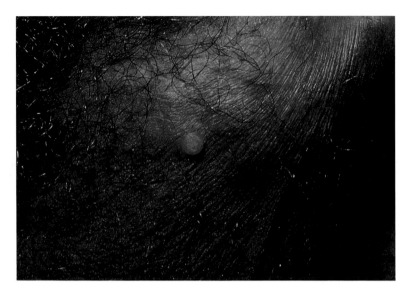

Figure 15.15. Sebaceous cyst on the skin of the scrotum.

genital warts and unnecessarily treated. Another disease which should be distinguished from pearly penile papules is lichen nitidus, but these usually can be found on the shaft of the penis, in the groin, or the lower abdomen, or elsewhere. On biopsy these lesions closely resemble lichen planus.

Treatment

Treatment is not necessary. If desired, they can be surgically removed.

Sebaceous Cysts

Sebaceous cysts are the retention cysts which usually appear on the face, neck and trunk, but may also occur on the scrotum or the labia majora (Figure 15.15). True sebaceous cysts are very rare and many of them when examined histologically turn out to be the epidermal cysts. They appear as small spherical tumors which, if punctured, reveal a viscous content. Some of them may have noticeable small black dots which correspond to the former opening. They are usually asymptomatic unless secondarily infected.

Diagnosis: the appearance and location of the sebaceous cyst is characteristic.

Differential diagnosis includes nodular lesions of scabies, molluscum contagiosum, calcinosis cutis, tuberous xanthoma, and histiocytoma.

Treatment

The cyst can be surgically removed if desired.

Steatocystoma Multiplex

Steatocystoma multiplex is a variant of sebaceous cysts. It appears as small, moderately firm yellowish cystic nodules most commonly seen on the genitalia

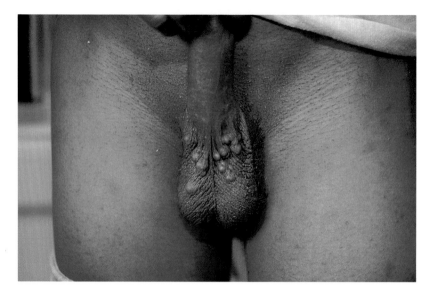

Figure 15.16. Steatocystoma multiplex on the skin of the scrotum.

(Figure 15.16) but may also occur on the head or trunk. The cysts adhere to the overlying skin, and their wall is complexly folded and contains sebaceous glands. On incision the cysts yield an oily fluid.

Diagnosis is based on the characteristic clinical picture and can be confirmed by biopsy.

Differential diagnosis includes hypertrophic papules of secondary syphilis, nodular scabies, molluscum contagiosum, epidermoid cysts, idiopathic scrotal calcification, and tuberous xanthomas.

Treatment

Treatment is not necessary. If secondarily infected, the cysts can be excised and the patient should receive systemic antibiotics until the signs of inflammation disappear.

Epidermal Cyst

Epidermal inclusion cysts are benign, asymptomatic lesions which result from the implantation of epidermis into dermis. They may also arise from the upper portion of a hair follicle. The epidermal lining of the cyst is identical to that of the surface epidermis. It produces keratin, which forms the content of the cyst.

Clinically, epidermal cysts appear as flesh-colored nodules. On palpation the lesions feel firm but not hard, suggesting the semisolid content of the cysts. They vary in size from several millimeters to several centimeters in diameter. They may be located anywhere including the genital region (Figure 15.17), but are most frequent on the head and trunk.

Diagnosis can be made clinically. If the central core is patent it can be also

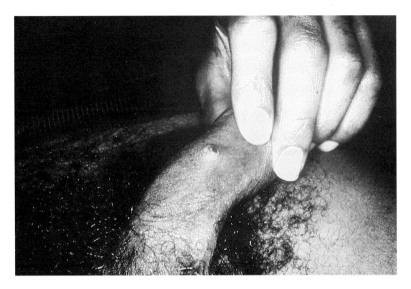

Figure 15.17. Epidermal cyst on the skin of the penis.

confirmed by squeezing the cyst and expressing whitish-gray material which is the macerated keratin. Biopsy is unnecessary but may confirm diagnosis.

Differential diagnosis includes lipoma, nodular scabies, molluscum contagiosum, histiocytoma.

Treatment

Epidermal cyst can be excised or removed by curettage. It is important that the entire cyst with its lining be removed in order to prevent recurrence. Frequently no therapy is necessary.

PREMALIGNANT AND MALIGNANT TUMORS

Leukoplakia

The term leukoplakia has been used to describe a persistent white patch on a mucous or mucocutaneous surface. Lesions of leukoplakia have been found mainly on the lips and oral mucosa and also on the inner aspect of the labia majora, on the labia minora, and on other surfaces of the vulva as well as on the penis (Figure 15.18).

Clinically, the patches are hyperkeratotic, white, and slightly elevated. They are usually well defined with a little tendency to extend peripherally.[25] The lesions are believed to be potentially malignant, and a small percentage may progress to squamous cell carcinoma.

Diagnosis is based on the clinical picture, confirmed by biopsy.

Differential diagnosis includes candidiasis, lichen planus, lichen sclerosus et atrophicus (may coexist with leukoplakia), and morphea.

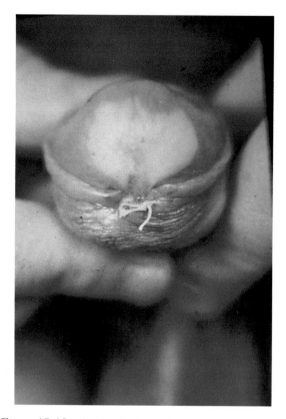

Figure 15.18. Leukoplakia on the glans of the penis.

Treatment

Cryosurgery with liquid nitrogen or shave excision are the methods of choice. One percent fluorouracil solution may be applied for 2 to 3 weeks or until erythema and erosions become marked.[25] Lesions suspected of being squamous cell carcinoma are best excised.

Lichen Sclerosus et Atrophicus of the Penis

Lichen sclerosus et atrophicus (LSA) of the penis (balanitis xerotica obliterans) is most common in middle-aged men, but it can occur in children or elderly men.[26-28] The etiology of the condition is still unknown, and the disorder affects whites more frequently than other races. The lesions of LSA appear as small, pale or white plaques on the glans of the penis (Figure 15.19), the skin of the prepuce (the terminal part of it is most commonly affected), and very rarely on the scrotum. The lesions around the meatus may result in urethral stricture, causing disturbances in the flow of the urine. The lesion on the prepuce may produce contracture of the foreskin or adhesion of the prepuce to the glans, resulting in a need for circumcision. On the margin of the lesion there may be telangectasias and petechiae. The disease is chronic, and at the beginning of the process men have no complaints but

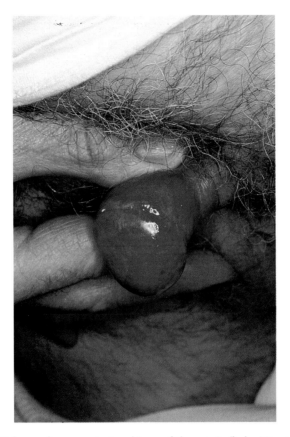

Figure 15.19. Lichen sclerosus et atrophicus of the penis (balanitis xerotica obliterans): note the pale plaques on the glans and numerous telangiectasias and petechiae.

mild irritation. There were few reports of LSA in which squamous cell carcinoma has occurred.[29,30]

Diagnosis is based on the clinical picture but should be confirmed by biopsy.

Differential diagnosis includes any form of balanitis, vitiligo, leukoplakia, lichen planus, Bowenoid papulosis, squamous cell carcinoma, and Paget's disease. If maceration and/or ulceration occurs, the disease should be distinguished from sexually transmitted diseases (STDs) that produce genital ulcerations (syphilis, herpes, chancroid, donovanosis, and lymphogranuloma venereum).

Treatment

Treatment should be started with topical application of low potency steroid creams twice daily. If there is no improvement medium or high potency steroid should be applied twice daily for a period not exceeding 10 days. Persistent lesions can be cured with an intralesional injection of steroids or by freezing the lesion with liquid nitrogen. For those men who as a result of contracture of the prepuce develop phimosis or suffer from urethral stricture, surgical intervention is required. Application of 2% testosterone ointment has also been used with good results.[31]

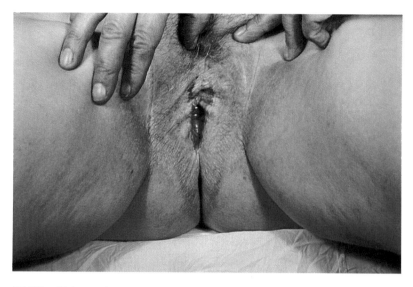

Figure 15.20. Lichen sclerosus et atrophicus of the vulva (kraurosis vulvae): whitish atrophic wrinkled plaques around vulva; telangiectasias.

Lichen Sclerosus et Atrophicus of the Vulva

Lichen sclerosus et atrophicus (kraurosis vulvae) is more frequent in women than men. It occurs most commonly in women at or after menopause but may occur at any age.[26,28,32,33] If present before puberty, LSA may completely resolve without treatment.[26]

LSA in women may be asymptomatic or cause itching, irritation, and result in dyspareunia. The lesions which are first white atrophic plaques usually appear in the vulva and the perianal area (Figure 15.20). Individual lesions may aggregate, causing larger wrinkled plaques. Beyond the margins of the atrophic plaques, telangiectasias and small petechiae may be seen. Atrophic tissue, which especially in longstanding lesions is fragile, may erode, macerate, or become lichenified. Repeated cycles of erosion and healing may result in contraction of the introitus, which interferes with intercourse. LSA may result in atrophy of the labia minora and clitoris. Although LSA has a predilection for the vulva and perianal area, the lesion can also be found on the trunk and extremities and rarely on the tongue and buccal mucosa. Squamous cell carcinoma has been reported in patients with chronic LSA.[32,34]

Diagnosis can be made by clinical observation but biopsy is necessary for histologic confirmation.

Differential diagnosis includes leukoplakia, candidal vulvitis, vitiligo, morphea, squamous cell carcinoma, and Paget's disease. In the case of erosive lesions, any STD which produces genital ulcerations should also be distinguished.

Treatment

The treatment is the same as in men (see page 369).

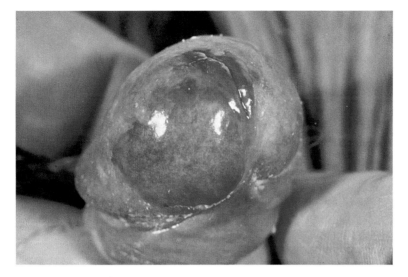

Figure 15.21. Erythroplasia of Queyrat.

Erythroplasia of Queyrat

Erythroplasia of Queyrat (EQ) represents Bowen's disease of the mucous membranes.[25] The disease occurs rather late in life, with men much more commonly affected than women. Affected men nearly always are uncircumcised. The lesion takes the form of a moist, slightly raised, well-defined, red, smooth, or velvety plaque which bleeds easily (Figure 15.21). It may slowly increase in size or remain unaltered. The lesion may slightly itch or burn. In men the glans of the penis, the inner surface of the prepuce, and the corona and in women the labia minora are the most common sites. Histology is that of Bowen's disease and, like Bowen's disease of the skin, EQ has the potential for degeneration into squamous cell carcinoma.[25,35] Erythroplasia of Queyrat is frequently undistinguishable both clinically and histologically from genital intraepithelial neoplasia (GIN) caused by human papilloma viruses. Some authors believe it is a variant of GIN.[36]

Diagnosis is based on clinical appearance and histological features.

Differential diagnosis: LSA, balanitis, balanitis plasmocellularis of Zoon, primary syphilis, and squamous cell carcinoma.

Treatment

Erythroplasia of Queyrat can be treated with 5-Fluorouracil, cryotherapy or local excision. The method of choice seems to be topical application of 5-Fluorouracil cream under the occlusion. In case of suspicion of malignant transformation, surgical excision is recommended.

Bowen's Disease

Bowen's disease may appear on any part of the body, including the penis, vulva, or perianal region. It appears as a slightly elevated, irregular, reddish-brown

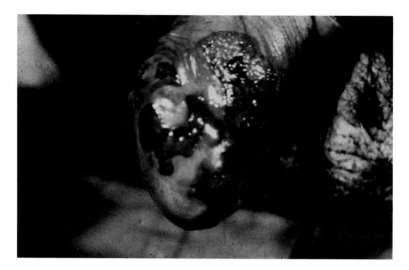

Figure 15.22. Bowen's disease of the penis: irregular, elevated plaques with well-defined borders.

scaling plaque with well-defined borders (Figure 15.22). It may persist for years or grow very slowly by lateral extension. After months or years, the process may invade the dermis, causing induration and ulceration of the lesion.[25] Histologically Bowen's disease is an intraepithelial carcinoma or carcinoma "in situ," which may precede a squamous cell growth.[37,38] Some investigators have found that patients with Bowen's disease have a higher than expected incidence of unrelated internal malignancy.

Diagnosis is based on clinical appearance and chronic course and can be supported by histology.

Differential diagnosis includes eczema, psoriasis, neurodermatitis, seborrheic dermatitis, fixed drug eruption, LSA, GIN, and squamous cell carcinoma.

Treatment

Bowen's disease on the genitals can be treated with topical application 5% 5-Fluorouracil cream under the occlusion twice daily for 4 to 8 weeks. Treatment should be discontinued when erosion and superficial necrosis occur. The cream should be applied to the tissue surrounding the lesion to destroy clinically inapparent disease.[25] A small lesion can be treated with cryosurgery, laser or electrodesiccation and curettage. In case of a malignant transformation surgical excision with wide margin is recommended.

Paget's Disease

Paget's disease is a precancerous condition which usually occurs on the nipple of the breast in women; however, it may affect other parts of the body including the genital area. Extramammary Paget's disease is rare and occurs most often in elderly patients. The disease may be associated with internal malignancy such as adenocarcinoma or carcinoma of the rectum (Figure 15.23) and carcinoma of the cervix.[25,39,40]

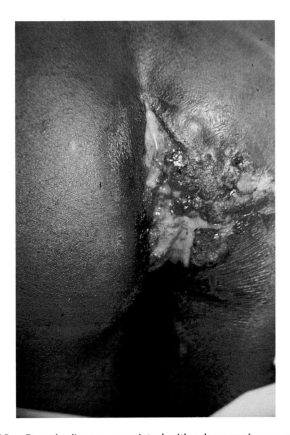

Figure 15.23. Paget's disease associated with adenocarcinoma of the colon.

The lesion appears as an irregularly shaped, scaly, reddish, infiltrated plaque. Supeficial weeping and crusting erosions strongly resemble eczema. Early lesions are small and unilateral but may increase in size to involve large areas. If genitalia are involved in men the scrotum is the most commonly involved. In women the labia majora is the most common site. In both sexes the disease may be present in the perianal region and in the groin.

Diagnosis is made by biopsy.

Differential diagnosis includes eczema, erythroplasia of Queyrat, Bowen's disease, leukoplakia, lichen planus, tinea, and cutaneous candidiasis. Erosive lesions should be distinguished from STDs which produce genital ulceration.

Treatment

Surgery is the treatment of choice. There is a report of successful treatment of Paget's disease of the vulva with topical bleomycin.[41]

Squamous Cell Carcinoma of the Vulva

Squamous cell carcinoma (SCC) is more likely to occur in middle-aged or postmenopausal women. It often arises from leukoplakia or another premalignant condition that appears in the vulva. There is also a strong association between

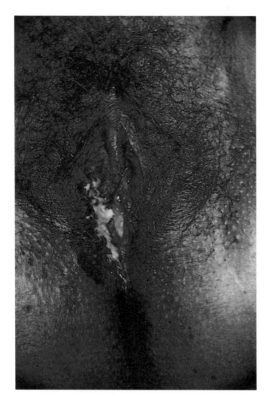

Figure 15.24. Squamous cell carcinoma of the vulva: papillary growth resembling warts on the right labium majoris.

vulvar warts caused by certain types of human papillomavirus (HPV-16, HPV-18) and squamous cell carcinoma of the vulva.[36,42,43]

The lesion usually develops on the inner surface of the labia majora but may occur everywhere in the vulva (Figure 15.24). They appear as ulcerative nodules or papillary growths resembling genital warts, but they almost always have an infiltrated base and are hard on palpation. The process is chronic, and the first metastases are most likely to appear in regional lymph nodes.

Diagnosis is established by biopsy.

Differential diagnosis includes all STDs that cause genital ulceration plus other conditions discussed in the following subsection.

Treatment

Surgical excision is the usual therapeutic approach.[44] Regional lymph nodes should be examined and removed if necessary. Radiation therapy was also used for some lesions.

Squamous Cell Carcinoma of the Penis

Squamous cell carcinoma of the penis occurs usually in middle-aged or elderly men; uncircumcised men are predominantly affected.[45-47] It is believed that chronic

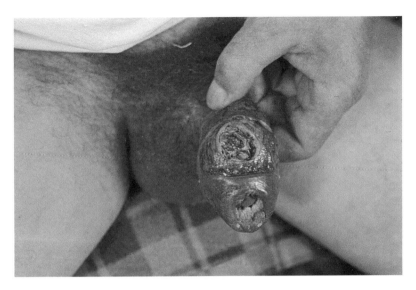

Figure 15.25. Squamous cell carcinoma of the penis: hard ulcerative masses penetrating through the glans of the penis.

or recurrent balanitis, particularly in the presence of predisposing factors such as lichen sclerosus et atrophicus, play a certain part in its causation. Also, the premalignant lesions that occur on the penis, such as the erythroplasia of Queyrat, Bowen's disease, GIN, and Paget's disease, may result in SCC. There is growing evidence that certain types of human papillomavirus (HPV-16, HPV-18) play a significant role in the etiology of SCC of the penis.[42,43,48]

The lesions usually develop under the prepuce and appear as reddish plaques or small warty nodules that are firm and indurated. Erosion and ulceration may be present, although the lesions are generally asymptomatic. When SCC increases in size, it may penetrate through the prepuce, causing a fungating mass covered with purulent or bloody exudate. The process is chronic, producing hard infiltrative masses over the years with ulcerating, oozing surfaces and raised rolled borders (Figure 15.25). The lesions may metastasize, with inguinal nodes primarily involved.

Diagnosis is established by biopsy.

Differential diagnosis includes all STDs which manifest with genital ulcers, and the duration of the lesion is an important clinical clue. It should also be distinguished from erythroplasia of Queyrat, Bowen's disease, Paget's disease, leukoplakia, Buschke-Löwenstein tumors, condylomata acuminata, balanitis, and balanoposthitis.

Treatment

Surgical excision is the method of choice. Small localized lesions can be treated with radiotherapy. In case of metastases to the inguinal nodes they should be removed along with the primary tumor.

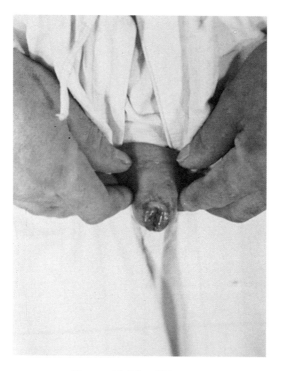

Figure 15.26. Phimosis.

MISCELLANEOUS SKIN DISEASES

Phimosis

The normal foreskin can be retracted behind the glans of the penis and returned to its normal position without difficulty. Phimosis (Figure 15.26) develops when retracting the foreskin over the glans is impossible. This can be due to congenital narrowing of the distal part of the prepuce or can be acquired, caused by an acute or chronic inflammatory process in the prepuce or the glans.

When phimosis occurs, normal cleanliness is difficult or impossible, causing secretions to accumulate. This may eventually become infected and aggravate the existing problem. Severe phimosis may lead to difficulties in micturition and erection. Sexual intercourse may be painful or impossible. Occasionally, urine retention has been reported. The following conditions are known to contribute to acquired phimosis: primary and secondary syphilis, genital herpes, chancroid, donovanosis, bacterial, fungal, or viral balanoposthitis, bacterial infection of the penis (folliculitis, furuncles, cellulitis, abscess), and contact dermatitis.

Treatment

The treatment of phimosis rests on the treatment of underlying diseases (syphilis, chancroid, etc.). Even though phimosis can be secondary to viral or fungal infections, systemic administration of antibiotics is justified because of the

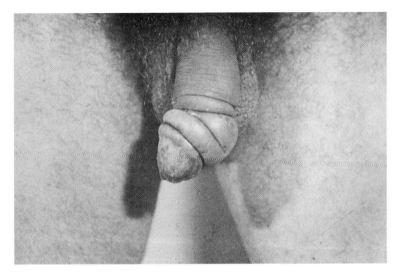

Figure 15.27. Paraphimosis.

bacterial involvement in the inflammatory process under the prepuce. Subpreputial irrigations with saline repeated several times a day may be helpful in promoting resolution. Patients with congenital phimosis should pay special attention to the hygiene of the penis. In case of recurrences caused by infectious agents or in congenital phimosis, circumcision is recommended.

Paraphimosis

Paraphimosis (Figure 15.27) develops when the foreskin, retracted behind the glans of the penis, cannot be returned to its normal position. The opening of the foreskin acts as a constricting ring round the shaft of the penis. The retracted foreskin and the glans of the penis become edematous and tender. The blood circulation is disturbed in both the foreskin and the glans, causing the latter to look cyanotic.

If paraphimosis remains uncorrected, linear ulceration may develop on the prepuce along the tight, constricting ring. The condition becomes extremely painful, and if the foreskin cannot be manually replaced over the glans, surgery may be needed.

Paraphimosis frequently occurs during intercourse in men with partial or complete congenital phimosos or results from an underlying inflammatory process in the prepuce or the glans of the penis.

The following conditions are known to produce paraphimosis: congenital or acquired phimosis, primary syphilis, genital herpes, donovanosis, balanoposthitis (regardless of cause), trauma, and contact dermatitis.

Treatment

In case of paraphimosis proper anatomical conditions should be restored as soon as possible since prolonged paraphimosis may result in partial or sometimes total necrosis of both the glans and the foreskin. This can be accomplished by gentle (the condition is very painful), prolonged but firm pressure on the edematous glans which usually enables the constricting ring to be brought back over the glans of the penis. In some cases, general anaesthesia may be required to make this possible. In patients in which this manipulation is fruitless, incision of the constricting ring may be required.

Circumcision should be considered since the recurrence is frequent but should not be performed until the inflammation subsides. Underlying diseases (syphilis, genital herpes, chancroid, etc.) should be treated without delay.

Psoriasis

Psoriasis is a common (1–2 percent of people worldwide are affected) chronic skin disease of unknown etiology. The typical lesion is a sharply demarcated, elevated papule or erythematous patch with irregular borders and silvery-white scales that can vary in amount. Pinpoint bleeding and the Koebner phenomenon may be present; nail abnormalities also occur.

Predilection sites are the elbows, knees, scalp, and sacral area, but the lesion may occur anywhere on the skin, including the genital region.[16,49] In the groin or the genitals (Figure 15.28) there may be less scaling than in the typical lesion of psoriasis elsewhere (Figure 15.29), and maceration may be the predominant feature. Pinpoint bleeding can be more difficult to demonstrate than in other areas of the skin, and the genital lesions are usually more resistant to treatment.

Differential diagnosis includes seborrheic dermatitis, lichen planus, intertrigo, secondary syphilis, and tinea cruris.

Treatment

Psoriasis can be treated with topical agents such as tar and anthralin preparations, steroid ointments and ultraviolet light. Systemic agents (methotrexate, psolrens and UVA) are usually reserved for patients with severe or widespread disease and those who respond poorly to topical treatment. Some topical agents, like tar or anthralin preparations, should be avoided in anogenital lesions because of their irritating properties. Administration of systemic cytotoxic drugs and/or PUVA (psoralens plus ultraviolet A) are not indicated in psoriasis localized to anogenital lesions. Psoriasis on the genitalia is best treated with topical application (also under occlusion) of medium or high potency steroid ointments.

Vitiligo

Vitiligo is an acquired loss of skin pigmentation due to the absence or marked decrease in melanocytes and melanin in the epidermis. The cause of the disease is unknown, and since there is an association with certain autoimmune diseases, it has been suggested that autoimmune destruction of melanocytes may be involved in the pathogenesis of the condition.[50-52]

The lesion appears as white, depigmented macules with well-defined borders (Figure 15.30). The loss of pigmentation may be inapparent in fair-skinned patients

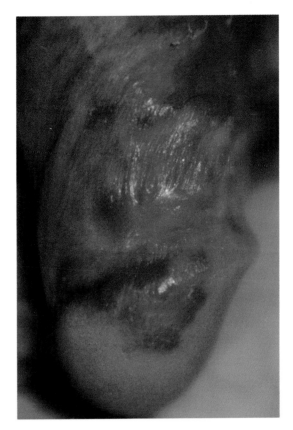

Figure 15.28. Psoriatic lesions on the glans and skin of the penis. In this distribution scaling is less prominent.

but is very distinctive in blacks or dark-skin caucasians. Hair follicles within the depigmented areas may have tiny areas of pigmentation around the hair, but otherwise pigment is lacking. The depigmented areas often have hyperpigmented borders, which is most apparent in fair-skinned individuals. With time, the depigmented areas of skin may become more extensive, but after several months the lesions become static. The condition may be limited to the genitals or associated with lesions elsewhere on the body.[49]

Diagnosis is based on the characteristic appearance of lesions.

Differential diagnosis: vitiligo in the genitalia is not likely to be confused with other conditions; however, diseases such as pityriasis versicolor, leprosy, and tinea may at times be considered.

Treatment

Treatment is not necessary. If desired, the lesion can be covered with cosmetics to match the normal-colored skin. Several therapies aimed at repigmentation of the lesions (PUVA) produced suboptimal results. The use of topical high-potency steroids has been successful in some patients.

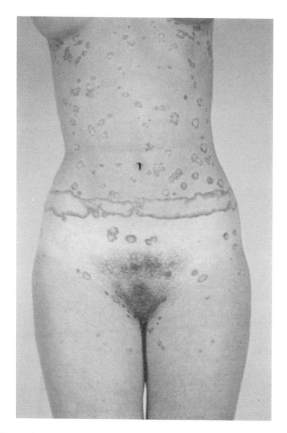

Figure 15.29.   Typical psoriasis on the trunk spreading to the genital area. Note the Koebner phenomenon in the belt area.

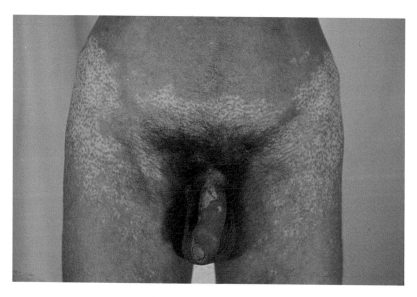

Figure 15.30.   Vitiligo.

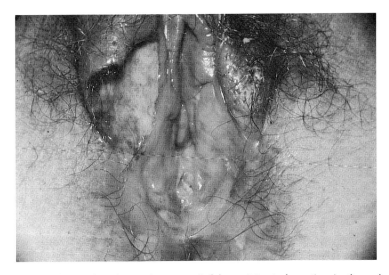

Figure 15.31. Behçet's syndrome: painful persistent ulceration in the vulva.

Behçet's Syndrome

Behçet's syndrome is a rare, chronic, relapsing condition of unknown etiology. It is believed that it can be of viral origin or that the manifestations are secondary to vascular immune complex depositions.[53] The cardinal features of Behçet's syndrome are severe and persistent oral and genital ulceration followed by eye lesions and arthropathy.[54,55] In males, painful genital ulcers most typically appear on the scrotum and penis.[16] In females, the labia majora are frequently affected (Figure 15.31) but lesions may also occur on the vagina and cervix. In both sexes ulceration may occur around the anus and in the perineum.

The lesions may be multiple or solitary. They are superficial, tender ulcerations, frequently with necrotic bases and surrounded with a red halo which on a mucous membrane gives them an aphthouslike appearance. In some cases the lesions can be destructive, leaving scars on healing.

The eye findings usually follow oral and genital lesion and include (in decreasing order) iridocyclitis, conjunctivitis, corneal ulceration, and choroiditis. In severe cases eye lesions may lead to blindness.

Arthritis is usually preceded by arthralgia. The most frequently involved joints are knees, ankles, fingers, wrists, elbows, and feet. It usually resolves without sequelae, and in only a small proportion of patients there may be radiologic evidence of cartilage destruction and/or bone erosions.

Other manifestations of the syndrome include the signs of neurologic involvement with changes in CSF, thrombophlebitis, intestinal ulceration, epididymitis and orchitis, aneurysms of systemic and pulmonary circulations, pneumonitis, pericarditis, and glomerulonephritis.

Other skin lesions that may occur with Behçet's syndrome include erythema nodosum–like lesions, vesicular, papular, and pustular rashes, pyodermas, and acneiform lesions.

Behçet's syndrome is a chronic condition with exacerbations and remissions, and it is quite common to see the patients with incomplete forms of the disease—for example, recurrent ulceration on the genitalia or in the mouth only—while the other manifestations do not develop until after many months or years.

Diagnosis is a clinical one. Laboratory tests are not specific, and histology resembles the lesions seen in a delayed hypersensitivity reaction to an intradermal antigen.

Differential diagnosis includes infection caused by herpes simplex, aphthosis, secondary syphilis, chancroid, Stevens-Johnson syndrome, systemic lupus erythematosus, and Reiter's syndrome.

Treatment

There is at present time no specific or consistently reliable therapy for Behcet's syndrome. The mainstay therapy for many manifestations of the syndrome are systemic corticosteroids and anti-inflammatory agents. Prednisone is administered initially in a 50 to 60 mg dose per day tapered over several days to a maintenance dose between 5 to 20 mg per day. Several cytotoxic agents such as chlorambucil, azathioprine as well as cyclosporine colchicine, thalidomide, dapsone, chloroquine, acyclovir, alfa-interferon and 13-cis retinoic acid have been reported to be helpful with or without simultaneous administration of systemic corticosteroids.[56] Oral or genital ulcers may benefit from application of topical steroid creams.

Adverse Drug Eruptions

Adverse drug eruptions in the anogenital region include generalized drug reactions in which involvement of the genital region is only a part of the generalized skin rash and localized drug eruptions (fixed drug eruption) limited to the genitals.[16]Contact dermatitis, urticaria, erythema multiforme, or Stevens-Johnson syndrome caused by drugs are discussed elsewhere.

Generalized drug reactions from the standpoint of the venereologist are most commonly caused by penicillin or other antibiotics and trimethoprim-sulfamethoxazole. The skin lesions that appear in the anogenital region are part of a generalized eruption which may have different characteristics.[57]

Localized drug eruption or fixed drug eruption appears as a single (occasionally multiple) lesion which is usually a well-defined erythematous light red or brown plaque (Figure 15.32, Figure 15.33). The lesion may be irritating, and if pigmentary changes occur, they may persist for a long time. The lesion recurs shortly after reexposure to the allergenic drug.

Diagnosis is based on a history of recent drug intake and the presence of characteristic skin lesions.

Differential diagnosis in generalized drug eruption should include viral exanthems, toxic erythemas, and secondary syphilis. Generalized drug eruption is pruritic and usually starts proximally and proceeds distally, with the legs being the last to be involved. Fixed drug eruption on the genitalia should be be distinguished from hyperpigmentation that may occur after disappearance of primary chancre, annular lesions of lichen planus, and balanitis circinata.

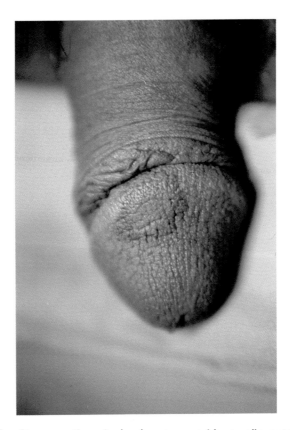

Figure 15.32. Drug eruption: single plaque caused by an allergy to tetracycline.

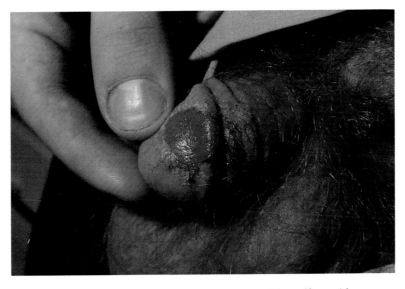

Figure 15.33. Fixed drug reaction caused by sulfonamides.

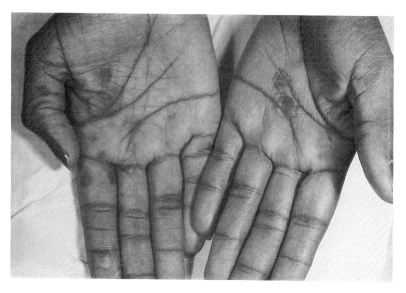

Figure 15.34. Erythema multiforme: typical "iris" lesion on the palms caused by drugs.

Treatment

Withdrawal of the offending drug is in many instances all that is necessary. Symptomatic treatment with antihistamines (hydroxizine) may sometimes be necessary to reduce itching. Topical steroids may be used for a short period of time.[58]

Erythema Multiforme

Erythema multiforme is a disease which may be provoked by viral (herpes simplex) and bacterial infections, by drugs, and less frequently by other stimuli.[59-61] The lesions are primarily seen on the hands and feet (Figure 15.34) but may also occur on the skin and mucous membranes of the anogenital region (Figure 15.35). Cases in which the eyes and the mucosal surfaces of the mouth and genitals are involved are called "Stevens-Johnson syndrome."

The skin lesions initially present as erythematous papules or plaques which spread to form characteristic "iris" or "target" lesions.[16] The latter is a round dusky red plaque with concentric and annular borders and a cyanotic, purpuric, or vesicular center. There may be various degrees of exudation.

Diagnosis is based on the presence of characteristic iris lesions and a history of antecedent factors (most frequently infection by herpes virus or streptococci or ingestion of drugs).

Differential diagnosis should include all sexually transmitted diseases producing genital lesions (genital herpes, chancroid, syphilis, scabies). Balanitis or balanoposthitis vulvitis or vulvovaginitis; Behçet's syndrome; contact dermatitis and fixed drug eruptions.

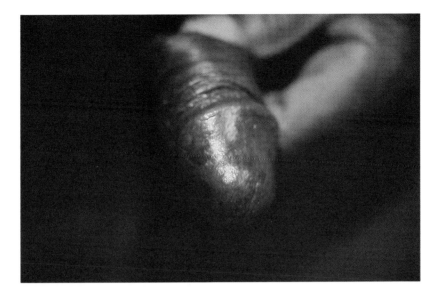

Figure 15.35. Erythema multiforme: annular lesion on the glans of the penis.

Treatment

Withdrawal of the offending drug or treatment of a precipitating infection is important. Although there is no convincing evidence that any form of therapy alters the course of this disease acyclovir 200 mg orally 5 times a day for 5 to 7 days should be administered in cases in which herpes simplex infection is believed to be the precipitating factor.[62,63] Erythromycin 250 mg orally 4 times a day for 7 days is used if streptococci or other bacteria are the cause. Systemic administration of corticosteroids is controversial but is still employed in severely ill patients or in Stevens-Johnson syndrome. Local measures are seldom necessary. Topical therapy consists of antiseptic dressings and steroid creams. Pruritis can be controlled by oral administration of antihistamines (hydroxizine).

Contact Dermatitis

Contact dermatitis in the anogenital region may result from application of various chemicals used in contraceptives, cosmetic lubricants, "aphrodisiacs" or medicines administered in the form of vaginal or anal suppositories.[61] (Figure 15.36). It can also be due to materials used in condoms or pessaries. Clothing and detergents used to wash them may provoke contact dermatitis in the anogenital region similar to that in other areas of the body.[49] The latter produce skin lesions not necessarily on the genitals but on the skin of pubic region, on the buttocks, and in the belt area.

Treatment

Offending substances should be removed and contact with them in the future avoided. In acute dermatitis with weeping lesions wet compresses with saline or

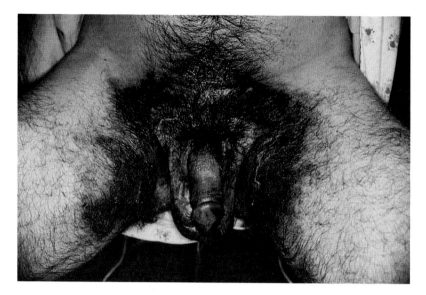

Figure 15.36.   Severe contact dermatitis caused by cosmetics.

Burow's solution are indicated. When the lesion is dried up steroid creams with or without antimicrobial agents should be used. Loose-fitting undergarments and avoidance of binding clothing is recommended.

Traumatic Lesions

Traumatic lesions of the genitals are not uncommon. They may appear as a result of sexual intercourse or accidental injury or may be self-inflicted during masturbation or by mentally disturbed patients.

Mechanical Injury

In the male the prepuce and the frenulum is most frequently affected. Especially the latter is often torn during intercourse, producing bleeding which the patient notices immediately after intercourse. Oral sex may result in abrasion caused by a sex partner's teeth (Figure 15.37) and rectal sex is more likely to result in traumatic lesions on the penis and eventually secondary bacterial infection. Even prolonged sexual activity may result in penile edema without obvious external lesions.

Secondarily infected traumatic lesions may lead in uncircumcised men to edema of the prepuce and subsequent phimosis or paraphimosis. Another example of traumatic lesions in men are those caused by zipper injuries.

In virgin women the hymen may split during first intercourse, causing bleeding and pain. Injuries to the clitoris, caused by neurotic women who insert foreign objects into the vagina, are less common.

Penile or clitoris tourniquet syndrome due to strangulation of these organs by hair has been reported.[64,66] In the first case of a two-and-a-half year old boy, several strands of hair wrapped around the penis and buried under the epithelium were

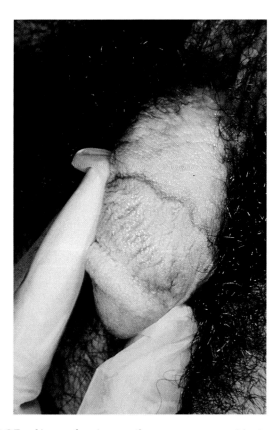

Figure 15.37. Linear abrasion on the prepuce caused by human teeth.

found to cause constriction. The penis was swollen and painful causing difficulties in voiding. Other foreign bodies such as threads, metal rings, and rubber bands may be the cause of similar conditions not only in children but in adolescents and adults as well.

Clitoral strangulation by hair has also been reported in women. Young patients presented with an enlarged, erythematous and extremely tender clitoris caused by hair wrappings.[65,66] In the majority of cases removal of foreign bodies is curative, however, in the case of late diagnosis certain complications (necrosis, deformities, transection of the urethra) may occur.

Another form of mechanical injury to the genitals is implantation of foreign bodies mainly into the skin of the penis. This has been done in order to improve sexual performance and subjugate the female partner. Practices not uncommon in the Orient are almost non-existent in the West. The materials used range from plastic, polished stones or liquid silicone, to pearls and ivory which is said to be favored by the Chinese. These devices are usually round or oval in shape and are called "bulleetus" in the Philippines or "chang ball" in Korea. Both terms mean "ball bearings".[67] The number of bulleetus worn by a man may vary, usually from two to five, however, as many as eighteen, arranged in a spiral form, were described. In most instances bulleetus do not produce symptoms except when becoming secondarily infected. Western physicians, however, are frequently surprised when accidentally discovering bulleetus during routine examinations of an Oriental patient.

Chemical Injuries

Chemical trauma in both men and women results most frequently from the application of strong antiseptics, deodorants, or medications. Even harsh soap applied to the genitals may cause local irritation and superficial skin lesions. Mentally disturbed patients may apply irritating chemicals to the genitals, causing severe irritation and chemical burns.

Diagnosis: even though patients attribute the lesions to trauma (it appears immediately after intercourse or after application of certain chemicals or medications), physicians should be alert to the possibility that the genital lesions may be the result of STD.

Diffential diagnosis should include all sexually transmitted diseases causing genital lesions. In the case of chemical burns (oozing erosive lesions), secondary syphilis, extensive genital herpes; Behcet's syndrome, Stevens-Johnson syndrome, pemphigus, and neurotic excoriations should be included.

Treatment

In case of mechanical injury, bleeding should be stopped by pressure applied to the lesion or by the suture if the damage is more extensive. However, the majority of traumatic lesions of the genitals will heal spontaneously. Secondary infection may be prevented by topical application of Bacitracin or Neosporin ointments.

In case of chemical injury the remnants of the offending substance should be washed off with saline or tap water. Oozing or wet lesions can be treated with compresses with saline or potassium permanganate solutions. Secondary infections can be prevented either by systemic administration of antibiotics or if the lesions are small with topical applications of Bacitracin or Neosporin ointment.

Lichen Planus

Lichen planus (LP) is a common skin disease of unknown etiology. Drugs such as antimalarials, gold, barbiturates, thiazide diuretics, phenolphthalein, and dapsone may cause lichen planus–like eruptions. LP may involve the penis or vulva as part of a widespread eruption or as a solitary manifestation. In genitalia the typical papular lesions have a tendency to assume an annular configuration.[16] In men the glans penis and the inner side of prepuce are most often involved (Figure 15-38). In females the lesions may be present on the vulva and the vaginal vault where they resemble lesions found commonly in the oral mucosa. LP lesions may be found in the anus as well.

The sites of predilection of LP are as follows: flexor surfaces of wrists, forearms, legs, oral mucosa, and genitalia. Characteristic features are itchy, red or violaceous, shiny, flat-topped papules. A fine white network (Wickham's striae) overlying the papules may be seen. The Koebner phenomenon is present in active phases.

Differential diagnosis includes secondary syphilis, GIN, drug eruptions, psoriasis, and lichen sclerosus et atrophicus.

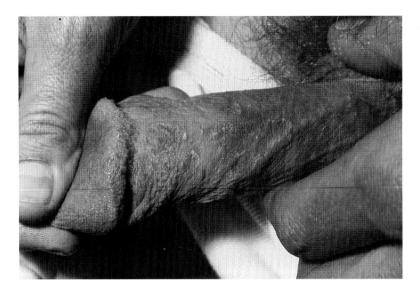

Figure 15.38. Lichen planus: annular violaceous lesion on the skin of the penis.

Treatment

Lichen planus is a self-limiting disease. Treatment is symptomatic and rests on the administration of topical corticosteroid creams starting with hydrocortisone, but if it is not effective, more potent, fluorinated corticosteroids should be tried. In case of severe pruritus antihistamines or tranquilizers may be helpful.

Pemphigus

Pemphigus is a rare blistering disease involving the skin and mucous membranes. This autoimmune disease predominantly occurs in middle and old age. The bullae are superficial and appear on normal skin or mucosa. They easily rupture, leaving large areas of denuded skin (Figure 15.39). The lesions are usually weeping and bleeding and heal with hyperpigmentation but without scarring. There is a positive Nikolsky's sign. (Pressure to the bulla causes the fluid to dissect the tissue and extension of the bulla).

Diagnosis can be confirmed by revealing deposits of immunoglobulins (predominantly IgG) and/or C-3 in the intercellular space by direct or indirect immunofluorescence. Tzanck test for acantholytic cells is positive.

Differential diagnosis includes genital herpes, in which lesions are more vesicular than bullous, herpes zoster, erosive papules of secondary syphilis, Stevens-Johnson syndrome, pemphigoid, dermatitis herpetiformis, and porphyria cutanea tarda.

Treatment

Pemphigus is a serious dermatologic disease requiring hospitalization. Large doses of systemic corticosteroids should be administered as soon as the diagnosis is

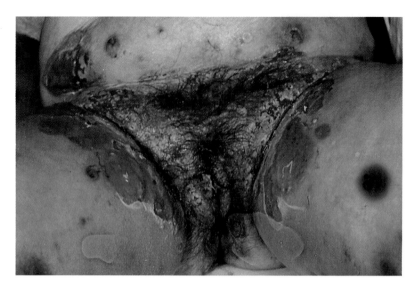

Figure 15.39. Large areas of denuded skin in the genital area caused by pemphigus.

made. Other agents presently used include methotrexate, cyclophosphamide, azathioprine,[63] gold, dapsone and plasmapheresis. Skin lesions should be treated as burns to prevent secondary infection with wet packs and Silvadene or other creams containing antiseptics.

Bullous Pemphigoid

Bullous pemphigoid is a chronic disease characterized by large, flaccid, often fluid-filled or hemorrhagic blisters on an erythematous base. The disease usually involves elderly patients. The lesions appear mainly on the upper arms and inner thighs but may appear also in the anogenital area (Figure 15.40). Lesions on mucous membranes are rare but should be considered during diagnosis.

Diagnosis: stable blisters on an erythematous base. Histology (subepidermal blister) and immunofluorescence (direct and indirect) shows a band of immunoglobin and complement present at the epidermal-dermal junction.[69]

Differential diagnosis: pemphigus, dermatitis-herpetiformis, genital herpes, and secondary syphilis.

Treatment

Combined systemic administration of steroid (prednisone) and immunosuppression (azathioprine, methotrexate, cyclophosphamide) usually controls pemphigoid effectively.[70,71] Local measures include topical application of antiseptic creams or compresses to prevent secondary infection.

Plasma Cell Balanitis of Zoon

Plasma-cell balanitis of Zoon (benign erythroplasia of the penis) is a rare form of benign erythroplasia.[72] It appears as a chronic moist shiny red plaque on the

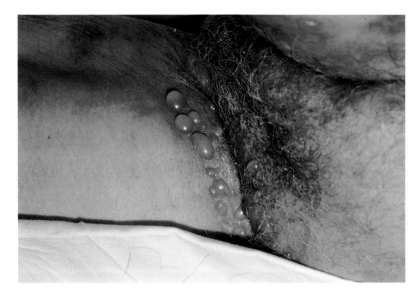

Figure 15.40. Bullous pemphigoid: stable blister on the left labium majoris and the groin.

glans of the penis or the inner surface of the prepuce (Figure 15.41). Lesions may also appear on the vulva and in the oral mucosa of both sexes.

Diagnosis is based on clinical appearance confirmed by biopsy, which reveals a dense infiltrate of plasma cells in the upper dermis.

Differential diagnosis includes erythroplasia of Queyrat, Bowen's disease, bowenoid papulosis (GIN), balanitis, drug eruption, lichen planus, and psoriasis.

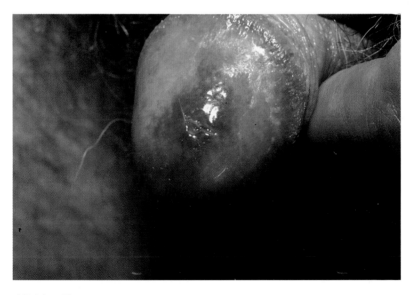

Figure 15.41. Plasma-cell balanitis of Zoon: moist shiny red plaque on the glans of the penis; biopsy confirms diagnosis.

Treatment

Topical application of low potency corticosteroid (hydrocortisone) cream is usually sufficient. Superficial electrodessication or cryotherapy is an alternative to topical treatment with corticosteroids.

Seborrheic Dermatitis

Although the lesions of seborrheic dermatitis can be localized anywhere in the body, the typical locations are in the seborrheic areas, such as the scalp and scalp margins, eyebrows, base of the eyelashes, nasolabial folds, and the sternum. The disease is characterized by the presence of asymptomatic, ill-defined erythematous lesions covered with yellowish fatty scales. The lesions of seborrheic dermatitis can be also found in the genitalia and perineum of either sex.[49] In the anogenital region they may look the same as in the other parts of the body or may appear as sharply defined erythematous plaques with scaly borders. In the groin the appearance may be of intertrigo.[16] Extensive and flourishing seborrheic dermatitis can be the skin harbinger of AIDS.[73,74] (See Figure 14.6, Chapter 14, p. 316.)

Diagnosis is based on clinical features, which are quite characteristic, and the presence of lesions in a typical distribution elsewhere on the body.

Differential diagnosis of seborrheic dermatitis in the anogenital region should include psoriasis, intertrigo, tinea, secondary syphilis, contact dermatitis, and pityriasis versicolor.

Treatment

Topical application of low or medium potency corticosteroid creams is the method of choice in the treatment of seborrheic dermatitis in the anogenital region. However, in the case of weeping eczematous lesions, wet compresses with antiseptics are recommended. If secondary infection is suspected topical antimicrobial preparations should be added.

REFERENCES

1. Rodin P, Kolator B: Carriage of yeasts on the penis. *Br Med J* 1:1123–1124, 1976.

2. Davidson F: Yeasts and circumcision in the male. *Brit J Vener Dis* 53:121–122, 1977.

3. Waugh MA, Evans EGV, Nayyar KC, et al: Clotrimazole (Canesten) in the treatment of candidal balanitis in men with incidental observations on diabetic candidal balanoposthitis. *Br J Vener Dis* 54:184–186, 1978.

4. Morrissey R, Xavier A, Nguyen N, et al: Invasive candidal balanitis due to a condom catheter in a neutropenic patient. *South Med J* 78:1245–1246, 1985.

5. Lucks DA, Venezio FR, Lakin Ch M: Balanitis caused by group B streptococcus. *J Urol* 135:1015, 1986.

6. Brook I: Balanitis caused by group B B-hemolytic streptococci, *Sex Transm Dis* 7:195–196, 1980.

7. Burdge DR, Bowie WR, Chow AW: *Gardnerella vaginalis*—associated balanoposthitis. *Sex Trans Dis* 13:159–162, 1986.

8. Kinghorn GR, Jones BM, Chowdhury FH: Balanoposthitis associated with *Gardnerella vaginalis* infection in men. *Br J Vener Dis* 58:127–129, 1982.

9. Cree GE, Willis AT, Phillips KD, et al: Anaerobic balanoposthitis. *Br Med J* 84:859–860, 1962.

10. Peutherer JF, Smith IW, Robertson DHH: Necrotising balanitis due to a generalized primary infection with herpes simplex virus type 2. *Br J Vener Dis* 55:48–51, 1979.

11. Soendjojo A, Pindha S: *Trichomonas vaginalis* infection of the median raphe of the penis. *Sex Transm Dis* 8:255–257, 1981.

12. Willmott FE: Genital yeasts in female patients attending a VD clinic. *Br J Vener Dis* 51:119–122, 1975.

13. Diddle AW, Gardner WH, Williamson PJ, et al: Oral contraceptives medications and vulvovaginal candidiasis. *Obstet Gynecol* 34:373–377, 1969.

14. Rees E: Gonococcal bartholinitis. *Br J Vener Dis* 43:150–156, 1967.

15. Davis JA, Rees E, Hobson D: Isolation of *Chlamydia trachomatis* from Bartholin's duct. *Br J Vener Dis* 54:409–413, 1978.

16. Felman YM, Nikitas JA: Nonvenereal anogenital lesions. *Cutis* 26:347–423, 1980.

17. Witkowski JA, Agache PG: Hidradenitis suppurativa. In Rook A, Parish L Ch, Beare JM: *Practical Management of the Dermatologic Patient.* Philadelphia, J.B. Lippincott Co., 1986, 89–91.

18. Thomas R, Barnhill D, Bibro M, et al: Hidradenitis suppurativa: A case presentation and review of the literature. *Obstet Gynecol* 66:592–595, 1985.

19. Moschella SL: Hidradenitis suppurativa. In: Maddin S: *Current Dermatologic Management,* ed. 2. St. Louis, CV Mosby, 1975, pp. 176–177.

20. Nasemann T, Sauerbrey W, Burgdorf WH: Fundamentals of Dermatology, New York Springer-Verlog, 1983, p. 73.

21. Habif TP: Superficial fungal infections In: *Clinical Dermatology,* St. Louis, CV Mosby, 1985, pp. 207–239.

22. Lookingbill DP, Marks JG: Principles of Dermatology. Philadelphia, WB Saunders Co, 1986, p. 118.

23. Bernstein JE, Robinson TWE: Herpes zoster. In: Rook A, Parish L Ch, Beare JM: *Practical Management of the Dermatologic Patient,* Philadelphia, JB Lippincott Co, 1986, p. 87–88.

24. Ackerman AB, Kornberg R: Pearly penile papules-acral angiofibromas, *Arch Dermatol,* 108:673–675, 1973.

25. Habif TP: Premalignant and malignant skin tumors. In: *Clinical Dermatology,* St. Louis, CV Mosby, 1985, pp. 423–452.

26. Clarck JA, Muller SA: Lichen sclerosus et atrophicus in children: A report of 24 cases. *Arch Dermatol,* 95:476–479, 1967.

27. Steigleder G, Schlater M: Lichen sclerosus et atrophicus. In: Arands R, Gumpost SL, Popkin GL, *Cancer of the Skin.* Philadelphia, WB Saunders, 1976, pp. 635–645.

28. Harrington CJ, Dunsmore IR: An investation into the incidence of autoimmune disorders in patients with lichen sclerosus et atrophicus. *Br J Dermatol,* 104:563–566, 1981.

29. Bart R, Kopf A: Tumor conference #18: Squamous cell carcinoma arising in balanitis xerotica obliterans. *J Dermatol Surg Oncol* 4:556–558, 1979.

30. Weber P, Rabinovitz H, Garland L: Verrucous carcinoma in penile lichen sclerosus et atrophicus. *J Dermatol Surg Oncol* 13:529–532, 1987.

31. Friedrich EG, Kalra PS: Serum levels of sex hormones in vulvar lichen sclerosus and the effect of topical testosterone. *N Engl J Med* 310:488–491, 1984.

32. Saurmond D: Lichen sclerosus et atrophicus of the vulva. *Arch Dermatol* 90:143–152, 1964.

33. Laude TA, Narayanaswamy G, Rajkumah S: Lichen clerosus et atrophicus in an eleven year old girl: report of a case. *Cutis* 26:78–80, 1980.

34. Hart W, Norris H, Helwig E: Relation of lichen sclerosus et atrophicus of the vulva to development of carcinoma. *Obstet Gynecol* 45:369–377, 1975.

35. Stratigos JD, Felman YM, Balanitis: In Rook A, Parish L Ch, Beare JM. *Practical Management of the Dermatologic Patient.* Philadelphia, J.B. Lippincott Co., 1986, pp. 19–22.

36. Obalek S, Jablonska S, Orth G: HPV-associated intraepithelial neoplasia of external genitalia. *Clin Dermatol* 3:104–113, 1985.

37. Callen JP, Headington J: Bowen's and non-Bowen's squamous intraepithelial neoplasia of the skin. *Arch Dermatol* 116:422–426, 1980.

38. Kimura S: Bowenoid papulosis of the genitalia. *Int J Dermatol* 21:432–436, 1982.

39. Chanda JJ: Extramammary Paget's diseases: Prognosis and relationship to internal malignancy. *J Am Acad Dermatol* 13:1009–1114, 1985.

40. Powell FC, Bjornsson J, Doyle JA, et al: Genital Paget's disease and urinary tract malignancy. *J Am Acad Dermatol* 13:84–90, 1985.

41. Watring WG, Roberts JA, Lagasse LD, et al: Treatment of recurrent Paget's disease of the vulva with topical bleomycin. *Cancer* 41:10–11, 1978.

42. Gissmann L, Gross G: Association of HPV with human genital tumors. *Clin Dermatol* 3:124–129, 1985.

43. Mroczkowski TF, McEwen C: Warts and other human papillomavirus infections. *Postgrad Med* 78:91–98, 1985.

44. Wolcott HD, Gallup DG: Wide local excision in the treatment of vulvar carcinoma in situ: A reappraisal. *Am J Obstet Gynecol* 150:695–698, 1984.

45. Lenowitz H: Cancer of the penis. *J Urol,* 56:458, 1966.

46. Narayana AS, Olney LE, Leoning SA, et al: Carcinoma of the penis; analysis of 219 cases. *Cancer* 49:2185–2191, 1982.

47. Onuigbo WB: Carcinoma of skin of penis. *Br J Urology,* 57:465–466, 1985.

48. Barrasso R, DeBrux J, Croissant O, et al: High prevalence of papillomavirus-associated penile intraepithelial neoplasia in sexual partners of women with cervical intraepithelial neoplasia. *N Engl J Med* 317:916–923, 1987.

49. Williams TS, Callen JP, Owen LG: Vulvar disorders in prepubertal female. Ped Ann 15:588–605, 1986.

50. Korkij W, Soltani K, Simjee S, et al: Tissue-specific autoantibodies and autoimmune disorders in vitiligo and alopecia areata. *J Cutan Pathol,* 11:522–530, 1984.

51. Soubiran P, Benzaken S, Bellet C, et al: Vitiligo: Periferal T-cell subset imbalance as defined by monoclonal antibodies. *Br J Dermatol* 113 (suppl 28):124–127, 1985.

52. Gould IM, Gray RS, Urbaniak SJ, et al: Vitiligo and diabetes mellitus. *Br J Dermatol* 113:153–155, 1985.

53. Jorizzo JL, Hudson RD, Schmalstieg FC: Behçet's syndrome: Immune regulation, circulating immune complexes, neutrophil migration and colchicine therapy. *J Am Acad Dermatol* 10:205–214, 1984.

54. Wong RC, Ellis CN, Diaz LA: Behçet's disease. *Int J Dermatol,* 23:25–32, 1984.

55. Jorizzo JL, Taylor RS, Schmalstieg FC, et al: Complex aphthosis: A forme fruste of Behçet's syndrome. *J Am Acad Dermatol* 13:80–84, 1984.

56. Cawson RA, Aram H: Behçet's syndrome. In Rook A, Parish L Ch, Beare JM: *Practical*

Management of the Dermatologic Patient. Philadelphia, J.B. Lippincott Corp. 1986 p. 23–24.

57. Millikan LE, Mroczkowski TF: Immunology of adverse drug eruptions. *Clin Dermatol,* 4:30–40, 1986.

58. Millikan LE, Kocsard E: Drug reactions. In Rook A, Parish L Ch, Beare JM: *Practical Management of Dermatologic Patient.* Philadelphia, J.B. Lippincott Corp., 1986 pp. 55–57.

59. Ting HC, Adam BA: Erythema multiforme: Epidemiology, clinical characteristic and natural history in fifty-nine patients, *Aust J Dermatol* 25:83–88, 1984.

60. Leigh IM, Mowbray JF, Levene GM: Recurrent and continuous erythema multiforme—a clinical and immunological study. *Clin Exp Dermatol* 10:58–67, 1985.

61. Goette DK, Odom RB: Vaginal medication as a cause for varied widespread dermatitides. *Cutis* 26:406–409, 1980.

62. Lemak MA, Duvic M, Bean SF: Oral acyclovir for the prevention of herpes-associated erythema multiforme. *J Acad Dermatol* 15:50–54, 1986.

63. Fisher M, Katz S. Fever and rash. In Lebwohl M. Difficult diagnoses in dermatology. New York, Churchill Livingstone, 1988 pp. 133–185.

64. Garty BZ, Mimouni M, Varsano I: Penile tourniquet syndrome. *Cutis* 31:421–432, 1983.

65. Press S, Schachner L, Paul P: Clitoris tourniquet syndrome. *Pediatrics,* 781–782, 1980.

66. Chapman HL: Digital strangulation by hair wrapping. *Can Med Ass* 98:125, 1968.

67. Sugathan P: Bulleetus. *Int J Dermatol* 26:51, 1987.

68. Smolle J: The treatment of pemphigus: A review of 44 cases, *Hautartzt,* 36:96–102, 1985.

69. Weigand DA: Effect of anatomic region on immunofluorescence diagnosis of bullous pemphigoid. *J Am Acad Dermatol* 12:274–278, 1985.

70. Ahmed AR, Maize JC, Provost TT: Bullous pemphigoid: Clinical and immunologic follow up after successful therapy *Arch Dermatol,* 113:1043–1046, 1977.

71. Habif TP: Vesicular and bullous diseases. In *Clinical Dermatology.* St. Louis, CV Mosby, 1985, pp. 325–340.

72. Stern JK, Rosen T: Balanitis plasmacellularis circumscripta (Zoon's balanitis plasmacellularis). *Cutis,* 25:57–60, 1980.

73. Eisenstat B, Wormser GP: Seborrheic dermatitis and butterfly rash in AIDS. *N Engl J Med* 311:189, 1984.

74. Mathes BM, Douglass MC. Seborrheic dermatitis in patients with acquired immunodeficiency syndrome. *J Am Acad Dermatol* 13:947–951, 1985.

INDEX